RESOURCE CENTER FOR DEVELOPMENTAL DISABILITIES
~~MENTAL HEALTH MATERIALS CENTER, INC.~~
~~30 EAST 29th STREET, NEW YORK, N.Y. 10016~~

MAIDSTONE FOUNDATION
1225 Broadway
New York, NY 10001
212 8895760

THE PRADER-WILLI SYNDROME

THE PRADER-WILLI SYNDROME

Edited by
**Vanja A. Holm, M.D.,
Stephen Sulzbacher, Ph.D.,**
and
Peggy L. Pipes, R.D., M.P.H.
Child Development and
Mental Retardation Center
University of Washington
Seattle

Technical Editor
Michael J. Steffes

```
PRADER-WILLI SYNDROME ASSOC.
5515 MALIBU DRIVE
EDINA, MN    55436
```

University Park Press
Baltimore

UNIVERSITY PARK PRESS
International Publishers in Science, Medicine, and Education
300 North Charles Street
Baltimore, Maryland 21201

Copyright © 1981 by University Park Press

Typeset by Action Comp. Co., Inc.
Manufactured in the United States of America by The Maple Press Company.

All rights, including that of translation into other languages, reserved. Photomechanical reproduction (photocopy, microcopy) of this book or parts thereof without special permission of the publisher is prohibited.

Prader-Willi Syndrome is based on the National Prader-Willi Syndrome Workshop held at the Lake Wilderness Conference Center of the University of Washington, Maple Valley, Washington, June 13-15, 1979.

Library of Congress Cataloging in Publication Data

Main entry under title:

The Prader-Willi syndrome.

    Most of the chapters were presented at a conference sponsored by the University of Washington in 1979.
    Bibliography: p.
    Includes index.
    1. Prader-Willi syndrome—Congresses. I. Holm, Vanja A., 1928-
II. Sulzbacher, Stephen. III. Pipes, Peggy L. IV. Washington (state) University. [DNLM: 1. Prader-Willi syndrome. WM 300 P896 1979]
RJ520.P7P72   616'.047   80-25352
ISBN 0-8391-1638-1

Contents

Contributors viii
Foreword
   Nancy M. Robinson xiii
Preface xv

chapter 1
The Prader-Willi Syndrome   Historical Perspective
   Michael J. Steffes, Vanja A. Holm, and Stephen Sulzbacher 1

chapter 2
Federal Programs for the Developmentally Disabled
   Gerald D. LaVeck 17

part I   **ETIOLOGY AND DIAGNOSIS**

chapter 3
The Diagnosis of Prader-Willi Syndrome
   Vanja A. Holm 27

chapter 4
**A View of the Etiology and Pathogenesis
of Prader-Willi Syndrome**
   James W. Hanson 45

chapter 5
Diagnosis and Therapy in the First Phase of Prader-Willi Syndrome
   Hans Zellweger 55

chapter 6
Clinical Experience with 23 Cases of Prader-Willi Syndrome
   *Henry G. Dunn, W. Jun Tze, Robert M. Alisharan, and
   Michael Schulzer* 69

part II   **OBESITY MANAGEMENT**

chapter 7
Nutritional Management of Children with Prader-Willi Syndrome
   Peggy L. Pipes 91

chapter 8
Nutrition, Metabolism, Body Composition, and Response to the Ketogenic Diet in Prader-Willi Syndrome
Ralph A. Nelson, Diane M. Huse, Ralph T. Holman,
Barbara O. Kimbrough, Heinz W. Wahner,
C. Wayne Callaway, and Aldine B. Hayles................... 105

chapter 9
Surgical Treatment of Morbid Obesity in Prader-Willi Syndrome
Robert T. Soper, Edward E. Mason, Kenneth J. Printen,
and Hans Zellweger 121

chapter 10
Elevated Adipose Tissue Lipoprotein Lipase in the Pathogenesis of Obesity in Prader-Willi Syndrome
Robert S. Schwartz, John D. Brunzell, and Edwin L. Bierman . . . 137

part III **BEHAVIORAL AND SOCIAL ASPECTS**

chapter 11
Behavioral and Cognitive Disabilities in Prader-Willi Syndrome
Stephen Sulzbacher, Keith A. Crnic, and Jeff Snow 147

chapter 12
Cognitive Processing in Children with Prader-Willi Syndrome
Judith L. Warren and Earl Hunt 161

chapter 13
Speech and Language Characteristics of Children with Prader-Willi Syndrome
Cynthia Branson 179

chapter 14
A Behavioral Approach to Treatment of Prader-Willi Syndrome
Barringer D. Marshall, Jr., Charles J. Wallace, John Elder,
Karen Burke, Tim Oliver, and Richard Blackmon............. 185

chapter 15
Maintenance of Programmed Weight Loss in Patients with Prader-Willi Syndrome
Glenn Hirsch and Karl Altman............................. 201

chapter 16
A Retrospective Study of the Behavior of Prader-Willi Syndrome versus Other Institutionalized Retarded Persons
Ruth Turner and Rogelio H. A. Ruvalcaba 215

chapter 17
Relaxation Training with Youngsters with Prader-Willi Syndrome
  Stevan L. Nielsen and Stephen Sulzbacher 219

chapter 18
Implications of Prader-Willi Syndrome for the Individual and Family
  Jurgen Herrmann 229

chapter 19
Social Work Intervention Strategies for Families with Children with Prader-Willi Syndrome
  Judith M. Leconte 245

part IV MEDICAL ASPECTS

chapter 20
Medical Management of Prader-Willi Syndrome
  Vanja A. Holm 261

chapter 21
Physical Growth in Prader-Willi Syndrome
  Jane K. Nugent and Vanja A. Holm 269

chapter 22
Endocrine Profiles and Metabolic Aspects of Prader-Willi Syndrome
  W. Jun Tze, Henry G. Dunn, and Raphe L. Rothstein 281

chapter 23
Scoliosis in Prader-Willi Syndrome
  Edwin L. Laurnen 293

chapter 24
Physical Exercise for Children and Adults with Prader-Willi Syndrome
  Paula M. Carman 299

chapter 25
The Prader-Willi Syndrome   Directions in Future Research
  Stephen Sulzbacher, Vanja A. Holm, and Peggy L. Pipes 313

The Prader-Willi Syndrome   An Annotated Bibliography 317

Index 339

Contributors

Robert M. Alisharan, M.B., F.R.C.P.(C)
Fellow in Paediatric Endocrinology
Faculty of Medicine
The University of British Columbia
Vancouver, British Columbia
Canada

Karl Altman, Ph.D.
Assistant Professor of Community Health (Psychology)
Director of Psychology Intern Training
University of Kansas Medical Center
Kansas City, Kansas 66103

Edwin L. Bierman, M.D.
Professor of Medicine
University of Washington School of Medicine
Seattle, Washington 98195

Richard Blackmon
Research Assistant
Clinical Research Unit
Camarillo Neuropsychiatric Institute
Camarillo, California 93010

Cynthia Branson, M.A.
Lecturer in Speech and Hearing Sciences
University of Washington
Seattle, Washington 98195

John D. Brunzell, M.D.
Associate Professor of Medicine
University of Washington School of Medicine
Seattle, Washington 98195

Karen Burke, B.S.
Research Associate
Clinical Research Unit
Camarillo Neuropsychiatric Institute
Camarillo, California 93010

C. Wayne Callaway, M.D.
Assistant Professor of Medicine
Mayo Medical School
and
Director of the Nutrition Consulting Service
Mayo Clinic
Rochester, Minnesota 55901

Paula M. Carman, M.O.T., O.T.R.
Acting Instructor
Division of Occupational Therapy
Department of Rehabilitation Medicine
University of Washington School of Medicine
Seattle, Washington 98195

Keith A. Crnic, Ph.D.
Assistant Professor of Psychiatry and Behavioral Sciences
University of Washington School of Medicine
Seattle, Washington 98195

Henry G. Dunn, M.B., F.R.C.P. (Lond.), F.R.C.P.(C)
Professor and Head, Division of Neurology
Department of Paediatrics
Faculty of Medicine
The University of British Columbia
Vancouver, British Columbia
Canada

John Elder, Ph.D.
Psychologist
Clinical Research Unit
Camarillo Neuropsychiatric
 Institute
Camarillo, California 93010

James W. Hanson, M.D.
Associate Professor of Pediatrics
Division of Medical Genetics
The University of Iowa Hospitals
 and Clinics
Iowa City, Iowa 52242

Aldine B. Hayles, M.D.
Professor of Pediatrics and
 Medicine
Mayo Medical School
and
Consultant
Pediatrics and Medicine
Mayo Clinic
Rochester, Minnesota 55901

Jurgen Herrmann, M.D.
Associate Professor of Pediatrics
The Medical College of Wisconsin
and
Director, Birth Defects Center
Milwaukee Children's Hospital
Milwaukee, Wisconsin 53233

Glenn Hirsch, M.A.
Division of Psychology
Children's Rehabilitation Unit
University of Kansas Medical
 Center
Kansas City, Kansas 66103

Vanja A. Holm, M.D.
Assistant Professor of Pediatrics
University of Washington School
 of Medicine
Seattle, Washington 98195

Ralph T. Holman, Ph.D.
Professor of Biochemistry
and
Executive Director
Hormel Institute
University of Minnesota
Austin, Minnesota 55912

Earl Hunt, Ph.D.
Professor of Psychology
Chairman, Department of
 Psychology
University of Washington
Seattle, Washington 98195

Diane M. Huse, M.S., R.D.
Instructor in Clinical Nutrition
Mayo Medical School
and
Nutritionist
Mayo Clinic
Rochester, Minnesota 55901

Barbara Olson Kimbrough, M.D.
Resident
Ophthalmology
Mayo Clinic
Rochester, Minnesota 55901

Edwin L. Laurnen, M.D.
Clinical Associate Professor of
 Orthopedic Surgery
University of Washington School
 of Medicine
Seattle, Washington 98195

Gerald D. LaVeck, M.D.
Clinical Professor of Epidemi-
 ology and Pediatrics
University of Washington School
 of Medicine
and
Medical Consultant
U.S. Public Health Service,
 Region X
Seattle, Washington 98101

Judith M. Leconte, M.S.W.
Clinical Instructor
School of Social Work
University of Washington
Seattle, Washington 98195

Barringer D. Marshall, Jr., M.D.
Supervisor
Clinical Research Unit
Camarillo Neuropsychiatric
  Institute
and
Staff Psychiatrist
Camarillo State Hospital
Camarillo, California 93010

Edward E. Mason, M.D.
Professor of Surgery
The University of Iowa
  Hospitals and Clinics
Iowa City, Iowa 52242

Ralph A. Nelson, M.D., Ph.D.
Professor of Nutrition
School of Clinical Medicine
University of Illinois
and
Director of Research
Carle Foundation Hospital
Urbana-Champaign, Illinois
  61801

Stevan L. Nielsen, B.S.
Doctoral Candidate
Department of Psychology
University of Washington
Seattle, Washington 98195

Jane K. Nugent, M.D.
Assistant Professor of Clinical
  Pediatrics
Upstate Medical Center
Syracuse, New York 13210
and
Associate Director of Pediatric
  Education
Wilson Memorial Hospital
Johnson City, New York 19404

Tim Oliver, R.N.
Charge Nurse
Clinical Research Unit
Camarillo Neuropsychiatric
  Institute
Camarillo, California 93010

Peggy L. Pipes, R.D., M.P.H.
Lecturer, School of Nutritional
  Sciences and Textiles
University of Washington
Seattle, Washington 98195

Kenneth J. Printen, M.D.
Professor of Surgery
The University of Iowa Hospitals
  and Clinics
Iowa City, Iowa 52242

Nancy M. Robinson, Ph.D.
Associate Professor of Psychiatry
  and Behavioral Sciences
University of Washington School
  of Medicine
Seattle, Washington 98195

Raphe L. Rothstein, M.D., F.R.C.P.(C)
Assistant Professor of Paediatrics
Faculty of Medicine
The University of British
  Columbia
Vancouver, British Columbia
Canada

Rogelio H. A. Ruvalcaba, M.D.
Professor of Pediatrics
University of Washington School
  of Medicine
and
Clinical Director
Rainier School
Buckley, Washington 98321

Michael Schulzer, M.D., Ph.D.
Associate Professor
Departments of Medicine and
  Mathematics
The University of British
  Columbia
Vancouver, British Columbia
Canada

Robert S. Schwartz, M.D.
Assistant Professor of Medicine
University of Vermont
Burlington, Vermont 05405

Jeff Snow, M.A.
Education Consultant
Clinical Training Unit
Child Development and Mental
  Retardation Center
University of Washington
Seattle, Washington 98195

Robert T. Soper, M.D.
Professor of Surgery
Director, Pediatric Surgery
  Service
The University of Iowa Hospital
  and Clinics
Iowa City, Iowa 52242

Michael J. Steffes, M.A.
Editor
Clinical Training Unit
Child Development and Mental
  Retardation Center
University of Washington
Seattle, Washington 98195

Stephen Sulzbacher, Ph.D.
Associate Professor of Psychiatry
  and Behavioral Sciences and
  of Pediatrics
University of Washington School
  of Medicine
Seattle, Washington 98195

Ruth Turner, Ed.D.
School Psychologist
Sumner School District
Sumner, Washington 98390
(formerly Clinical Psychologist,
  Rainier School, Buckley,
  Washington)

W. Jun Tze, M.D., F.R.C.P.(C)
Associate Professor and Head
Division of Endocrinology
Department of Paediatrics
Faculty of Medicine
The University of British
  Columbia
Vancouver, British Columbia
Canada

Heinz W. Wahner, M.D.
Professor of Laboratory Medicine
Mayo Medical School
and
Head
Section of Diagnostic Nuclear
  Medicine
Mayo Clinic
Rochester, Minnesota 55901

Charles J. Wallace, Ph.D.
Associate Director, Mental Health
Clinical Research Center for the
  Study of Schizophrenia
and
Staff Psychologist
Camarillo State Hospital
Camarillo, California 93010

Judith L. Warren, Ph.D.
Senior Fellow in Department of
  Obstetrics and Gynecology
and in
Department of Psychiatry and
  Behavioral Sciences
University of Washington School
  of Medicine
Seattle, Washington 98195

Hans Zellweger, M.D.
Professor Emeritus of Pediatrics
The University of Iowa Hospitals
  and Clinics
Iowa City, Iowa 52242

Foreword

This report of a 1979 conference on Prader-Willi syndrome represents communication among a heterogeneous band of researchers with a joint interest in a puzzling and unusual disorder. The sophistication of the investigations within their several disciplines is a result of the dedication with which the authors have pursued the joint goals of understanding and intervention. To some extent they have succeeded; yet, the puzzle remains unsolved.

This volume presents up-to-date and comprehensive sets of findings that suggest that Prader-Willi syndrome can and should be identified very early in a child's life, and that with sufficient vigor and resolve its management can yield substantially positive results. The crippling effects of two cardinal symptoms, obesity and behavioral disorder, can be modified; life can be lengthened; cognitive deficits may even be reduced. The studies reported here can serve as guidelines for other clinical researchers who are willing to accept the demanding, unrelenting challenge of treating a most difficult and intractable disorder. I have seen the monthly clinic at the University of Washington's Child Development and Mental Retardation Center, and it is obvious that the professionals involved conduct both research and service there with the highest standards of the clinician-scientist, and with clarity, wisdom, patience, firmness, and good humor. To the authors of these papers, both the University of Washington group and their guests, my hat is off.

Nancy M. Robinson, Ph.D.

Preface

Prader-Willi (P-W) syndrome is a disorder characterized by poor muscle tone and feeding problems in infancy, and by obesity, short stature, disorders in sexual development, and behavioral and cognitive disabilities throughout the remainder of life. These medical and behavioral problems result in very complex needs that require the services of professionals from many fields, including medicine, nutrition, psychology, education, social work, occupational and physical therapy, and speech pathology. Unfortunately, the information available to help professionals in planning for and providing these services has in most cases been scattered and limited in extent. This book summarizes research and clinical experience from all these fields. All the chapters contain new information, in some cases making important revisions in the picture of this syndrome and in the needs it creates. Knowledge about this syndrome continues to grow rapidly. Some current research indicates that a high proportion of cases of P-W syndrome might be caused by the absence of minute portions of chromosome 15. If these exciting findings are confirmed, only parts of the discussions of etiology and diagnosis might be of historical interest by the time this book is in print. However, the great majority of the information is still applicable. Since previous publications addressed themselves for the most part to medical or nutritional problems, readers will find the information on behavioral problems especially pertinent.

The bulk of the book is divided into four sections dealing with etiology and diagnosis, obesity management, behavioral and social aspects, and medical aspects of the syndrome. One of the functions of the first chapter in each section is to provide an introduction to the issues dealt with in that section. Chapter 1, which deals with the historical perspective, contains background information relevant to the whole book. An annotated bibliography is included to aid those who wish to read further.

Although this book is intended primarily for professionals, we have made an attempt to reach a wider audience, especially parents of P-W syndrome children and caregivers in group homes and other community facilities. We think that they will find much of the information useful.

Most of the chapters were presented at a conference on P-W syndrome sponsored by the University of Washington and funded by the U.S. Health Services Administration, Bureau of Community Health Services, Office of Maternal and Child Health (Grant no. MCT-000986-01-0). The conference and, to an even greater extent, this book represent a synthesis of work relating to P-W syndrome by clinical researchers from throughout the United States and Canada.

Although each of the editors has been involved in all parts of the book, Vanja Holm has been primarily responsible for the sections on diagnosis and medical management, Stephen Sulzbacher for the behavioral section, and Peggy Pipes for the obesity management section.

We are grateful to the Office of Maternal and Child Health for providing the funding for the conference out of which this book grew and for many of the expenses of editing and producing it as well. Their support was essential.

Credit is also due the Child Development and Mental Retardation Center of the University of Washington and its director, Dr. Irvin Emanuel, for providing the clinical facilities and academic working atmosphere for much of the pioneering work reported here. We also appreciate the efforts of the personnel, particularly Jean Reeves, involved in running the Prader-Willi Syndrome Clinic at the center.

We would like to thank the contributors of the individual chapters, who often took time from very busy clinic schedules to complete them. For help and encouragement with this project in its initial stages we are grateful to Dr. Gerald LaVeck. Susan Chapman made a major contribution to the success of the conference out of which this book grew. Finally, we would like to express our appreciation to Ken Westby for doing an excellent job of typing the manuscript.

We hope that our efforts and those of the contributors lead to further improvements in the diagnosis and treatment of Prader-Willi syndrome. This is certainly our paramount wish in producing this book.

This book is dedicated to the memory of
Daniel Neason (1966–1980),
one of our earliest patients
for whom we had high hopes,
and
Paula Carman (1945–1980),
a beloved colleague whom we miss.

chapter 1

THE PRADER-WILLI SYNDROME
Historical Perspective

Michael J. Steffes, Vanja A. Holm, and Stephen Sulzbacher

> In this chapter the historical background of the Prader-Willi syndrome is discussed, including two possible cases from the 17th and 19th centuries. —*Eds.*

We can assume that Prader-Willi (P-W) syndrome individuals existed long before the syndrome was identified in 1956, and they were given a specific diagnostic label. Since the discovery was so recent, it is especially interesting to see whether indications of the syndrome can be found earlier. Humankind's long-standing interest in obesity and hyperphagia can be seen in art, mythology, folklore, and literature. Characters such as Falstaff, Mr. Pickwick, or, for that matter, Santa Claus, still appeal to the imagination. However, one would not expect a search in these areas to reveal individuals who could be specifically identified as having P-W syndrome because they have not been concerned primarily with the kind of precise physical description necessary for medical or scientific purposes.

This makes it all the more surprising that in two portraits of a 17th century Spanish girl, the clinical features of P-W syndrome are clearly in evidence (Figures 1.1 and 1.2). The subject of the paintings was 6-year-old Eugenia Martínez Vallejo, known as "La Monstrua" because of her great obesity. The paintings were done by Juan Carreño de Miranda, painter to the Spanish court, at the order of King Charles II about 1680. Eugenia had been summoned to the court by the king, who was noted for his fondness for human oddities, when news of her unusual appearance reached him (Beruete y Moret, 1909). At the time, she weighed about 120 pounds (Moreno Villa, 1939). The excessive obesity at such an early age, in addition to the small triangular mouth and the small hands and feet, strongly suggests P-W syndrome. The distribution of adipose tissue is typical for the syndrome. Naturally one cannot make a precise clinical diagnosis on the basis of two paintings and a few scraps of historical information, but there is no likely alternate explanation for this girl's appearance. We can, of course, assume that many other cases of P-W syndrome existed

1

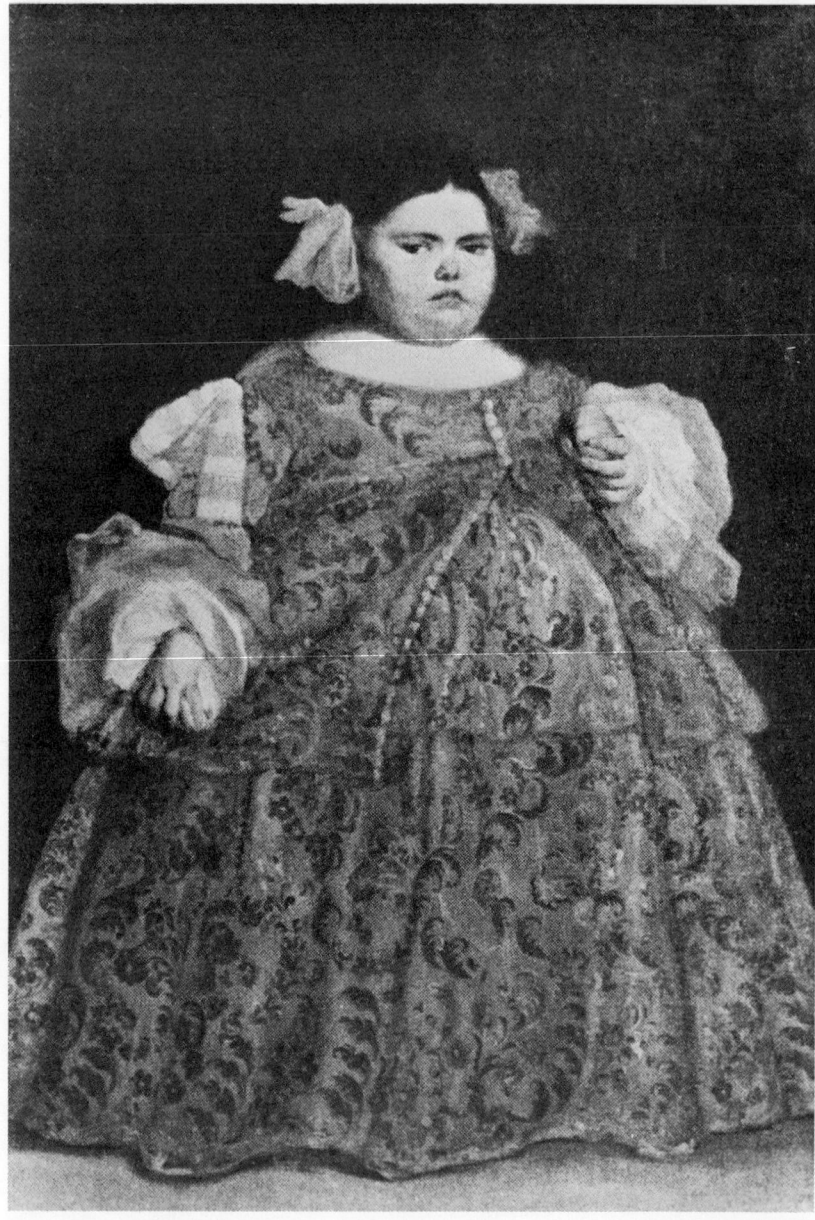

Figure 1.1. Juan Carreño de Miranda, *Eugenia Martínez Vallejo, "La Monstrua"* (Museo del Prado).

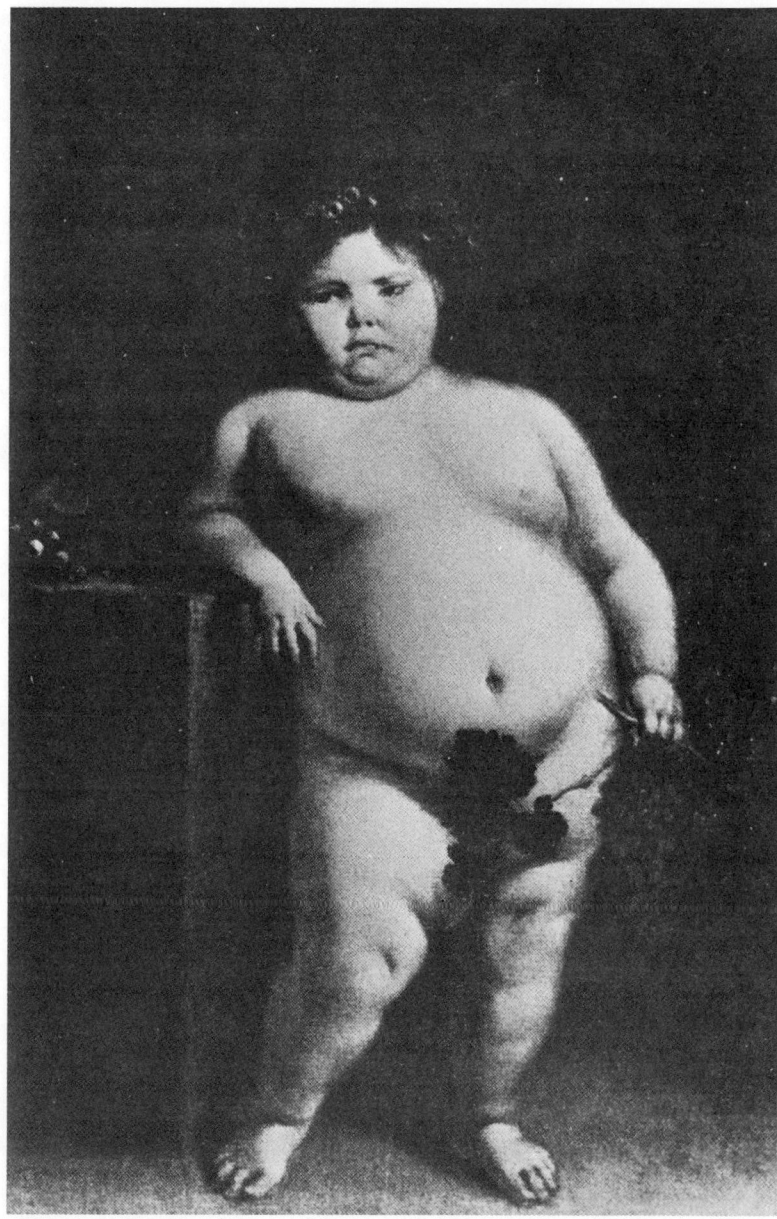

Figure 1.2. Juan Carreño de Miranda, *Eugenia Martínez Vallejo as Silenus* (Museo del Prado).

throughout history. This particular one is recorded for us because of King Charles's peculiar tastes.

It is remarkable that this unusual combination of symptoms did not attract the attention of the medical profession earlier. Many extremely obese individuals have been mentioned in early medical literature. Unfortunately, descriptions are seldom complete enough to determine whether or not the patient had any features of P-W syndrome other than obesity and, in a few cases, hyperphagia. Information on the early years of these patients is seldom available, making it impossible to tell whether the initial stage of poor muscle tone and feeding difficulties was present.

One 19th century investigator did, however, leave a very full description of a patient who appears to meet most of the diagnostic criteria for P-W syndrome. J.L.H. Down, now remembered chiefly for the syndrome named for him, described a case of what he called "polysarcia" in 1887. Since the patient was mentally retarded, had small hands and feet, had little body hair, did not menstruate, and weighed 210 pounds at a height of 4 feet 4 inches, McKusick (1978) has suggested that she had P-W syndrome. In addition to the characteristics cited by McKusick, Down mentioned that she had been "delicate and thin" up to the age of 7, which suggests the early hypotonic stage of P-W syndrome. She continued to gain weight even when restricted to a diet which left others only "fairly nourished." Again, this is typical of the syndrome. It is heartening to note that this patient successfully reduced her weight from 210 pounds to 133 pounds while in an institution following a carefully supervised diet prescribed by Down.

Down did not, however, distinguish this case from other kinds of excessive obesity. He considered it a typical example, although this patient had little in common with those he mentioned at the beginning of his article—the middle-aged, the well-to-do, and the indolent. This patient was young, poor, and had never eaten a luxurious diet. In spite of all the evidence, caution is advised before confidently assuming that this girl is the first case of P-W syndrome in medical literature. Brain (1967) calls her disease "adiposogenital dystrophy," a term which merely indicates that the patient is obese and has small genitals.

Adiposogenital dystrophy is sometimes used synonymously with Fröhlich's syndrome, although in Fröhlich's patient the disorder occurred with a tumor of the pituitary gland (Bruch, 1939); the diagnosis should only be used for these cases or, at most, cases of adiposogenital dystrophy in which organic brain disease is present (Zellweger & Schneider, 1968). Prior to the work of Prader, Willi, and their colleagues (1963), these would have been the best medical diagnoses available for P-W syndrome individuals. Neither adiposogenital dystrophy nor Fröhlich's syndrome involves hyperphagia. Unfortunately, there has been a great deal of confusion about the proper use of the term "Fröhlich's syndrome," leading one author to suggest some time ago that it had outlived its clinical usefulness (Bruch, 1939).

HISTORY

Diagnosis

In 1956, Prader, Labhart, and Willi published a brief article describing a new syndrome characterized by obesity, short stature, cryptorchidism, and mental retardation, with lack of muscle tone in infancy. (See Chapter 5 for a brief description of the work which led to the discovery of the syndrome.) With their colleague, Fanconi, they presented information regarding the syndrome at the 8th International Pediatric Congress in Copenhagen in 1956. The most distinctive feature of the syndrome is the hyperphagia, or voracious appetite, over which the P-W person has little control and which leads to the characteristic excessive obesity.

After the first publications of Prader et al., clinicians all over the world recognized that an appropriate diagnosis had been found for many of the obese boys with small genitals, whom they had seen. Case reports of the new syndrome were soon published from England (Laurance, 1961), Canada (Dunn, Ford, Auersperg, & Miller, 1961), the United States (Zellweger, Smith, & Cusminsky, 1962), France (Gabilan, 1962), Spain (Sánchez Villares, Martín Esteban, & Durantez Mayo, 1964), Sweden (Forssman & Hagberg, 1964), the Netherlands (Monnens & Kenis, 1965), and Belgium (Hooft, Delire, & Casneuf, 1966). In addition to the characteristics noted in the original description, many observers found small triangular mouths, almond-shaped eyes, small hands and feet, and incomplete puberty. As a group, P-W syndrome individuals have very distinct clinical features.

As physicians continued to work with this puzzling condition, the information they acquired began to appear in more detailed studies. In 1963, Prader and Willi published a paper analyzing 14 cases. They confirmed their earlier work, and described diminished fetal movements, an IQ of 40 to 50, and a tendency to diabetes. Laurance followed up his original report of cases in 1967, confirming and elaborating on the original findings. He also speculated that eventually subgroups within the syndrome could be distinguished, either on an etiological or a pathological basis. In 1968, three important articles on the syndrome appeared—by Gabilan and Royer, Zellweger and Schneider, and Dunn. All discussed their experience with the syndrome since their original reports.

Gabilan and Royer discussed 11 cases. A major contribution of their study was the extensive work they had done on the orthopedic problems of the syndrome. They had observed scoliosis, lordosis, coxa valga, hip dislocation, and epiphysiolysis, which they considered should be added to the descriptions of anomalies in the syndrome. They also observed dental problems and a tendency to strabismus. They noted that two patients were brother and sister and in another case the parents were related, suggesting the possibility that the syndrome is recessively inherited.

The next important study to appear was Zellweger and Schneider's report of 14 cases. They reported that laboratory studies had not revealed consistent abnormalities. They also clearly differentiated between the two stages of the syndrome, the infant hypotonic stage and the obese second stage. A full discussion of differential diagnoses during these two stages was included. During the earlier stage, it was necessary to distinguish P-W children from those with neuromuscular disorders, such as congenital muscular dystrophy, neonatal myasthenia, prenatal onset Werdnig-Hoffman disease, brain injuries, intracranial hemorrhages, and cerebral malformations. (See Chapter 5 for a fuller discussion.) The second stage could be confused with Laurence-Moon-Biedl syndrome or with Fröhlich's adiposogenital dystrophy. The authors pointed out that while P-W syndrome and Laurence-Moon-Biedl syndrome share common features—mental retardation, obesity, and hypogonadism—they differ in that the Laurence-Moon-Biedl syndrome includes retinitis pigmentosa and polydactyly. In adiposogenital dystrophy, mental retardation is not always present and the infantile hypotonia does not occur. Zellweger and Schneider also speculated about the possibility of a disorder in the hypothalamus as the cause of the syndrome. This remains a convincing hypothesis. They also urged caution in considering the syndrome hereditary, in spite of some evidence that could be so interpreted.

Dunn began his article with an extensive review of the literature to date, although publication times were too close for him to make use of the two previously described articles, and then reported his own nine cases. He suggested that in addition to the characteristics delineated by Prader et al. (1956), the following be added to descriptions of the syndrome: normal or somewhat large head circumference, delayed dentition, dental caries and defective enamel, fair hair, blue eyes, phimosis, and strabismus. He also noted a slowing down of behavioral development in early childhood. Again, extensive laboratory studies revealed no consistent abnormalities. Only two of his nine cases were pre-diabetic. Three of the patients had chromosome abnormalities, one of them an XYY karyotype.

The next major article about the syndrome was published by Hall and Smith (1972). They tabulated abnormalities occurring in 32 P-W patients. Hypotonia, feeding problems and delayed developmental milestones in infancy, male hypogenitalism, and obesity were the only characteristics found in 100% of their cases. Poor fetal vigor, mental deficiency, personality problems, short stature, delayed bone age, acromicria, and male cryptorchidism occurred in 50% or more of the cases discussed. The article is particularly noteworthy for correcting the impression sometimes left by earlier publications that the P-W temperament is always pleasant and affable. Hall and Smith pointed out that after early childhood, temper tantrums and stubborness often occur, and "by late adolescence and adulthood almost all of the individuals had serious personality problems" (p. 288).

Obesity Control

It has been clear from the beginning that excessive obesity is the major health problem of P-W individuals, often leading to early death from heart disease or other complications. A number of different approaches to the management of P-W obesity have been tried—appetite-depressing drugs, experimental diets, gastric bypass surgery—but a carefully planned low calorie diet with some behavioral controls is still the preferred method (Pipes, Chapter 7, this volume). As early as 1964, Evans reported success in reducing obesity with a reasonably palatable and nutritionally sound diet. He was not, however, able to maintain long term weight loss.

It was only in 1973 that a method of long term, outpatient diet therapy, maintaining health and growth in P-W syndrome children while reducing or preventing obesity, was published (Pipes & Holm; see also Holm & Pipes, 1976). This approach to obesity control resulted from work with the first child who had been referred to the Child Development and Mental Retardation Center at the University of Washington in 1969. He was 18 months old when his family moved to Seattle. The diagnosis had been made at age 7 months by an astute pediatrician. He had recovered from the "failure to thrive" stage (Figure 3) and was well proportioned at 15 months. At 18 months his height and weight were in the 25th percentile. In an effort to prevent the development of obesity, described as inevitable for this syndrome in the literature of that time, a diet was prescribed that was sufficient in calories for normal children of the same age and size. In spite of this intervention, he gained weight rapidly and was above the 95th percentile at 27 months of age (Figure 4). His energy intake in relation to weight lost or gained was assessed, leading to the discovery that children with P-W syndrome have lower energy needs than normal children (Pipes & Holm, 1973). This finding was confirmed by experience with other young P-W syndrome children. The ideal of this dietary method is to prevent the occurrence of obesity caused by foraging and gorging—it is necessary that all food not included in the diet be made inaccessible by

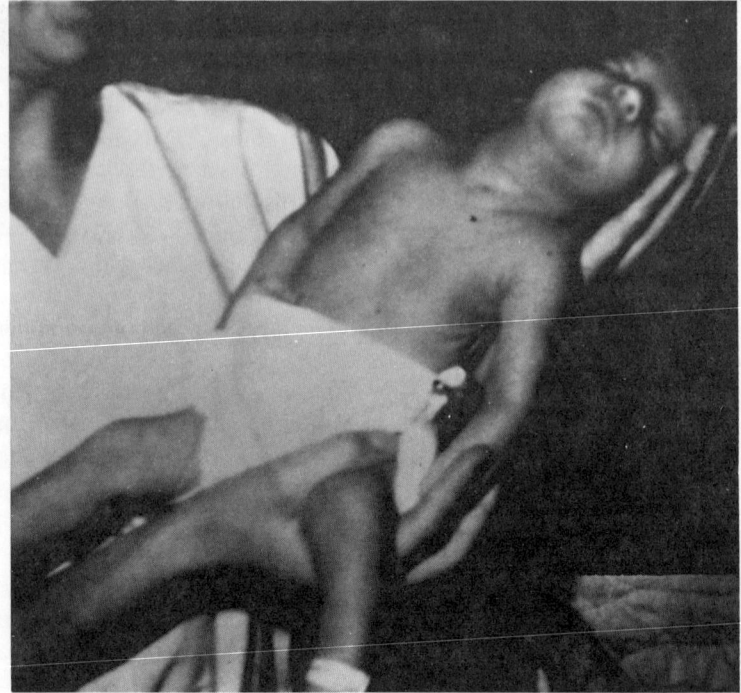

Figure 1.3. A Prader-Willi syndrome child in the infant hypotonic stage.

locking cupboards and refrigerators. This, as well as the careful measurements necessary for this dietary plan, makes that full cooperation by the patients' families essential for success.

However, it is extremely difficult to continue to maintain stringent control over access to food for older P-W persons because of their greater freedom of movement. Ideally the P-W persons themselves should take responsibility for controlling their own obesity. In some cases this may well be possible. However, the extreme strength of the compulsion to eat, coupled with the fact that many P-W individuals are mentally retarded, makes it difficult in most cases. Behavior modification programs now exist for developing better eating habits and show some promise of beneficial long term results (Hirsch & Altman, Chapter 15, this volume; Marshall, Wallace, Elder, Burke, Oliver, & Blackmon, Chapter 14, this volume). There is now a much better chance, especially since a number of P-W individuals have been prevented from becoming obese in childhood, that the "inevitable" fate of people with this syndrome—early death from complications of extreme obesity—can be prevented in some cases.

Interdisciplinary Management

Growing awareness of the complexity of the needs of persons with P-W syndrome led in 1972 to the start of the first clinic exclusively for the syndrome at the Child Development and Mental Retardation Center (CDMRC) at the University of Washington. The CDMRC—like other University-Affiliated Facilities—is committed to interdisciplinary intervention for children with developmental disabilities (Allen, Holm, & Schiefelbusch, 1978). It soon became apparent that children with P-W syndrome needed the services of an entire developmental team. Obesity control alone necessitated involvement of the nutritionist, the pediatrician or internist, and the behavioral management specialist. Hypotonia and inactivity required advice and treatment by occupational and physical therapists. Developmental delays prompted psychological assessment. Speech and language problems led to evaluations and suggestions from speech pathologists. There were special educational considerations requir-

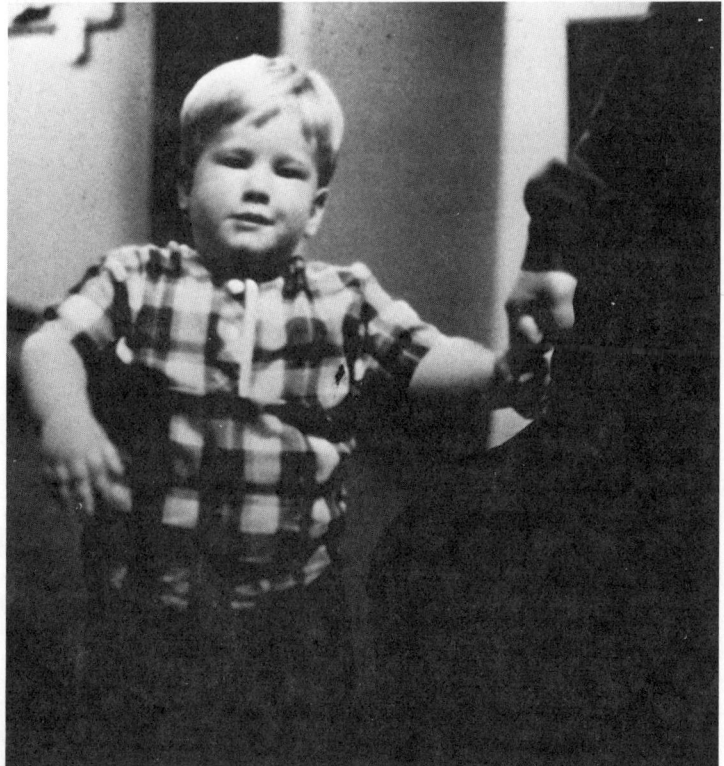

Figure 1.4. The child shown in Figure 1.3 at 27 months.

ing advice from educators. A multitude of physical problems made it necessary for pediatricians dealing with P-W syndrome to seek endocrinological, orthopedic, and other consultations. Finally, it was realized that families, schools, caseworkers, and, in fact, everyone dealing with these children, faced a variety of overwhelming behavioral, emotional, and social problems. It became clear that family support services from social workers and advice on behavioral management from psychologists were needed.

The interdisciplinary group at CDMRC chose to create a specialty clinic for this syndrome for two reasons. First, the symptom complex in P-W syndrome is unique. As professionals began to acquire experience with P-W children, it seemed reasonable to allow one individual in each discipline a chance to develop expertise by repeated exposure to these symptoms. Second, it was assumed that the parents of P-W children would be likely to benefit from meeting other parents facing similar child-rearing problems; a specialty clinic would facilitate such parent association.

Partly as a result of reports in the popular press, P-W syndrome is now more commonly diagnosed. Thus, services for P-W persons in similar interdisciplinary settings in other parts of the country are now being provided.

Research in Other Areas

To date, the bulk of the research on P-W syndrome has centered on diagnosis and, to a lesser extent, obesity control. The interdisciplinary approach has led to the accumulation of extensive clinical experience in other areas such as psychology, education, social work, speech therapy, and physical therapy. In regard to these areas, clinical experience at the University of Washington indicates that the needs of P-W persons differ from those of other handicapped persons. The research that has begun confirms this. Recently it has been found that the ways in which P-W persons process information and retrieve it from their memories are different both from those of normal persons and from those of other mentally handicapped people (Warren & Hunt Chapter 12, this volume). This study included a P-W person of normal IQ who nonetheless shared the cognitive deficits of retarded P-W individuals. This indicates that the educational needs of all P-W persons may be unique. Sulzbacher, Crnic, and Snow (Chapter 11, this volume) discuss relationships between weight and IQ and have tentatively concluded that prevention of obesity results in a higher IQ for P-W children. To date, psychology is the only non-medical area in which research has begun. The clinical experience that is being accumulated should be important in determining the design of future research (see also Sulzbacher, Holm, & Pipes, Chapter 25, this volume).

THE PRADER-WILLI SYNDROME ASSOCIATION

The importance of the family to the person with P-W syndrome cannot be exaggerated. A normal child owes much to his or her parents, a mentally retarded person with minor physical abnormalities owes still more. The P-W person, whose life may be shortened if the obesity is not controlled, depends on the parents to an even greater degree. The behavior problems mentioned earlier can make living with an older P-W child extremely difficult. It is only too easy to give in to the insatiable appetite before the threat of tantrums. Also, it is exhausting to have to exercise constant vigilance and ingenuity to prevent foraging for food and other unauthorized eating. It is clear that the family with a P-W child has special needs. In part these are met by careful professional nutritional supervision for the child. Yet many of the strains put on these parents are only increased by the need to carry out very precise dietary programs. The ignorance of the general public, and of many professionals as well, of the specialized needs of persons suffering from this rare disorder contributes to parents' problems. In addition to professional services, there is a need for parents to have contact with other parents who share similar problems and frustrations. This was accomplished to some degree by local groups who met informally, such as the one at the University of Washington P-W Syndrome Clinic. However, there was neither ongoing organization nor contact with those in different geographical areas.

In the spring of 1975 a national organization, the Prader-Willi Syndrome Parents and Friends, later named the Prader-Willi Syndrome Association, was founded for parents and others interested in the welfare of people with the syndrome. Since some of the parents who founded it lived in Massachusetts and others lived in the state of Washington, a wide geographic distribution was assured from the start. Publication of a newsletter, *The Gathered View*, was begun. In the earliest years of the association, this publication was its major activity and provided, as it still does, valuable information for parents of P-W children. It also serves as a much needed vehicle for communication among them.

Later the association was incorporated, bylaws were adopted, and tax-exempt status was obtained. A handbook for parents was produced, meeting the need for concise, reliable information in non-technical language (Neason, 1978). As the syndrome and the association received publicity, the central office, staffed on a volunteer basis by one family, answered an enormous number of requests for information. Also in 1978 the association began to disseminate information in Spanish with a synopsis of the parents' handbook.

Various local groups, some predating the founding of the association, are affiliated with the national organization. Those in Seattle, Sacramento, and Cambridge, Massachussetts, were among the earliest. There are also groups in Minnesota, Los Angeles, and Vancouver, British Columbia. A group has begun in Australia and there are individual members in England and Germany.

The Prader-Willi Syndrome Association held its first annual conference in Minneapolis in 1979. In addition to a business meeting, there were presentations by researchers and other professionals working with the syndrome. Two of the papers presented at this conference were later expanded for this book (Herrmann, Chapter 18; Zellweger, Chapter 5). The conference also provided an opportunity for parents from around the country to meet, become acquainted, and share concerns. For some parents this was the first time they had seen a P-W person other than their own child. A number of adults with P-W syndrome attended.

THE NATIONAL PRADER-WILLI SYNDROME WORKSHOP

The Prader-Willi Syndrome Association conference was preceded by a few weeks by another conference on the syndrome, sponsored by the University of Washington. About 60 people from throughout the United States and Canada attended. This conference provided an opportunity for clinical researchers to share their work with other professionals. A wide range of papers was presented, most of them printed in this volume, and open discussions were held to better define diagnostic criteria and treatment techniques. The publication of this volume, making accessible to the general public the results of the conference, represents the achievement of one of the major goals of the University of Washington's Prader-Willi Syndrome project.

CONCLUSION

At this point, more than a beginning has been made in efforts to resolve problems relating to P-W syndrome. The identification of the syndrome has made possible meaningful research. P-W persons are no longer puzzling, obese individuals with various other abnormalities, but now can be identified as a group with specific common characteristics. Once this enormous first step had been taken it was possible for clinicians to refine further the clinical picture and to begin research concerning possible causes of the syndrome and methods of therapy. Knowledge of the syndrome has rapidly increased (see the annotated bibliography at the end of this volume). Therapeutic methods now available make it possible to ameliorate the condition of P-W people, although this is still far from easy for those involved.

The development of a viable organization devoted to the interests of persons with the syndrome is also an important step. The Prader-Willi Syndrome Association has survived its difficult early years and now seems to be firmly established. At this point, providing information and offering mutual support for parents remain the principal functions. Other activities will probably evolve as the organization grows.

One major question that remains to be resolved is whether or not facilities and services for P-W people should be separate or integrated ("mainstreamed"). Until the public schools and social service agencies become more aware of the specialized needs of P-W persons and make greater efforts to meet them, it will be possible to make a case for special facilities. Understandably, however, the economic burden of separate facilities—schools, summer camps, vocational training programs, sheltered workshops, recreation programs, group homes—for a relatively small population such as this is unreasonably great. In the long run, the desirable direction seems clear. P-W persons, like all others, should be integrated into society as fully as possible. The gain to the individual which would result is surely the most important consideration. Parents in the United States are fortunate in that Public Law 94-142 (Education for All Handicapped Children Act) obliges the public school system to provide appropriate education for every child in the least restrictive environment, regardless of the kind of handicap or severity of the condition. Private social services are not under the same constraints, yet it is to be hoped that as they become more knowledgeable about this condition, and as pressure from individuals and organized groups increases, they will begin to make provision for P-W persons.

Therefore, it is clear that while much progress has been made, much remains to be done. Medical and nutritional problems will remain the center of concern, but other areas must also be developed. Many questions that have long been resolved with other handicapping conditions are just beginning to take shape with respect to Prader-Willi syndrome.

REFERENCES

Allen, K.E., Holm, V.A., & Schiefelbusch, R. *Early intervention: A team approach.* Baltimore: University Park Press, 1978.
Beruete y Moret, A. de. *The school of Madrid.* London: Duckworth; New York: Scribner's, 1909.
Brain, Lord. Chairman's opening remarks: Historical introduction. In G.E.W. Wolstenholme & R. Porter (Eds.), *Ciba foundation study group no. 25; Mongolism.* Boston: Little, Brown & Co., 1967.
Bruch, H. The Fröhlich syndrome: Report of the original case. *American Journal of Diseases of Children,* 1939, *58,* 1282-1289.
Down, J.L.H. *On some of the mental affections of childhood and youth.* London: J.H. Churchill, 1887.

Dunn, H.G. The Prader-Labhart-Willi syndrome: Review of the literature and report of nine cases. *Acta Paediatrica Scandinavica,* 1968, Suppl. 186, 1-38.
Dunn, H.G., Ford, D.K., Auersperg, N., & Miller, J.R. Benign congenital hypotonia with chromosomal anomaly. *Pediatrics,* 1961, *28,* 578-591.
Evans, P.R. Hypogenital dystrophy with diabetic tendency. *Guy's Hospital Reports,* 1964, *113,* 207-222.
Forssman, H., & Hagberg, B. Prader-Willi syndrome in boy of ten with prediabetes. *Acta Paediatrica,* 1964, *53,* 70-78.
Gabilan, J.C. Syndrome de Prader, Labhart et Willi. *Journées pédiatriques,* 1962, *1,* 179-185.
Gabilan, J.C., & Royer, P. Le syndrome de Prader, Labhardt et Willi (étude de onze observations). *Archives Françaises de Pédiatrie,* 1968, *25,* 121-149.
Hall, B.D., & Smith, D.W. Prader-Willi syndrome: A resumé of 32 cases including an instance of affected first cousins, one of whom is of normal stature and intelligence. *The Journal of Pediatrics,* 1972, *81,* 286-293.
Holm, V.A., & Pipes P.L. Food and children with Prader-Willi syndrome. *American Journal of Diseases of Children,* 1976, *130,* 1063-1067.
Hooft, C., Delire, C., & Casneuf, J. Le syndrome de Prader-Labhardt-Willi-Fanconi: Étude clinique, endocrinologique et cytogénétique. *Acta Paediatrica Belgica,* 1966, *20,* 27-50.
Laurance, B.M. Hypotonia, obesity, hypogonadism and mental retardation in childhood. Proceedings of the 32nd Annual Meeting, British Paediatric Association, Cambridge. *Archives of Disease in Childhood,* 1961, *30,* 690.
Laurance, B.M. Hypotonia, mental retardation, obesity, and cryptorchidism associated with dwarfism and diabetes in children. *Archives of Disease in Childhood,* 1967, *42,* 126-139.
McKusick, V.A. *Mendelian inheritance in man: Catalogs of autosomal dominant, autosomal recessive, and x-linked phenotypes* (5th ed.). Baltimore: The Johns Hopkins University Press, 1978.
Monnens, L., & Kenis, H. Enkele onderzoekingen bij een patient met het syndroom van Prader-Willi. *Maandschrift voor Kindergeneeskunde,* 1965, *33,* 482-498.
Moreno Villa, J. *Locos, enanos, negros y niños palaciegos: Gente de placer que tuvieron los Austrias en la corte Española desde 1563 a 1700.* Mexico: La Casa de España en Mexico, 1939.
Neason, S.A. *Prader-Willi syndrome: A handbook for parents.* Long Lake, Minn.: Prader-Willi Syndrome Association, 1978.
Pipes, P.L., & Holm, V.A. Weight control of children with Prader-Willi syndrome. *Journal of the American Dietetic Association,* 1973, *62,* 520-524.
Prader, A., Labhart, A., & Willi, H. Ein Syndrom von Adipositas, Kleinwuchs, Kryptorchismus und Oligophrenie nach myatonieartigem Zustand im Neugeborenenalter. *Schweizerische Medizinische Wochenschrift,* 1956, *86,* 1260-1261.
Prader, A., Labhart, A., Willi, H., & Fanconi, G. Ein Syndrom von Adipositas, Kleinwuchs, Kryptorchismus und Idiotie bei Kindern und Erwachsenen, die als Neugeborene ein myatonie-artiges Bild geboten haben. *Proceedings of the VIII International Congress on Paediatrics., Copenhagen, 1956.*
Prader, A., & Willi, H. Das Syndrom von Imbezillität, Adipositas, Muskelhypotonie, Hypogenitalismus, Hypogonadismus und Diabetes mellitus mit "Myatonie"—Anamnese. *Second International Congress on Mental Retardation, Vienna, 1961* (Part I, p. 353). Basel and New York: S. Karger, 1963.
Sánchez Villares, E., Martín Esteban, M., & Durantez Mayo, O. Amiotonia con-

genita con sindrome de Prader-Willi incompleto. *Boletín de la Sociedad Castellano-Astur-Leonesa de Pediatría,* 1964, *5,* 191-208.

Zellweger, H., & Schneider, H. Syndrome of hypotonia-hypomentia-hypogonadism-obesity (HHHO) or Prader-Willi syndrome. *American Journal of Diseases of Children,* 1968, *115,* 588-598.

Zellweger, H.U., Smith, J.W., & Cusminsky, M. Muscular hypotonia in infancy: Diagnosis and differentiation. *Révue Canadienne de Biologie,* 1962, *21,* 599-612.

chapter 2

FEDERAL PROGRAMS FOR THE DEVELOPMENTALLY DISABLED

Gerald D. LaVeck

> Following is the text of Dr. LaVeck's remarks at the National Prader-Willi Syndrome Workshop, held at the University of Washington, June 13-15, 1979. As a representative of the funding agency, Dr. LaVeck described the context within which to view funding for workshops of this nature.—*Eds.*

The Prader-Willi syndrome is not common but its impact on those persons affected and their parents is significant. The federal government, specifically the Office for Maternal and Child Health (OMCH) in the Bureau of Community Health Services (BCHS), provided financial support for this workshop. Why should the Department of Health and Human Services (HHS) be interested in a relatively rare syndrome and be willing to provide this support? Is not HHS concerned with major problems like cancer, heart disease, arthritis, and stroke?

The support of this workshop to develop guidelines for the management of these special children and to discuss areas of research is just one example of many hundreds of awards that are made by various components of HHS to fund research, training, and services to benefit handicapped children. Many federal programs are directed toward handicapped children. Selected health-related programs are discussed here.

HISTORICAL BACKGROUND

Although the Maternal and Child Health and Crippled Children's Programs were created in 1935 under Title V of the Social Security Act, the American people became more aware of the problems of mental retardation during the early 1960s. A condition that dims the lives and limits the productivity of as many as six million children and adults, costs billions of dollars, and creates tens of millions of heartaches cannot be viewed with complacency by a nation that prides itself on scientific and social initiative. In recognition of these facts, President Kennedy in 1961 appointed a panel of 27 scientists, educators, and other leaders to study the problem and formulate a "Proposed Program of National Action to Combat

Mental Retardation." The report of the panel (1962) and the subsequent passage of two major legislative measures were signals for an intensified and coordinated effort on the part of national, state, and local agencies and civic and professional groups to plan for all aspects of the problem of mental retardation.

In preparation for the new legislation that was passed late in 1963, a new institute was created at the National Institutes of Health (NIH). The National Institute of Child Health and Human Development became responsible for generating new knowledge in the biological and social sciences pertaining to mental retardation and related aspects of human development. The Mental Retardation Facilities and Community Mental Health Centers Construction Act of 1962, passed by Congress in October, 1963, provided much needed construction money. This law authorized grants for construction of 1) centers for research on mental retardation and related aspects of human development and 2) University Affiliated Facilities. In addition, community mental health centers were created. Although mental health centers are not primarily concerned with children with developmental disabilities, they represent an important resource for children with emotional problems associated with developmental problems. Legislation at about the same time resulted in funds for states to plan programs to improve services for retarded individuals.

About this time, the Maternity and Infant Care (MIC) and the Children and Youth (C&Y) projects were established. MIC projects, which are now required in every state, provide medically and financially eligible pregnant women with obstetrical care and followup on their high risk babies during the first year of life. The purpose of this legislation was to reduce mental retardation and infant mortality.

The legislation providing construction grants culminated in the building of 12 mental retardation research centers, nearly all in university settings, of which the Child Development and Mental Retardation Center (CDMRC) at the University of Washington is one. Support from many sources is necessary to facilitate investigations of problems that will lead to new knowledge about the prevention and amelioration of mental retardation. Some of the research centers are large complexes, involving major departments and graduate schools of the university and providing a broad spectrum of biomedical, behavioral, and social science research. Others are more specialized facilities, narrower in scope, and more highly concentrated on a particular aspect of the problem. Research training is also conducted in most of these centers. The centers rely particularly on financial support from NIH.

A total of 21 University Affiliated Facilities (UAFs) were designated in addition to the research centers. Many of these UAFs are located at universities with research centers. This is true at the University of Washington where a UAF is part of the CDMRC. In contrast, at the University of Oregon Health Sciences Center there is a UAF but not a research center. The original purpose of the UAFs was to provide clinical facilities for a complete range of services for mentally retarded persons. Such services were to include inpatient and outpatient services; aid in demonstrations of services for diagnosis, treatment, education, training, and care for mentally retarded persons; and clinical training of physicians and other specialized personnel. The original legislation was clearly oriented toward medical training. Now UAFs are interdisciplinary with a wide variety of disciplines participating in training programs. A heavy service component in some UAFs meets the needs of many children with developmental disabilities. Children with developmental problems are assessed in UAFs where they receive care or are referred to appropriate community facilities for services.

OFFICE FOR MATERNAL AND CHILD HEALTH

The BCHS is located in the Health Services Administration. One of the major organizational components of the BCHS is the OMCH. The OMCH is responsible for the administration of the formula grants that go to all states to support Maternal and Child Health and Crippled Children's Services. The program is administered through the 10 Regional Offices scattered throughout the country, including one in Seattle. These programs have been in existence since 1935 and are often referred to as Title V programs. For many years the Children's Bureau administered Title V. Through a series of reorganizations, the major component of the Children's Bureau eventually became the OMCH.

In addition to its concern for crippled children, this organization established diagnostic evaluation clinics for mentally retarded persons in the 1950s. Currently, the OMCH makes awards to institutions of higher learning for the conduct of training, supports services in various settings for genetic counseling, supports laboratories for cytogenetics and biochemical genetics, and funds special conferences such as the Prader-Willi Syndrome Workshop to further our knowledge concerning specific developmental problems. Other activities include special emphasis on adolescents, improved pregnancy outcome, and projects designed to reduce infant mortality.

In the early years of the UAFs, the services offered as a part of training were assessment of children to determine how severely they were affected and referral elsewhere for whatever management might be available. Now much more emphasis is given to management and outreach training and development of resources. In addition, a number of new federal programs have emerged which should complement the activities of UAFs and expand the services available to children. Following is a brief discussion of some of these new health programs.

Genetic Diseases Act

The Genetic Diseases Act (PL 94-278) was passed in April, 1976, although the first appropriation ($4 million) was not provided until fiscal year (FY) 1978. Late in 1978 the legislation was extended and amended and appropriations have increased.

The act provides for health services such as testing, counseling, diagnosis, and information and educational programs for genetic diseases. Over 30 programs have been approved under this legislation. Most programs are statewide or regional in scope, often including a number of states. For example, the state of Washington was the recipient of an award that was made to the Title V Agency to provide regional services.

The Genetic Diseases Act requires that testing and counseling programs be established and operated in conjunction with existing health programs. That is, a purpose of the act is to foster collaboration and coordination and establish linkages with existing programs, especially maternal and child health programs. For example, the BCHS has continued to encourage expansion of newborn metabolic screening and to consolidate and develop regional efforts. Screening has been supported in many states through Title V formula grants or special project grants. In this region, Oregon has a program in which all newborn infants in Oregon, Idaho, Alaska, Nevada, and Montana are screened for six specific metabolic disorders. The two diseases that are more prevalent are phenylketonuria (PKU) and hypothyroidism. If these disorders can be detected early in the newborn period, appropriate treatment can be given to prevent the subsequent development of mental retardation. The state of Washington has its own screening program for PKU and hypothyroidism. In Washington approximately one in 4,000 infants has hypothyroidism. Although the follow-up period is still short, all detected cases are being treated and the children are developing normally. Many children with PKU are referred to the CDMRC or to faculty members at the university and to the Children's Orthopedic Hospital and Medical Center. The UAF follows up all children with congenital hypothyroidism identified by newborn screening.

Another example of a linkage relates to the UAF. There is an agreement between the genetics program and the UAF in Seattle. Children with genetic diseases who are in need of further evaluation because of developmental disabilities are referred to the UAF. Those at the UAF who need genetic counseling or sophisticated diagnostic procedures are referred to the appropriate genetic counseling clinic or to consultants. Genetic counseling clinics are available in Seattle, Walla Walla, Tacoma, and Spokane. Additional clinics will be developed in the state. Also, the

UAFs are in a position to emphasize training in genetic diagnosis and counseling which will further the statewide efforts in this field.

The Crippled Children's Division at the University of Oregon Health Sciences Center includes a UAF and a statewide genetics program, the latter established before new legislation was passed. The state of Washington provides services for Alaska, Idaho, and Montana, whereas Oregon serves Idaho and Alaska. Thus, in the northwest programs that are regional in scope and that focus on developmental and genetic defects are being developed.

Supplemental Security Income—Disabled Children's Program (SSI-DCP)

Public Law 94-566 provides legislative authority for the SSI-DCP as an amendment to Title XVI of the Social Security Act. This state formula grant program is also administered by the BCHS through a written agreement with the Social Security Administration. The purpose of the SSI-DCP is to provide for the delivery of medical, social, developmental, educational, and rehabilitative services to blind and disabled children under 16 years of age, who are receiving Supplemental Security Income benefits. The SSI-DCP must locate these children, get them into the health care system, and make certain that needed care is rendered on an individual basis. In almost all of the states, the SSI-DCP is administered by Crippled Children's Services agencies. Each child and his or her parents are counseled as to the services the program has to offer. An individual service plan (ISP) is developed for each child and the care provided under each plan is monitored. This, and the requirement for interagency collaboration, are having a revitalizing effect on the Crippled Children's Service programs.

Written agreements must be developed between the SSI-DCP and such state programs as developmental disabilities, vocational rehabilitation, Medicaid, education for the handicapped, mental health, and services to the blind. The purpose of this collaboration is to make possible the maximum utilization of existing resources, make available a complete range of services for handicapped children, prevent duplication of services, and coordinate the implementation of ISPs.

A multidisciplinary approach to the development of an ISP is required. A number of agencies will often be involved in developing and implementing a plan for the child. Many UAFs will become involved in developing and establishing ISPs since developmental and neurological defects are the most common chronic problems encountered in the SSI-DCP. The first full year of the SSI-DCP was 1978, and as of late 1980 most state programs were not yet fully operational due to legislative delays.

Establishing interagency collaboration will be a long process, but it is essential to the provision of services and to the development of ISPs.

It is estimated that over 200,000 referrals were made to all state SSI-DCPs in FY 1980. The success of the effort will depend on the degree to which interagency collaboration is achieved, written agreements are developed by each state program, and existing resources, such as UAFs, are used. Pratt (Note 1) describes three models that are used by different state SSI-DCPs. Model A operates by having a state staff manage the program and contract with one or more outside agencies to perform the counseling, while preparing and monitoring the service plans, and scheduling or delivering the services. With model B, the state SSI staff provide the initial counseling, write the service plan, and purchase care that cannot be provided by cooperative agency agreements. Finally, with model C, the SSI staff manage the program, provide counseling, help assess children, write ISPs, and deliver some services not provided by cooperative agreements.

Neonatal Intensive Care Units

Complications of pregnancy that result in early death of the fetus or infant are also those that can result in permanent handicap for the developing child. These include mental retardation, epilepsy, cerebral palsy, hearing and vision impairments, and other handicaps. We cannot focus exclusively on biological problems, however. Evidence is accumulating that inadequate mothering is likely to follow when bonding fails to occur. Deficiencies in maternal-child bonding are thought to be associated with adverse developmental outcome for the child.

The disadvantages of low birth weight are clear. Yet, most babies weighing over 1,500 g at birth live and develop into normal children, and the outlook for those weighing less than 1,500 g has improved as measured by survival rate. It is thought that much of this progress is the result of better coordination between obstetrics and pediatrics and improved methods of care in the neonatal intensive care unit (NICU).

A recent study by Pape, Bunic, Ashby, and Fitzhardinge (1978) recorded all 43 infants of birth weight less than 1,000 g who were admitted to an NICU in Toronto during 1974 and followed up for 2 years. Seven (16%) had retrolental fibroplasia; four (9%) had major neurological defects; nine (21%) had developmental delay with a developmental quotient (DQ) of less than 80. Defects of the nervous system were closely associated with a neonatal history of intracranial hemorrhage or seizures or both. Eighty-two percent of the children were the product of high risk pregnancies. Prior to 1970 approximately 75% of these very small infants died and only 15% survived as normal children. In the study of Pape et al., 53% died and 33% survived without handicaps, a twofold increase in the number of normal survivors.

There is reason to believe that maternal, fetal, and neonatal mortality and morbidity rates can be reduced. This might be facilitated by identifying patients at high risk early in pregnancy and providing optimal care for the mother, fetus, and infant. We do not know precisely the benefits of modern perinatal medicine. Data supporting this approach are not as firm as many of us would like. However, evidence is accumulating that improved pregnancy outcome may be a consequence of early identification of high risk mothers and fetuses and the application of appropriate treatment methods as described by the American Academy of Pediatrics (1977).

Finally, it is important to follow up those infants who have received intensive care. Infant mortality is falling. Perhaps much of this progress is because of better coordination and methods of perinatal care. However, few follow-up studies have been conducted long enough to document clearly the prognosis for the development of survivors of new methods of intensive care. Many NICU follow-up programs have begun.

Thus a new major focus of attention for UAFs is NICU babies who are at high risk for developmental problems. Identifying high risk children, providing appropriate intervention, and counseling parents can prevent problems associated with the unexpected recognition of deficiencies in development at later age.

CONCLUSION

A few major health programs that were recently initiated or have received special attention lately have been reviewed. In particular, some new health-related efforts requiring linkages with UAFs to maximize effectiveness have been outlined. The UAFs not only provide needed services to developmentally disabled persons but also serve as a catalyst for research. Workshops like the Prader-Willi Syndrome Workshop, which bring together researchers from all parts of the country, are essential for dissemination of newly discovered information and also help to stimulate additional research. The future looks bright for improved services for handicapped children because of these integrative efforts.

REFERENCE NOTE

1. Pratt, W.M. *The management framework for SSI/DC Programs: Evaluation team perspective.* Paper presented at the National Meeting of SSI/DC Programs, Chicago, September 1978.

REFERENCES

American Academy of Pediatrics, Committee on Fetus and Newborn. *Standards and recommendations for hospital care of newborn infants.* Evanston, Ill.: Author, 1977.

Pape, K.E., Bunic, R.J., Ashby, S., & Fitzhardinge, P.M. The status at two years of low-birth-weight infants born in 1974 with birth weights of less than 1001 gm. *The Journal of Pediatrics*, 1978, *92*, 253-260.

President's Panel on Mental Retardation. *A proposed program for national action to combat mental retardation.* Washington, D.C.: U.S. Government Printing Office, 1962.

part I
ETIOLOGY AND DIAGNOSIS

chapter 3
THE DIAGNOSIS OF PRADER-WILLI SYNDROME

Vanja A. Holm

> This chapter discusses the diagnosis of Prader-Willi syndrome, adding new information to established diagnostic criteria. This includes diagnosing this obesity syndrome in patients who are not currently obese, revising estimates of the incidence of scoliosis upward and of diabetes mellitus downward, and the discovery that many persons with this syndrome lack the ability to vomit and sensitivity to pain. This chapter is intended as a diagnostic standard until definite biomedical correlates have been developed.—*Eds.*

The diagnosis of Prader-Willi (P-W) syndrome, like many other syndromes, is much less precise than many medical diagnoses. It compares to the diagnosis of Down syndrome before the discovery of the chromosomal abnormality that causes that condition. Before 1959 the physical stigmata of mongolism, as it then was called, were the only guidelines to diagnosis. This is still the situation with P-W syndrome, with the added complication that the physical stigmata, especially in infancy and early childhood, are even less prominent than in Down syndrome. In P-W syndrome, as is true of most other syndromes, one finds a spectrum, i.e., some afflicted persons have most of the characteristic findings, others only a few. Clinicians do not always agree on minimal criteria for diagnosis.

The following outline of the symptomatology of P-W syndrome and guidelines to diagnosis truly represent a consensus. The information has been compiled from the literature, from studies reported in other chapters of this book, and from a questionnaire study carried out in 1977. The diagnosis of P-W syndrome in the latter study was made by a number of physicians across the country. Consensus is further ensured by the fact that these diagnostic criteria were presented to and discussed with physicians actively involved with P-W patients and participating in the University of Washington's Prader-Willi Syndrome Workshop.

The prevalence of P-W syndrome is still unknown. Consensus of opinion among the physicians consulted indicates that a figure of 1:10,000 is a reasonable estimate. It is among the five most common syndromes in most birth defects clinics and many clinicians agree that it is one-fifth to one-tenth as common as Down syndrome.

Background information about the questionnaire study will be provided before specific diagnostic criteria are discussed.

QUESTIONNAIRE STUDY

Questionnaires were mailed to parents and professionals who had written to the University of Washington Prader-Willi Syndrome Clinic with questions about the syndrome. (See questionnaire in Appendix A.) Of 106 returned questionnaires, 98 contained enough information on persons diagnosed as having P-W syndrome by other physicians to satisfy standards for clinical diagnosis of P-W syndrome used in 1977.

The mean age of the patient population was 14.1 years (range 1.0–32.1). Seventy-five percent were living in single families (68% with both biological parents), 12% were in residential schools and group homes, and the rest were in a variety of living situations, including 7% in institutions. Eighty percent of the information was provided by parents; the rest came from professional caregivers. Fifty-six percent of the P-W persons were males, and 95% were white. It should be noted that the information might be considered selective: The data came from people who chose to contact our clinic. The results may not accurately reflect the distribution of symptoms in the total population of P-W persons.

DIAGNOSTIC CRITERIA

Symptoms present in P-W syndrome have been divided into four categories: 1) symptoms essential for diagnosis; 2) symptoms occurring in 50% to 95% of the cases; 3) those occurring in 10% to 50% of the cases; and 4) rare but important symptoms occurring in less than 10% of the cases.

Symptoms Essential for Diagnosis of P-W Syndrome

Most precepts in medicine have exceptions. An occasional person might have so many other symptoms of P-W syndrome that the diagnosis is evident without one of the symptoms listed in this category. However, the following symptoms should be considered obligatory before a firm diagnosis of P-W syndrome is made.

Infantile, Supraspinal (or Central) Hypotonia This symptom occurred in 100% of the P-W persons in the questionnaire study. Of these, 44% had severe, 29% moderate, 23% extreme, and 4% mild hypotonia. Hypotonia-related symptoms, i.e., symptoms that seem to be due directly to hypotonia, include:

1. Abnormal delivery. In the questionnaire study, 22% of the P-W persons had been born by breech and 18% by cesarean section (see also Nugent & Holm, Chapter 21, this volume).
2. Poor suck. This was present in 97% of the cases.

3. Feeding problems in infancy requiring special nipples, gavage feedings, etc. Ninety-eight percent of the responders noted this problem.
4. Delayed motor landmarks. From the questionnaire study, the average age at independent sitting was 13 months, walking 28 months, tricycle riding 4.2 years, bicycle riding 9 years. The oldest child still unable to walk was 5¼ years of age. Only 17 individuals in this study were able to bicycle.

Zellweger (Chapter 5, this volume) discusses the differential diagnosis of the floppy infant. The terminology he uses to describe hypotonia was agreed upon at the workshop. "Infantile" implies that the symptom is most marked in infancy. Even though it improves with age, it is still a mild handicap in older children with P-W syndrome (Carman, Chapter 24, this volume). "Supraspinal" (or central) indicates that studies of the neuromotor unit are normal. Such studies are frequently done in infancy in the P-W child. The typical P-W motor milestones arrived at from the questionnaire study agree with informal observations reported by clinicians familiar with the syndrome.

Hypogonadism This terminology is retained, even though "abnormal development of physical sexual characteristics" would be a more accurate description of the symptomatology. Hypogonadism is considered an essential symptom. However, physicians might have difficulties in recognizing hypogonadism in young children. Girls might have small labia minora, a highly subjective finding. Boys usually have small penile size. By measuring the length of the penis and comparing it to available growth charts (Smith, 1976), this observation becomes an objective one. Undescended testes during childhood are very common in P-W syndrome, but the exact incidence is not known. Masculinization and feminization in adolescence are usually delayed and incomplete. In the experience of most of the clinicians at the workshop, adolescent sexual development might also be disordered. Early pubarche is common. One occasionally sees cases where sexual development is out of order in other ways (Kauli, Prager-Lewin, & Laron, 1978; Smith, Neeman, Wulff, & Seely, 1970).

Parental recognition of hypogonadism is limited, as reflected in the questionnaire study. Fifty-two percent knew that their sons' testes were undescended. Four percent felt that male sexual development was normal. Twelve percent made similar observations about their daughters. According to parental report, of 19 girls over 16 years of age, 11 had never had menstrual periods. Of those who did, mean age of menarche was 17 years, ranging from 13 to 28.

Tze, Dunn, and Rothstein (Chapter 22, this volume) state that hypogonadism in P-W syndrome seems to be hypothalamic. Studies of the hypothalamic-pituitary axis might in the future aid in the diagnostic assessment of hypogonadism in young children, especially prepubertal girls. At the present time the assessment of hypogonadism is clinical, by history and physical examination only.

It is assumed that all persons with P-W syndrome are sterile, because no such persons have been known to be sexually active. The question of whether or not a P-W person could be fertile is of interest. If a pregnancy should occur, the outcome would be of great interest. A minor chromosomal abnormality or a spontaneous mutation of a dominant gene has not yet been ruled out as a cause of P-W syndrome, even though the most commonly held theory is that the defect is a polygenically inherited central nervous system malformation involving the hypothalamus (Hanson, Chapter 4, this volume). A report of the outcome of pregnancies from an institution in England is of interest. Of two women supposedly diagnosed as having P-W syndrome, one gave birth to a similarly afflicted child as well as one normal and two otherwise abnormal infants. The other woman was reported to have a normal child (Laxova, Gilderdale, & Ridler, 1973). If the diagnosis of P-W syndrome was correct in these women, it would indicate that the etiology of P-W syndrome might be a chromosomal abnormality or a dominant gene. Outcome of any pregnancy involving a P-W partner should be thoroughly documented and reported in the medical literature.

Obesity Obesity after early infancy, occurring without intervention, is an essential symptom. Obesity is always preceded by a period of "failure to thrive." Clinically the length of that period seems to correlate with the degree of hypotonia. Although the onset of obesity varies from 6 months to 5 to 6 years, in most cases it occurs around 2 years of age (Nugent & Holm, Chapter 21, this volume). The severely hypotonic child frequently becomes obese late, but maternal attitudes toward infant feeding and family eating patterns strongly influence the onset of this symptom.

Investigation of caloric intake invariably shows that caloric intake per centimeter of height is less in this syndrome than in a normal population of the same age (Pipes, Chapter 7, this volume). This finding can be used to confirm that the obesity is "P-W-like." Schwartz, Brunzell, and Bierman (Chapter 10, this volume) confirm that a greatly elevated level of lipoprotein lipase is found in fat biopsy, when this test is available.

The diagnosis of P-W syndrome in the person who is not obese deserves further comment. Diagnosis is seldom a problem in older individuals. One gets a history of previous obesity followed by a weight loss, usually achieved after heroic efforts. A need for unusually limited caloric intake both to lose and maintain weight provides additional strong support. Distribution of subcutaneous fat tissue constitutes an additional clue. Even though the face and upper trunk might look lean—incidentally, many of the "classical" facial features disappear when a P-W person looses weight—there is still excessive fat on the lower trunk, buttocks, and thighs.

Hypotonic boys with hypogonadism are often recognized as possible or likely victims of P-W syndrome in infancy. The diagnosis is also recognized with increased frequency in hypotonic females still in the failure to thrive stage. What criteria for "obesity" for the purpose of diagnosis should be used in these situations? It is absurd to propose that one wait to see whether the child actually becomes obese. Growth in height and weight can be followed carefully in these children. A sudden increase in weight percentile is usually noted during the preschool years and this proven tendency toward rapid weight gain can be used as a diagnostic criterion for obesity in this age group. The author has seen a great many young children with P-W syndrome who have never been allowed to become obese and who have, as they became older, showed so many of the other physical and behavioral characteristics of the syndrome that the diagnosis never was in doubt. In fact, we have yet to see a young child suspected of having P-W syndrome in whom subsequent events showed this early suspicion to be erroneous.

Dysfunctional Central Nervous System (CNS) Performance Mental retardation was previously considered an integral part of the definition of P-W syndrome. Most clinicians at the conference agreed that cognitive functioning of many youngsters with this syndrome is typical for those with learning disabilities, even though some afflicted individuals test in the mentally retarded range. The description "dysfunctional CNS performance" was agreed upon by parents and professionals at the conference as a fair description of the cognitive and learning styles of P-W persons.

Support for these clinical impressions was obtained from the questionnaire study. Developmental landmarks, as reported by the parents, indicate that the mean age of the first smile is 4 months, use of single words 21 months, sentences 3.6 years, and ability to read 7.5 years. The oldest child who did not use single words was 5 years old. This concurs with Branson's (Chapter 13, this volume) observation of an occasional case of severe expressive aphasia or apraxia in this condition. It was noted that the most advanced age at which a P-W person learned to read was 13.6 years. Reading was commonly mentioned among academic strengths. Arithmetic was frequently noted as an academic weakness; the mean age of being able to do simple one- and two-digit addition and subtraction was 8.4 years, with the oldest child learning these skills at 15 years. At least five individuals older than 15 years were unable to perform these tasks.

IQ information was available in 76 cases from the P-W questionnaire study. The test had been obtained at a mean age of 10 years (range 1.3 to

24 years). Twelve percent were in the normal range, 29% in the borderline range, 41% mildly retarded, and 12% moderately retarded. In a few cases, range of intelligence function could not be determined from the information provided. Educational placement, either past or present, was in regular educational programs in 6% of the cases and an additional 5% were in regular educational programs with special help. Twelve-and-one-half percent were either in learning disabilities classrooms or in educational programs for the "neurologically impaired." Fifty-eight percent were in other special education classes, with an additional 7% in preschools for handicapped children. A small number of children were in private schools, repeating classes in regular education, etc. Considering the IQs found in this population, academic achievement in the 34 youngsters who were over 16 years of age is disappointing. Mean grade level achieved was 3.3, ranging from kindergarten to 12th grade. Academic weaknesses most commonly mentioned were in arithmetic and writing. Strengths most commonly listed included puzzles, music, arts and crafts, and reading.

From information provided regarding highest independent living skills, the author judged whether the person's skill could be classified as appropriate, questionable, or delayed considering age. It was interesting that 72% were age-appropriate and only 14% delayed in feeding and meal preparation skills. In dressing and grooming, 60% were age-appropriate and 8% delayed. Fifty percent were age-appropriate and 27% delayed in their ability to get around independently in the neighborhood. The most difficult area seemed to be understanding of time and handling of money, where only 19% were age-appropriate and 63% delayed.

Thus, P-W syndrome is by no means always associated with mental retardation. Over 40% of afflicted individuals are *not* retarded. (Retardation is defined as 2 standard deviations or more below the mean on the IQ test used.) Prognostic interpretation from the above information would be that virtually all P-W persons eventually walk but might take as long as 6 years. All but a very few develop functional language, and those who do not probably have the capability of developing an alternative communication mode, like sign language. Reading and simple arithmetic are realistic academic goals and should be pursued. Considering available information on IQ (see also Sulzbacher, Crnic, & Snow, Chapter 11, this volume), the academic performance has been poor for individuals with P-W syndrome as has been the development of self-help skills (except feeding and food preparation!). Information presented here on academic achievement should not be used as prognostic indicators in P-W syndrome. Instead, it is hoped that the information now available will help educators program more effectively to help P-W individuals achieve better in the future.

Finally, there is no typical cognitive developmental pattern in P-W syndrome. There are some tendencies, however. Language tends to be a strength in the majority, with some spectacular exceptions, and reading skills are acquired at a nearly normal rate for many. Another peculiar strength seems to be the visual-perceptual skills required for puzzle assembling. (One P-W person was able to mix six 1,000 piece puzzles and put them together upside-down!) A weakness in many is number concepts. The only consistent problem in CNS performance discovered so far is the poor short term memory noted by Warren and Hunt (Chapter 12, this volume). The most meaningful statement one can make about cognitive function in the P-W syndrome population is that afflicted persons usually exhibit marked strengths and weaknesses which need to be individually analyzed for remediation. The clinical term coined here, *dysfunctional CNS performance,* imprecise as it may be, seems to be a fair description of intellectual functioning in P-W syndrome. We still do not know of any P-W person whose day-to-day cognitive functioning is normal.

Dysmorphic Facial Features The classical facial features described in P-W syndrome include narrow bifrontal diameter, almond-shaped eyes, and a triangular mouth. In the opinion of the clinicians at the workshop, most P-W persons show these characteristics. The findings are highly subjective and thought by some to be secondary to a CNS malformation (Hanson, Chapter 4, this volume). Most important, one would not expect a P-W person to show strong familial likeness.

Short Stature Considering Genetic Background If one uses Tanner's data of expected height growth from age 2 to 9 years considering mid-parental height (Tanner, Goldstein, & Whitehouse, 1970), one finds that nearly all children with P-W syndrome are short for their genetic background. Lack of a preadolescent growth spurt further contributes to the short stature in all adults with the syndrome (Nugent & Holm, Chapter 21, this volume).

Symptoms That Occur in 50% to 90% of the Cases

Small Hands and Feet Ninety-five percent of the persons in the questionnaire study were thought to have these characteristics. Most clinicians agree that approximately this percentage of P-W persons from midchildhood on have acromicria when appropriate measurements are taken and compared to available growth standards (Smith, 1976).

Skin Problems Of the 93 individuals for whom information is available, 91% had some kind of skin problem. The most common was skin picking, which occurred in 81%. Sixty-nine percent of the population were easily bruised. Other skin problems included persisting sores and infections. Acanthosis nigricans also has been described in this syndrome (Reed, Ragsdale, Curtis, & Richards, 1968).

Oral Pathology Of the respondents to the questionnaire study, 92 reported on oral findings. In 87% of the cases there was some form of oral pathology. Forty-seven percent reported unusual (sticky, foamy) saliva, 44% caries, and 39% abnormal bite. Many individuals had more than one oral problem.

Abnormal Cry in the Newborn Eighty-eight percent of the parents noted an abnormal cry in the newborn. Many commented that there was no cry or that the cry was weak while others described it as "squeaky," "kitten-like," or "whiny." It was the consensus of the clinicians that this symptom was *not* directly related to the hypotonia.

Scoliosis Laurnen (Chapter 23, this volume) found that 87% of people with P-W syndrome had significant scoliosis, i.e., a curve of 10° or greater. Only 12% of the parents from the questionnaire study were aware of the presence of scoliosis. This supports the contention that this symptom is severely underdiagnosed in P-W syndrome.

Strabismus This condition was reported in 64% of the patients. This incidence is similar to that observed by Hall (1972) in his clinic population.

Inability to Vomit Many respondents to the study provided the information that P-W persons known to them did not vomit under "normal" circumstances, e.g., with gastrointestinal flu or food poisoning. This information could not be quantified, since it had not been specifically requested. An informal polling of the parents participating in the parent meeting in Minneapolis in June, 1979 indicates that this problem occurs in approximately 75% of the cases of P-W syndrome.

Behavioral Problems Relating to Food Some authors, such as Nelson and his colleagues (Chapter 8, this volume), consider hyperphagia a universal symptom. However, the incidence of this symptom depends on the age of the patient population. It is unusual in very young children and increases with age. Responses to the questionnaire study indicate the following incidence of behavior problems: 80% gorge themselves, 79% forage for food, 74% have violent outbursts, 68% are preoccupied with food, 50% have temper tantrums, and 35% eat products generally considered inedible by others.

Behavioral problems and deviant social/emotional development are second only to obesity as a concern in any P-W population beyond the preschool age. Often the two go together.

Symptoms That Occur in 10% to 50% of the Cases

Abnormal Birth An abnormal birth was reported in 37% of the patients. Nineteen percent had been born by breech, 15 percent had been born by cesarean section, and an additional 3% had been born by section secondary to a breech position.

Myopia Twenty-four percent of the patient population in the questionnaire study were nearsighted. The author has seen several cases of non-familial high myopia in P-W syndrome.

Speech Articulation Problems This symptom was reported in 19% of the patients, which correlates well with the observation made by Branson (Chapter 13, this volume).

Decreased Pain Sensitivity This is a potentially important symptom which was reported by 18% of the responders. Clinical observation would suggest that it might be even more common than the study indicates.

Symptoms with Less Than a 10% Occurrence

Congenital Hip Dislocation This occurred in 8% of the patients. Many authors feel that this symptom is secondary to hypotonia. Knee and elbow dislocations also were noted in some patients.

Large Head Eight percent of the respondents noted a large head. Incidentally, less than one-third had observed the narrow bifrontal diameter, which most clinicians feel is present in a high percentage of cases. However, many of the clinicians noted occasional cases of non-familial large head circumference, present from birth, in patients who later have many of the typical findings of P-W syndrome. This has not been previously described in the literature.

Diabetes Mellitus Most discussions of P-W syndrome mention diabetes mellitus as an important symptom. In the questionnaire study it was present in only 7% of the cases. Most of the clinicians agreed that diabetes is quite unusual in P-W syndrome. In the author's experience, one individual in a patient population of almost 60 has developed diabetes. In fact, some of the clinicians felt that the incidence of diabetes is *less* in P-W syndrome populations than in normal populations with an equal degree of obesity.

Fractures after Minimal Trauma It is the impression of many clinicians that this is a common problem, but it occurred in only 5% of the population in the questionnaire study. An additional 15% of the population had had fractures following "normal" accidents, a fairly high number.

Seizure Disorders This additional symptom, probably falls in the percentage category of less than 10%. The incidence of seizures has been reported by others (Hall & Smith, 1972), but were not asked for in the questionnaire study.

SUMMARY

In this chapter, diagnostic criteria for P-W syndrome have been outlined. Noteworthy new information includes: 1) a definition of obesity in the non-obese P-W person, 2) the high incidence of scoliosis in this condition, 3) the finding of frequent inability to vomit combined with low pain sensitivity in some afflicted individuals, and 4) the suprisingly low incidence of diabetes mellitus considering the extreme obesity in this population. It is hoped that this information will aid physicians in making a clinical diagnosis of P-W syndrome until laboratory correlates become available. Early diagnosis is the mainstay in management of P-W syndrome, as is discussed in other sections of this book.

ACKNOWLEDGMENTS

I would like to thank those who filled out the questionnaires that formed the basis of this study and the physicians who took part in the diagnosis discussion at the University of Washington's Prader-Willi Syndrome Workshop: Audrey E. Griesbach, M.D., James W. Hanson, M.D., Barringer D. Marshall, Jr., M.D., Ralph A. Nelson, M.D., Jane K. Nugent, M.D., Rogelio H.A. Ruvalcaba, M.D., Robert T. Soper, M.D., and Andrée Walczak, M.D. I am grateful to Bryan D. Hall, M.D., A.B. Hayles, M.D., and Hans Zellweger, M.D., with whom I discussed the information in this chapter. I would also like to express my appreciation to the Department of Pediatrics faculty of the University of Washington School of Medicine for their contribution.

REFERENCES

Hall, B.D., & Smith, D.W. Prader-Will syndrome: A resumé of 32 cases including an instance of affected first cousins, one of whom is of normal stature and intelligence. *The Journal of Pediatrics,* 1972, *81,* 286-293.

Kauli, R., Prager-Lewin, R., & Laron, Z. Pubertal development in the Prader-Labhart-Willi syndrome. *Acta Paediatrica Scandinavica,* 1978, *67,* 763-767.

Laxova, R., Gilderdale, S., & Ridler, M.A.C. An aetiological study of fifty-three female patients from a subnormality hospital and of their offspring. *Journal of Mental Deficiency Research,* 1973, *17,* 193-225.

Reed, W.B., Ragsdale, W., Jr., Curtis, A.C., & Richards, H.J. Acanthosis nigricans in association with various genodermatoses. *Acta Dermato-Venereologica,* 1968, *48,* 465-473.

Smith, D.W. *Recognizable patterns of human malformation: Genetic, embryologic and clinical aspects* (2nd Ed.). Philadelphia: W.B. Saunders Co., 1976.

Smith J.D., Neeman, J., Wulff, J., & Seely, J.R. Clinical-metabolic study of the Prader-Willi syndrome. *Journal of the Oklahoma State Medical Association,* 1970, *63,* 234-238.

Tanner, J.M., Goldstein, H., & Whitehouse, R.H. Standards for children's height at ages 2-9 years allowing for height of parents. *Archives of Disease in Childhood,* 1970, *45,* 755-762.

Appendix A
QUESTIONNAIRE
I. Identifying Data

P-W PERSONS

Sex _____ Birth date _____ Birthplace _____

When, where and by whom was the diagnosis made? _____

_____

Has there ever been any doubt about the diagnosis? _____

Living situation (check which applies):

Biological parents	_____	Residential school	_____
Adoptive parents	_____	Group home	_____
Foster parents	_____	Institution	_____
One step-parent	_____	Other (describe)	_____
		_____	

II. Family History

MOTHER:
Race_____ Age (at time of birth of P-W person) _____

FATHER:
Race_____ Age (at time of birth of P-W person) _____

SIBLINGS (same parents as P-W person):

Sex	Year of Birth	State of Physical and Mental Health

HALF-SIBLINGS (please indicate if mother's or father's child):

Sex	Year of Birth	State of Physical and Mental Health	Mother's or Father's Child

The following space has been left for the same identifying information (sex, year of birth, and physical and mental health) on individual(s) known to you who is "blood"-related to the P-W person and who shows physical and/or mental characteristics similar to what is found in this condition (e.g., diabetes, learning problems, obesity, etc., as described in the accompanying statement). Please indicate the relationship between this person and the P-W person, but do *not* provide any names.

Sex	Year of Birth	State of Physical and Mental Health	Relationship to P-W Person

FAMILY HISTORY NOT KNOWN ____

III. Pregnancy and Birth History

(When answering the following questions, only mark items that seem to be different or unusual about this pregnancy, especially as compared to others of the same mother. Check the statements that seem applicable, describing when necessary.)

Labor was:
____Prolonged
____Unusually short
____Difficult

If either prolonged or unusually short, approximately how long? ____ (in hours)

The baby was delivered:
____Head first, face down (most common position)
____Head first, face up ("sunny side up")
____Breech (seat first)
____Footling (one or two feet first)
____Cesarean section (if the latter, why? _____)

The baby:
____Was resuscitated (oxygen given by mask or tube)
____Was kept in an incubator with oxygen (if so, how long? _____)
____Was kept in an incubator without oxygen (if so, how long? _____)
____Was hypotonic (limp, "floppy," with decreased muscle tone)
If yes, degree: Mild____ Moderate____ Severe____ Extreme____
____Had poor suck
____Had an unusual cry (if yes, try to describe _____)

Describe any other difficulties noted in the immediate neonatal period (first few hours of life):

Birth weight_____ Birth length_____

Head size at birth_____

NO INFORMATION REGARDING PREGNANCY AND BIRTH HISTORY IS AVAILABLE____

IV. Early Feeding History

How was this P-W person fed during the first months of life? Mark all statements that are applicable.

____The baby was breastfed (if so, how long? _____)
____Breastfeedings were tried but were unsuccessful (if so, why? _____)
____The baby was bottle fed from the beginning (if yes, were the nipples ordinary kind____ holes enlarged____ "premie" nipples____)
____The baby originally had to be gavage-fed (fed by tube) (if yes, how long? _____)

Which of the following statements regarding the P-W person's interest and attitudes toward food seems applicable during the first few months of life?

____The infant was an eager feeder
____The infant showed little interest in food (if yes, approximately how long did this last? _____)
____The infant had to be awakened to be fed (if yes, approximately how long did this last? _____

At about what age did this P-W person's feeding schedules and attitudes begin to seem appropriate (i.e., feeding skills, interest and amount of formula taken seemed like average infant or child of the same age)? ___

Use this place to describe additional observations (e.g., problems encountered, successful methods of treatment) made about feedings during the first few months of life.

NO INFORMATION REGARDING EARLY FEEDING HISTORY IS AVAILABLE____

V. Physical Growth

Please list *all* physical measurements known to you on this P-W person, whether they are home measurements, from physicians' records, baby books, etc. If the date and year when the measurement was obtained is known, please include this information; if the child's age only is known, substitute with that information. When possible, indicate how measurements were obtained (i.e., "rough home estimate," "doctor's records," "bathroom scale," "clinic evaluation," etc.). Include heights, weights, head circumferences, and any other physical measurements available from birth on to the present time. If space left available for this information is insufficient, please supply it on a separate sheet.

Date or Age   Height   Weight   Head Circumference   Other   How Obtained

If information regarding heights, weights, and other measurements is not available to you, but you would be willing to make this information available to us, indicate so by checking this blank____

Note that for us to obtain such information, the "Consent Form for Release of Information" included will have to be completed.

VI. Mental and Social Growth and Development

(Please go through the following list and fill in the answers which apply and of which you are reasonably confident about their accuracy.

This P-W person:

Smiled at age____

Sat unsupported at age____

Walked at age____

Could tricycle at age____

Bicycled at age____

Said first words at age____

Put two to three words together in short sentences at age____

Learned to read at age____

Could do simple one- and two-digit addition and subtraction at age____

This P-W person's highest (or present) academic achievement is as follows (indicate grade level or describe):

Reading _____

Arithmetic _____

Writing _____

This P-W person:

____Has special problems in this (these) area(s) of academic learning ____

_____

____Has special strengths in this (these) area(s) of academic learning ____

_____

____Has had successful vocational training in (type) _____

____Shows special skills and interest in _____

_____

This P-W person's highest independent living (self-help) skills are (describe):

Feeding and meal preparation _____

_____

Dressing and grooming _____

_____

Knowledge of time and money _____

_____

Ability to get around independently in the neighborhood _____

_____

Results of any formal testing (intelligence IQ tests, speech and language evaluation, social assessments, etc.) would be appreciated, *if* you know the outcome of such tests and *if* you care to share them with us.

Date	Name of Test	Results (e.g., "IQ" number, what you were told, "mental age," or category of functioning)

School experience:

Type of Program (e.g., regular, learning disabilities, MR)	From Age to Age	Experience of P-W Person Was Good, Indifferent, or Poor

VII. Medical Information

Please indicate which of the following medical conditions this P-W person has (or has had); when a condition is present, please give as much detail as possible, describe and indicate treatment and outcome in space made available on the right side of the questionnaire.

Description,
Treatment, and Outcome

1. Eyes
    a. Strabismus (crossed eyes, wandering or lazy eye)____
    b. Myopia (nearsightedness)____
       If present, at what age was it first noted?____
    c. Other eye or vision problems____
2. Ears
    a. Hearing loss____
       If present, indicate what kind (e.g., due to ear infections, fluid behind the drum, nerve loss, etc.)____
    b. Other ear or hearing problems____
3. Mouth
    a. Excessive dental caries____
    b. Orthodontic problems (for example, over- or underbite)____
    c. Unusual saliva, mouth odor or other problems____
    d. Voice or articulation differences____
4. Head and face
    a. Unusual head shape (e.g., narrow forehead, smaller head than usual)____
    b. Facial asymmetry (one half smaller than the other)____
    c. Other____
5. Heart and lungs
    a. Congenital heart disease____
       Indicate what kind, if known____
    b. Heart attack____
       If present, at what age?____
    c. Heart "trouble"____
       Indicate what kind and what symptoms were present ____

Description,
Treatment, and Outcome

    d. Shortness of breath____
    e. Frequent bronchitis or repeated pneumonias____
    f. Other____
6. Stomach and abdomen
    a. Acute stomach "upsets" (e.g., vomiting, diarrhea, etc.) as a result of overeating____
    b. Chronic stomach symptoms seemingly unrelated to food intake____
    c. Other____
7. Genitalia and secondary sexual development

MALE
    a. Size of male organs small for age____
    b. Undescended and/or small testes____
    c. Limited adolescent hair growth (face and body)____
       Please describe____
    d. Medication given for these symptoms____
       (Please indicate type of medication and results of treatment in as much detail as possible)

FEMALE
    a. Age of first menstruation____
    b. Irregular, sparse, or otherwise unusual periods____
    c. Limited breast development____
    d. Other unusual findings (e.g., early or limited pubic hair)____
       When present, please describe ____
    e. Medication given for these symptoms____
       (Please indicate what medications and the results of treatment in as much detail as possible)
8. Bones
    a. Small size of hands and/or feet____
    b. Back problems (scoliosis, swayback, etc.)____
    c. Fractures____
       Please indicate if there were unusual circumstances surrounding these, e.g., they occurred after limited trauma. We

would appreciate a description of which bones were fractured and if there were any problems with treatment or healing.
   d. Congenital hip dislocation (include treatment results)____
   e. Other bone problems____
9. Skin
   a. Habit of skin picking____
   b. Easy bruisability____
   c. Skin infections, sores, increased tolerance of pain and other symptoms____
10. Medical problems not listed above
    Diabetes____
    Other____

VIII. Behavior Characteristics

Please describe, at the end of this section, any unusual behavioral characteristics which relate to food or eating that appear to be typical of your P-W person, in addition to checking whether or not the following symptoms are present.

Does this P-W person show symptoms of:
____Gorging (eating large amounts of food, not stopping eating until all is gone)
____Stealing and/or hoarding of food and other items
____Consumption of unusual products (not considered edible by most people)

Please describe any prominent behavior characteristics of your P-W person in as much detail as you can in the space left below, in addition to indicating if the following symptoms are present.

Does this P-W person show:
____Excessive temper tantrums for age
____Temper outbursts
____Preoccupations or personal hangups (e.g., about special items, people, etc.)

IX. Problem Priorities

Please use the space below to list the problems, as you see them, that this P-W person has in approximate order of priority (the biggest problem listed first).

chapter 4

A VIEW OF THE ETIOLOGY AND PATHOGENESIS OF PRADER-WILLI SYNDROME

James W. Hanson

> In this chapter Dr. Hanson points out that, although we do not know the precise cause of Prader-Willi syndrome, it is now reasonably clear that all the problems characteristic of the disorder can be linked to a defect of the central nervous system, probably hypothalamic dysfunction. Discovery of the specific cause or causes would result in more precise diagnosis, more effective treatment methods, and, possibly, prevention. Still, there is much that can be done now for the Prader-Willi syndrome patient. Present knowledge indicates that families can be assured that the risk of recurrence of the syndrome within their families is slight.—*Eds.*

Many unanswered questions about Prader-Willi (P-W) syndrome continue to frustrate parents and doctors. The cause (etiology) of the observed abnormalities of growth and development in the P-W syndrome remains shrouded in uncertainty. Likewise, the mechanisms by which such factors may act on the developing baby (pathogenesis) have eluded discovery. Clinical investigations have so far failed to identify basic biochemical, anatomical, or physiological abnormalities by which this diagnosis can be confirmed. Thus, P-W syndrome remains a descriptive term for a group of persons who display a common set of features (Gorlin, Pindborg, & Cohen, 1976).

Furthermore, although P-W syndrome is one of the most frequently occurring recognizable patterns of altered growth and development encountered in genetic counseling clinics, there remains much confusion over the confines of this syndrome. Reliable incidence data are not available. Research activities continue to be descriptive in nature. With any such unsatisfatory state of affairs, treatment becomes supportive or symptomatic, rather than curative. Preventive measures are unknown, and at present prenatal medical intervention is not possible.

This assessment of our present knowledge about P-W syndrome may be unnecessarily pessimistic. As our understanding of P-W syndrome has improved, analogies have been recognized that are helping to determine useful areas of research and new approaches to patient care. It seems appropriate to review our present concepts of the syndrome in light of our present knowledge of human biology in hopes of further insights into this enigma. Before attempting this analysis, a general overview of birth defects and their origins is worthwhile.

ORIGINS OF BIRTH DEFECTS

Birth defect is a term generally used to describe an abnormality of form or function present at birth that is of serious significance for the health or happiness of an individual. The many causes of birth defects are summarized in Table 4.1. These include alterations of the genetic information of the body, adverse environmental factors, and combinations of the two that may interact to give rise to a problem. Several different genetic factors have been recognized. These include chromosomal abnormalities in which there are quantitative differences in the genetic material of the body, and single gene disorders in which there is a qualitative difference. There are also a host of environmental factors that may affect fetal growth and development.

These factors, both genetic and environmental, may act to give rise to two general classes of structural birth defects known as *deformations* and *malformations*. Examples of deformations are some types of clubfoot, where variations in stress inside the uterus have pressed (deformed) the ankle and foot into an abnormal position. Deformations result from some type of fetal constraint. This is in contrast to a malformation such as syndactyly (webbed fingers or toes) in which there is a failure of some intrinsic process within the embryo or fetus. Mechanisms such as cell death, hypoplasia, hyperplasia, asynchronous growth, and tissue dysplasia produce malformations.

Table 4.1. Factors that may cause birth defects

A. Genetic
   1. Chromosomal
   2. Single gene
   3. Polygenic
B. Environmental
   1. Infectious
   2. Physical
   3. Drug and chemical
   4. Maternal metabolic
C. Multifactorial combinations

It is important to recognize that each mechanism could affect the entire baby or, under special circumstances, could have a limited effect on one region of the fetal body. Furthermore, a defect that occurs early in prenatal life may have a cascade of effects on embryonic and fetal development and result in a broad pattern of defects at the time of birth.

Analysis of patterns of altered growth and development can lead to an improved understanding of the mechanisms (the embryonic and fetal events) that produce the abnormalities. An understanding of the mechanisms may lead directly to intervention (including treatment) or may contribute to recognition of possible causes and thus to prevention. With this background, let us return to the P-W syndrome.

PATHOGENESIS OF PRADER-WILLI SYNDROME

An analysis of the alterations of growth, performance, and morphogenesis in individuals with P-W syndrome suggests that a localized primary disturbance in the development of the brain may account for most or all of the observed abnormalities. The classical features of P-W syndrome can be divided into three categories: abnormalities of growth, abnormalities of central nervous system performance, and abnormalities of morphogenesis.

Abnormalities of Growth

The most striking abnormality of growth in P-W syndrome is the excessive weight gain which most commonly begins after the first year of life. Careful dietary studies have now clearly demonstrated that this problem of obesity is exogenous in origin. As expected under such circumstances, dietary restriction programs such as those carried out in Seattle and elsewhere have had substantial success in reducing the weight of affected individuals or in preventing excessive weight gain if instituted early in life (Holm & Pipes, 1976). However, the disturbances of growth in P-W syndrome also affect height gain so that short stature is characteristic of children with this condition. Heights above the 50th percentile are unusual. The origins of the short stature are not presently clear, although attempts to treat such individuals with anabolic steroids have met with some limited success in improving their overall growth and stature, suggesting a central mechanism such as a hormonal insufficiency (Nugent & Holm, Chapter 21, this volume).

Abnormalities of Central Nervous System Performance

Abnormalities of central nervous system performance in P-W syndrome are of several types also. These include alterations of learning potential, alterations in behavior, altered neuromotor function, central regulatory problems, seizures, and evidence of hypothalamic dysfunction.

Although not all children with P-W syndrome display frank mental retardation, most reported cases have scored below 80 on formal IQ tests, with the modal score being in the moderate range of mental deficiency. More recently, it has been recognized that some children with the syndrome may have IQ scores within or near the normal range. However, as suggested by Warren and Hunt (Chapter 12, this volume), there is an accumulating body of data to suggest that there may be a characteristic pattern of learning deficit, such as a defect of short term memory or a defect in visual processing of information. Such observations may have substantial implications for the education of children with this condition.

Children with P-W syndrome also often display rather characteristic behavior. Although most patients have been described as being friendly, cheerful, and good-natured, a small percentage develop serious behavioral problems and most are characterized as being very stubborn. Temper tantrums are frequent in many children with this condition. In addition, most of them display hyperphagia (excessive eating) and a tendency to fidget and pick or scratch at their skin.

Alterations of neuromotor function are a classical sign of P-W syndrome and often represent the initial complaint, since they are present in the newborn. A profound hypotonia, present at birth, results in difficulties in sucking and feeding and a severe delay in motor development. The hypotonia is supraspinal in origin and resolves spontaneously. Improvement commonly begins between 6 and 18 months of age, and serious degrees of hypotonia beyond 3 years are relatively unusual. Investigations of muscle physiology and pathology have not revealed significant evidence of major abnormalities, confirming the clinical impression that the primary abnormality is in the upper central nervous system. In later years functional signs of neuromotor difficulties include poor coordination, strabismus, and speech errors secondary to inaccurate tongue and mouth movements.

Another category of abnormalities of central nervous system performance includes problems of body regulation and homeostasis. It is common for parents and clinicians to note a tendency to fluctuations in body temperature. Many children with P-W syndrome have unexplained episodes of mild to moderate fever or have a persistent mild hypothermia. Furthermore, many of these children display unexplained lethargy. Such children are often characterized by their parents as being rather sleepy for no obvious reason.

Convulsions have been reported in a few cases. The etiology of these seizures is not clear and may be secondary to other complications of this disorder in some cases.

Evidence of hypothalamic dysfunction is presented in Chapter 22 of this volume (Tze, Dunn, & Rothstein). Certainly, the hypogonadism that children with P-W syndrome display appears most commonly to be hypogonadotropic in origin. Indeed, hypogonadism of other etiologies in a patient should bring this diagnosis into question. Other signs of hypothalamic dysfunction may include the problems in body homeostasis described above and other neuro-endocrine abnormalities.

Abnormalities of Morphogenesis

The third major category of abnormalities in P-W syndrome includes abnormalities of morphogenesis, specifically, craniofacial alterations and limb and skeletal abnormalities. The craniofacial features of P-W syndrome include a narrow bifrontal diameter with some slight upslant of the palpebral fissures (eye opening). The maxilla (upper jawbone) is narrow and the midface is often poorly developed. Such abnormalities have been associated with poor development of midline central nervous system structures in other malformation patterns.

Other craniofacial alterations suggest poor prenatal neuromuscular functioning. These include the rather triangular mouth which is secondary to poor development of the jaw. The poor mandibular (lower jaw) development may be secondary to reduced muscular stress in utero on the developing bony structures. The flat, mask-like, or expressionless (so-called myopathic) face sometimes seen in P-W syndrome can likewise be attributed to poor neuromuscular performance. Finally, the palate has often been described as narrow and high-arched. As has been shown previously (Hanson, Smith, & Cohen, 1976), this is a misinterpretation since the more striking features in most children with P-W syndrome are prominent lateral palatine ridges which tend to disappear as motor function improves after the neonatal period. This would suggest that alterations of prenatal tongue thrust account for this morphological abnormality.

Among the limb and skeletal features most characteristic of P-W syndrome are acromicria (small size of the distal portion of the limbs, including hands and fingers) and scoliosis (lateral curvature of the spine) (Laurnen, Chapter 23, this volume). These features may also be secondary to poor neuromuscular function in utero and during postnatal life as well, although specific information on this point is not presently available. Certainly, frank malformations of the vertebrae, pelvis, and ribs are not commonly found in P-W syndrome.

In any consideration of the abnormalities of morphogenesis, it is also important to note what ordinarily is not present. Thus, in the interest of accurate diagnosis, it should be pointed out that other abnormalities of morphogenesis involving other body systems are not ordinarily found in this disorder, although children with other malformations of the central nervous system, particularly those involving the so-called diencephalic structures, often show P-W-like functional disturbances, including obesity, hypogonadism, mental retardation, and hypotonia. One would not ordinarily expect to find a child with P-W syndrome displaying malformations of other body systems such as the heart, kidneys, other abdominal viscera, or limbs.

In order to synthesize a meaningful whole from such a mass of information from such diverse lines of investigation, one must understand that patterns of malformation and abnormal function in children may arise because of disturbances in various body systems or may arise because of a localized defect in morphogenesis of one particular region of the body. This may then have a cascade of effects on the subsequent development of other body systems and on the growth and performance of the newborn at a later date. In P-W syndrome, this latter would appear to hold true. Virtually all of the abnormalities observed in P-W syndrome point to a disturbance of development and function of the midline structures of the brain including the thalamus and hypothalamus (Clarren & Smith, 1977).

This concept has several important implications for an understanding of P-W syndrome. First, if one conceives of P-W syndrome as essentially a single localized defect in central nervous system development, this may imply that any factor that may damage that particular region of the nervous system prenatally could result in the pattern of abnormal growth and development at the time of birth that we refer to as P-W syndrome. This suggests at least the possibility of etiologic heterogeneity, that there may not be any single cause of P-W syndrome but rather a group of causes. By the same token, there may be many disorders that can superficially resemble P-W syndrome because they are associated with damage to the same region of the brain during prenatal life.

Localized defects in prenatal morphogenesis are generally critically time-dependent. That is, there are specific times during growth and development of the embryo and fetus when particular organ systems are most susceptible to damage. This may have important implications for prevention if we are able to identify the various environmental factors important in the causation of P-W syndrome. Knowledge as to the specific time during prenatal life when such damage could occur might allow us to remove these factors from contact with the pregnant population at those sensitive times of pregnancy.

Finally, the concept of a localized disturbance of growth and morphogenesis in the brain as being important in the pathogenesis of P-W syndrome helps to explain the variability of this condition. Obviously, the extent and severity of prenatal damage to the centers of the brain important in the development of this condition would affect the severity of manifestations in the child after birth. Children with more severe damage may show more obvious signs and symptoms of P-W syndrome and be more severely affected in every sense than children for whom the damage was less severe in degree or extent. This is supported by the apparent general correlation in severity of effects in various body systems in P-W syndrome. In the author's experience the children with the greatest learning problems seem to have more severe problems with obesity control and may have the poorest genital development. Thus, in P-W syndrome we should expect to see a spectrum of problems when all children with the syndrome are considered.

IMPLICATIONS FOR DIAGNOSIS, RESEARCH, AND PATIENT CARE

The foregoing discussion has several important implications for parents and those who care for children with P-W syndrome. These can be subdivided into three distinct areas: implications for diagnosis, implications for patient care, and implications for research.

Implications for Diagnosis

An accurate diagnosis, without which important areas of care may be omitted or inappropriate care given, is essential for the satisfactory care of children with P-W syndrome. It is important then to understand what constitutes an appropriate diagnostic workup and what features are necessary to establish a diagnosis of P-W syndrome. The components of the diagnostic evaluation of P-W syndrome are similar to those of children with other patterns of malformation and abnormal growth. History, physical examination, and laboratory tests should be used to identify abnormalities of growth, morphogenesis, and central nervous system performance consistent with the diagnosis. In addition, abnormalities in other body systems that might imply a different diagnosis should be sought, and appropriate diagnostic tests looking for specific etiological factors, such as chromosomal abnormalities, that might produce a similar condition (phenocopy) should be carried out. Included in this evaluation should be an examination of other family members for milder features of P-W syndrome or health problems that might indicate an alternative diagnosis of genetic origin. Several genetic conditions have many similarities to P-W syndrome. Included among these are boys with multiple X chromosomes (XXXY and XXXXY syndromes), the Bardet-Biedl syndrome, the Summitt syndrome, the Carpenter syndrome, and the Kallmann syndrome, to name but a few. Careful examination of patients with partial manifestations of P-W syndrome and the evaluation of other family members, as well as an understanding of the underlying pathogenetic mechanisms by which this condition arises, may allow us eventually to appreciate that many other children have been affected in a similar although milder way by the various contributing environmental or genetic factors that lead to P-W syndrome.

Implications for Patient Care

With regard to patient care, we should then stress that treatment must be individualized and designed to correct or ameliorate whatever abnormalities are present in a specific child. Thus, for some children treatment of scoliosis may be important. In others it may be important to correct strabismus, but in all it will be important to stress weight control and appropriate emotional care and education. For boys it is clearly important to follow genital development. It may be necessary to use testosterone treatment for satisfactory genital growth and improved adolescent maturation of various body structures. In some cases it is possible that girls may need appropriate endocrine therapy for ovarian dysfunction. Families need to understand the nature and origins of the condition affecting their child, they need to be informed concerning an appropriate program of care, and they should have unnecessary guilt and anxiety alleviated whenever possible.

In all instances genetic counseling for families should be an important part of the care program. In the absence of specific information concerning the cause(s) of P-W syndrome, figures for accurate recurrence risk are difficult to quote. Available empirical data based upon our present definition of P-W syndrome indicate a risk less than would be expected for monogenic disorders. However, occasional reports of affected siblings or other close relatives would suggest that the risk may well be somewhat increased for families in which the condition has occurred once. Past experience with P-W syndrome families and with other disorders stemming from a localized disturbance of morphogenesis would indicate that this risk may be around 3%. The risk for second degree or more distantly related relatives to have affected children would be expected to be correspondingly lower. For most families, this low risk of recurrence is probably not sufficiently great to enter in as a major factor in future reproductive decision making. However, this should be a decision made by each family in light of its own circumstances and family goals.

Implications for Research

Finally, with regard to research activities in the future, it now seems apparent that the central nervous system must be examined in a search for the basic functional problems in P-W syndrome. However, it will be important to evaluate large numbers of children with this condition and to describe their various physical and functional abnormalities with increased detail if we are to understand the confines of this condition. This may allow an improved understanding of possible etiological factors through epidemiological studies of factors associated with an increased risk of producing the various abnormalities found in P-W syndrome. Furthermore, such studies may allow us to elucidate times during pregnancy when such agents may produce the critical effect on the fetus or embryo.

SUMMARY

It would now appear likely that the various abnormalities of P-W syndrome can be attributed to a primary abnormality in the growth and development of midline structures of the central nervous system. There may be numerous causative factors that result in such a disturbance in the embryo or fetus. Many recognized genetic and environmental disorders that are associated with similar central nervous system abnormalities have features in common with P-W syndrome. Recognition of these factors is critical for accurate diagnosis and appropriate patient care, including genetic counseling. This should contribute to an improved understanding of the causes of P-W syndrome as well as to its management and prevention in the future.

REFERENCES

Clarren, S.K., & Smith, D.W. Prader-Willi syndrome: Variable severity and recurrence risk. *American Journal of Disease of Children,* 1977, *131,* 798-800.

Gorlin, R.J., Pindborg, J.J., & Cohen, M.M., Jr. Prader-Willi syndrome. In *Syndromes of the head and neck* (2nd ed.). New York: McGraw-Hill Book Co., 1976.

Hanson, J.W., Smith, D.W., & Cohen, M.M., Jr. Prominent lateral palatine ridges: Development and clinical relevance. *The Journal of Pediatrics,* 1976, *89,* 54-58.

Holm, V.A., & Pipes, P.L. Food and children with Prader-Willi syndrome. *American Journal of Diseases of Children,* 1976, *130,* 1063-1067.

chapter 5

DIAGNOSIS AND THERAPY IN THE FIRST PHASE OF PRADER-WILLI SYNDROME

Hans Zellweger

> In this chapter Dr. Zellweger discusses the differential diagnosis of the infant hypotonic stage of the Prader-Willi syndrome and makes recommendations for treatment. He also describes briefly the research that led to the discovery of the syndrome.—*Eds.*

A syndrome is a number of symptoms that occur together to characterize a specific disease or condition. The great phenotypic variability within mankind is due both to the enormous variation of the genotype of different individuals and to environmental influences that differ greatly from place to place. These variations account in part for the difficulties the diagnostician meets when endeavoring to delineate a given syndrome. This is often possible only after a great many cases have been studied over a great many years. The Prader Willi (P-W) syndrome is no exception. It took a number of years to reach a clear concept of this syndrome. There are still doubts whether P-W syndrome is a unique condition or a syndrome of heterogeneous origin.

The early history of P-W syndrome began in the 1940s when attempts were made at the Children's Hospital of the University of Zürich, by the author and others, to unravel the problem of the hypotonias of supranuclear or cerebral origin. At that time supranuclear hypotonias were classified as follows:

1. Parapostinfectious hypotonia (H)
2. H as early manifestation of degenerative brain disease
3. H after brain trauma, intracranial hemorrhage
4. H due to cerebral malformation
5. H due to dysfunction of the hypothalamo-pituitary axis
6. Essential or benign congenital H (Zellweger, 1946b, p. 430)

Those patients afflicted with hypotonias due to dysfunction of the hypothalamo-pituitary axis presented great feeding difficulties and severe hypotonia during infancy and later developed a voracious appetite with ensuing obesity. The patients in this study, as well as other patients with similar symptoms, were followed over many years by Prader in the Zürich Children's Hospital. Prader was interested in the endocrinological aspects of these patients. It was left to his astute clinical acumen and that of his co-workers to delineate a particular syndrome and publish the first description of it in 1956 under the title "A Syndrome of Obesity, Short Stature, Cryptorchidism, and Oligophrenia, with Amyotonia in the Newborn Period" (Prader, Labhart, & Willi, 1956). The first American case was described in 1962 (Zellweger, Smith, & Cusminsky). There are earlier published reports of cases similar to P-W syndrome, but these were not identified as such at the time (Dunn, Ford, Auersperg, & Miller, 1961; Ford, 1952, 1960; Jenab, Lade, Chiga, & Diehl, 1959).

Engel (1965) described a further case of P-W syndrome and coined the term HHO syndrome, indicating hypotonia, hypomentia, and obesity, respectively. A third H for hypogonadism was added 3 years later (Zellweger & Schneider, 1968), but the terms HHO and HHHO syndrome never became popular and were replaced by the now commonly used eponym Prader-Willi (or Prader-Labhart-Willi) syndrome. By 1979 more than 200 cases were published from different corners of the world. Many clinical centers have collected a series of 30 to 50 cases each, and several hundred, mainly from the United States, are listed in the files of the Prader-Willi Syndrome Association. The estimated incidence of P-W syndrome computed from the observations made at the Children's Hospital of the University of Zürich is about one in 25,000 live births (Zellweger & Soper, 1979). Nine out of 10 P-W patients are of subnormal intelligence; thus it can be concluded that P-W syndrome accounts for about 1% of all mentally retarded persons.

SYMPTOMS OF THE FIRST PHASE OF P-W SYNDROME

The symptomatology of P-W syndrome is well known (Table 5.1), yet there are still many cases where the diagnosis is not made before the patient has reached the second stage of the condition and developed considerable obesity. The first phase of P-W in particular, often escapes recognition. For this reason this chapter focuses on the course and symptomatology of the first phase of P-W syndrome and its differential diagnosis.

Pregnancies resulting in the birth of a P-W child are often complicated by hydramnios and decreased fetal movements toward the end of gestation. The duration of pregnancy varies more than usual; deliveries

Table 5.1. Clinical symptomatology of Prader-Willi syndrome

First phase
  Pre- and postnatal growth failure (more pronounced in males)
  Muscular hypotonia or atonia
  Hypo- or areflexia, including suck and swallowing reflexes
  Dolichocephaly with small bifrontal diameter
  Brachycephaly (in other cases)
  Facial diplegia with the typical triangular (fish) mouth
  Convergent squint, almond-shaped eyes, myopia
  Poorly modeled ears, narrow ear canals
  High palate
  Acromicria of hands and feet
  Thermolability, hypo- and hyperthermia
  Hypogonadism
    micropenis, scrotal hypoplasia, cryptorchidism in boys;
    small labia majora, absent labia minora in girls,
Second phase
  Delayed, rarely normal, psychomotor development
  Intelligence quotient from 20 to 90 and rarely higher
  Dysarthria
  Easygoing, affectionate character with lack of initiative
  Incontinent emotionality with outbursts of extreme joy but also streaks of stubbornness
  Later on, severe behavioral problems with meanness, verbal aggressiveness, and incoercible anger, almost rage
  Self-assaultiveness, trichotillomania, picking sores
  Short stature (height below 50th percentile)
  Hyperphagia
    a) Decreased perception of satiety
    b) Persistent painful hunger
  Obesity, notably of trunk and proximal parts of limbs
  Scoliosis, kyphosis
  Knock-knees, pedes valgoplani
  Congenital dislocation of hips
  Sleepiness
  Obesity-hypoventilation syndrome
  Increased glucose intolerance
  Aketotic diabetes mellitus
  Hypogonadism
    a) Hypogonadotrophic
    b) Hypergonadotrophic
  Male infertility
  Female primary or secondary amenorrhea
  Anovulatory menstrual cycles
  Incomplete development of secondary sex characteristics

before the 38th week and after the 42nd week are rather frequent. Breech deliveries occur with greater than usual frequency. The average birth weight is 300 grams below the average birth weight of controls matched for gestational age.

P-W patients are born with severe cerebral depression and remain in a depressed state for a considerable period of time. They are unresponsive, inactive, and severely hypotonic. The lack of muscular tone is in many instances severe enough to mimic flaccid paralysis. The tendon reflexes are absent or at least markedly decreased, which is rather unusual in the supranuclear hypotonias. Withdrawal reflex and Moro's response are likewise absent. The face is flat and expressionless. The mouth has a triangular shape and resembles an inverted V; this condition is sometimes called fishmouth or sharkmouth. Sucking and feeding difficulties may necessitate gavage feeding for an extended period of time. Other P-W children are fed with nipples with large openings, such as those commonly used for premature infants, or with a spoon or dropper. Feeding her P-W infant is a painstaking and frustrating experience for the mother and keeps her occupied for major parts of the day and night.

The muscular hypotonia of the first phase of P-W infants is comparable to that of some diseases of the lower motor unit, spinal cord lesions, and several cerebral hypotonias. A few symptoms that are diagnostic criteria or at least suggestive of P-W syndrome are mentioned as follows. There is conspicuous hypogonadism in the male P-W; the penis is small, the testicles are undescended in a great majority of cases, and the scrotum is hypoplastic. Often there is no scrotal sac but only a piece of corrugated skin in its place. The hypogonadism is less obvious in girls. Small labia majora and very small or absent labia minora suggest P-W syndrome if they occur in association with the above mentioned findings. Acromicria, i.e., small hands, fingers, feet, and toes, is characteristic of P-W syndrome, although it occurs in other conditions as well, notably Down syndrome. Laboratory findings include normal serum creatine kinase, electromyogram, motor nerve conduction velocity, and light microscopy of muscle. Histochemistry of muscle may reveal type II fiber atrophy consistent with disuse atrophy. Electron microscopic studies show such pathological alterations as disruption of myofilaments, accumulation of interfibrillary debris, and streaming of Z lines, although these changes are not pathognomonic for P-W syndrome. Moreover, they are not found in all cases of P-W syndrome (Afifi & Zellweger, 1969).

The duration of the first phase of the syndrome varies from a few months to approximately 2 years. Signs and symptoms of the second phase are listed in Table 5.1 and are discussed in this volume (Hanson, Chapter 4; Holm, Chapter 3).

DIFFERENTIAL DIAGNOSIS OF THE FIRST PHASE OF P-W SYNDROME

Diseases to be considered in the differential diagnosis of the first phase of P-W syndrome are diseases of the peripheral motor unit with congenital onset, birth traumatic spinal cord lesions, and some types of severe cerebral hypotonia.

Lower Motor Unit Conditions

Infantile Spinal Muscular Atrophy (ISMA) ISMA, also called Werdnig-Hoffmann disease, occurs more frequently than diseases of the peripheral motor neurone. Its incidence is about 1 in 20,000 infants. The disease is characterized by severe generalized muscle weakness, which is more severe proximally than distally. Paresis of intercostal muscles is present in some cases, yet the diaphragm muscle is preserved for a relatively long period of time, which results in abdominal or paradoxical respiration. Tendon reflexes are decreased or absent, but sucking and swallowing reflexes are preserved in most instances. Difficulties in sucking and swallowing appear only in the late stages of the disease, and some children die of pulmonary complications before these signs of bulbar palsy appear. The clinical symptoms of ISMA are not always noticed at birth. It often takes several months before parents become aware of their child's muscular weakness. In contrast to P-W syndrome children, ISMA children are not mentally depressed (except in rare cases of complicating anoxia). On the contrary, they are amazingly alert and socialize quite well even when they are severely paralyzed. Fasciculations are best seen in tongue and distal hand muscles and are characteristic of ISMA. They do not occur in P-W syndrome. Serum creatine kinase is normal during the early phases but may increase in chronic cases with superimposed myopathic changes. Motor nerve conduction velocity is normal, yet electromyograms show a neuropathic pattern with fibrillation and positive sharp waves when the muscle is at rest. The interference pattern is poor, and the discharges are of high voltage and long duration. Muscle biopsies show fascicles in various states of atrophy with interspersed large, rounded fibers. Histochemistry of the muscle shows fibertype grouping and often type II fiber predominance. The prognosis for ISMA is poor; the majority of patients die within the first 4 years. Patients without involvement of respiratory muscles survive longer and may develop arrested SMA. The SMAs are inherited with genetic heterogeneity well established. Autosomal recessive inheritance is most frequent. Autosomal dominance with and without presence of an activator allele is less common. X-linked recessive inheritance is decidedly rare and is more often seen in slowly progressing SMA (Zellweger, 1971; Zellweger, Schneider, & Schuldt, 1969).

Neuromuscular Glycogenosis (Gly II) This disease, also called generalized glycogenosis, glycogenosis type II, or Pompe's disease, has some clinical resemblance to ISMA, but muscle weakness is already apparent at birth or soon thereafter. Muscle atrophy is less pronounced and the muscles have a firm consistency, which is explained by glycogen deposits in the muscle. Difficulties with sucking and swallowing are recognized early in the course of the disease, just as in P-W syndrome, and fasciculations are absent. A major distinguishing feature is cardiomegaly, which is frequent in Gly II. The size of the heart may be excessive, filling major parts of the thoracic cage. The myocardium—as seen by echocardiography—is greatly thickened. The electrocardiogram shows high voltage ventricular complexes. Muscle biopsies show abundant glycogen deposits, which—if studied by electron microscopy—are inside and outside the swollen lysosomes. Gly II is a lysosomal disease, the missing enzyme being α-1-4,1-6-glucosidase. Muscle cells grown in tissue cultures show changes similar to those seen in muscle specimens obtained by biopsy (Askanas & Engel, 1977).

Benign Congenital Nonprogressive Myopathies Various types of the so-called benign congenital nonprogressive myopathies, such as congenital fiber type disproportion, type I fiber hypotrophy with central nuclei, central core disease, nemaline myopathy, and centronuclear myopathy (Brooke, 1978), may be present with severe hypotonia in infancy, although this is by no means a constant feature of these disorders. Some affected individuals show only mild hypotonia and insignificant weakness, and others have no clinical evidence of disease in spite of conspicuous pathology in the muscle. The benign congenital nonprogressive myopathies are inherited. Autosomal dominance is common, although autosomal recessive and X-linked recessive inheritance occur as well, notably for the centronuclear myopathies. Thus, genetic heterogeneity is undeniable, at least for some of these disorders (Schochet, Zellweger, Ionasescu, & McCormick, 1972). Neuroparalytic dislocation of the hips is occasionally encountered. External ophthalmoplegia and Marfanoid features characterize some instances of nemaline myopathy. Ophthalmoplegia occurs in the centronuclear myopathies as well. Creatine kinase may be normal or slightly elevated. Electromyograms show changes typical for myopathy. The specific diagnosis is made by histological, histochemical, and electron microscopic studies of muscle explants.

Muscular Dystrophies There are several muscular dystrophies that manifest muscular hypotonia in infancy. Some patients with Duchenne muscular dystrophy are hypotonic in infancy. The hypotonia is, however, not as severe as that in early P-W syndrome. On the other hand, there is a well known form of muscular dystrophy, the so-called severe congenital muscular dystrophy (SCMD), that shows extremely severe hypotonia and muscle weakness at birth. Infants afflicted with SCMD show muscle weakness similar to P-W syndrome. They are inactive and unable to move their extremities. Muscular atrophy is more pronounced than in P-W syndrome. Facial diplegia and difficulties with sucking and swallowing may be present, although not in all instances. Some patients with SCMD are born with arthrogryposis, a symptom of various muscular, neuronal, and supranuclear conditions; thus, muscle biopsy is indicated in every case of arthrogryposis. Serum creatine kinase is normal in cases where the dystrophic process has already reached the final stage. It may be slightly elevated in cases where the dystrophic process is ongoing. Highly elevated creatine kinase levels are uncommon in SCMD and are more suggestive of early Duchenne MD. The electromyogram is myopathic and the muscle biopsy shows features of muscle dystrophy with markedly increased endomysial fibrosis at times. Mental retardation is found in some cases, notably in a variant of SCMD common in Japan. Hypogonadism is not a feature of SCMD. SCMD is transmitted as an autosomal recessive trait and may thus affect more than one sibling of a given sibship. The prognosis for SCMD is poor; about 50% of the patients die in the first year of life. Survival into adulthood is exceptional.

Myasthenia Gravis This is a rare disease, occurring in about one in 20,000. Although it can begin at any age, onset in infancy is decidedly rare. However, about 10% to 15% of babies born to myasthenic mothers have a transient generalized, often severe, hypotonia with difficulties of sucking, swallowing, and respiration. This condition may last up to 3 months and may be life-threatening if not treated effectively with anticholinesterases. The maternal history of myasthenia gravis allows one to distinguish the child's hypotonia from P-W syndrome (Ionasescu, Zellweger, & Braga, 1977).

Peripheral Neuropathies The peripheral neuropathies, especially their most common variant Charcot-Marie-Tooth disease (CMT), begin in the second and third decade of life according to classical textbooks of neurology. However, onset in early childhood is not uncommon in the author's experience, and some cases show infantile hypotonia that may be as severe as the hypotonia of P-W syndrome. The infantile hypotonia of CMT is often a transient phenomenon, occurring, for example, during intercurrent infections (Zellweger, Schochet, Pavone, & Bodensteiner, 1971). CMT includes several variants. In some cases in which the primary lesion is axonal degeneration, the motor slow conduction velocity is normal or slightly subnormal. If, however, the primary lesion is in the myelin sheaths, very slow motor nerve conduction velocity is found. The early onset CMT with severe hypotonia in infancy belongs to the latter variant. Therefore, slow motor nerve conduction velocity allows the differentiation of this form of CMT from P-W syndrome. This CMT variant follows an autosomal dominant inheritance pattern with almost complete penetrance of the mutant gene.

Many of these conditions of the lower motor unit are accompanied by severe muscular hypotonia or atonia in the newborn period and in infancy. In contrast to P-W syndrome, cerebral depression is rarely a feature associated with these conditions. In addition, patients with these conditions show electro-physiological and pathological alterations in the muscle, which also allow them to be differentiated from cases of P-W syndrome. It may be more difficult to separate some of the conditions discussed below from those seen in P-W syndrome.

Spinal Cord Lesions

Severe muscular hypotonia or, rather, muscular atonia is found in cases of birth traumatic spinal cord lesions. These lesions occur almost exclusively after breech deliveries (Zellweger, 1945). If the child is extracted in a direction that deviates from the axis of the vertebral column, vertebral fractures, dislocations, hemorrhages into the vertebral canal, and even disruptions of the spinal cord may occur. In severe cases atonic paralysis and anesthesia below the lesion result. Lesions at the level of the upper cervical segments represent a life-threatening condition. Lesions in the lower cervical segments lead to flaccid quadriplegia, and if the fourth cervical segment is involved priapism results. If the reflex arch of the lower extremities is below the lesion, tendon and withdrawal reflexes are present in the legs, although the child does not have any sensory perception. Bladder and anal paresis are additional manifestations. These symptoms in combination with the loss of all sensory modalities allow one to distinguish birth traumatic spinal cord lesions from P-W syndrome. After some weeks muscle tone and motor function below the lesion may return, depending on the extent of the fiber disruption at the site of the lesion.

Cerebral Hypotonias

Cerebral or supranuclear hypotonias distinguished from P-W syndrome include Down syndrome, Zellweger syndrome, atonic diplegia, congenital myotonic dystrophy, and essential hypotonia.

Down Syndrome Patients with Down syndrome are often severely hypotonic, inactive, and areflexic in the newborn period. Sucking and swallowing reflexes are decreased. The infants appear to be cerebrally depressed, like infants with P-W syndrome; however, the phase of cerebral depression is shorter. Acromicria is also present. Hypogonadism is not a constant feature of infants with Down syndrome, although genital hypofunction is present in adolescents and adults. The presence of mongoloid features and the finding of an extra chromosome 21 or of parts of it lead to the correct diagnosis.

Zellweger Syndrome More difficult is the differential diagnosis between the first phase of P-W syndrome and the cerebrohepatorenal or Zellweger syndrome (ZS). High, receding forehead, hepatomegaly, hyperbilirubinemia, and hypoprothrombinemia in the first and second month, convulsions, glaucoma, cataracts, stippling of the patellae and acetabular synchondrosis, elevated serum iron and ironbinding capacity, and, occasionally, elevation of pipecolic acid in serum and/or urine help to differentiate the two conditions (Zellweger, 1979). However, not all of these signs and symptoms are found in every case of ZS. While the cerebral depression of P-W syndrome subsides after weeks or months, patients with ZS remain depressed, inactive, and severely hypotonic throughout their short life. Most ZS patients die within the first 6 months, survival beyond 1 year being exceptional. The oldest hitherto reported patient reached $2^{1}/_{2}$ years before he died. ZS is inherited as an autosomal recessive trait. Its occurrence in more than one sibling is not rare, yet ZS is often not recognized in the first case. In fact, the correct diagnosis of ZS is often reached only after the second or third case in a sibship.

Atonic Diplegia Persistent atonic diplegia is rather rare, yet a transient atonic phase is often seen in patients with cerebral palsy caused by prenatal brain lesions, perinatal anoxia, or birth trauma to the brain including intracranial hemorrhage. Some patients with initial atonia may show signs of spasticity, extrapyramidal hyperkinesis, or cerebellar ataxia later. Some of these patients are cerebrally depressed, at least in the beginning, yet in contrast to P-W syndrome they show hyperactive or exaggerated tendon reflexes after Monakow's diaschisis has subsided. A history of a traumatic delivery helps differentiate between P-W syndrome and atonic diplegia. There are, however, cases of cerebral depression and possible atonic diplegia that occur after a "normal" delivery. In these cases the brain has been damaged prenatally to such an extent that a so-called normal delivery is experienced as a traumatic event leading to cerebral depression and other neurological manifestations. These cases may be difficult to distinguish from early P-W syndrome. Electroencephalography, axial cerebral tomography, and various agglutination tests may be helpful in recognizing the underlying pathology in some instances. Absence of hypogonadism also helps in excluding P-W syndrome.

Congenital or Early Onset Myotonic Dystrophy (EOmyD) EOmyD presents a clinical picture that has great similarity to that of P-W syndrome. Polyhydramnios and scarcity of fetal movements are also frequently noted. Although it may surprise some readers that EOmyD is included under the supranuclear hypotonias, the severe cerebral depression, the atonia with preserved tendon reflexes, the mental retardation that is more severe than that in classical myD, and the absence of muscle pathology typical for myD, all suggest that EOmyD is categorically different from classical myD. Symptoms of myD appear later in these cases. Newborns and infants with EOmyD are severely hypotonic, or even atonic, and do not respond to external stimuli. Tendon, sucking, and swallowing reflexes are absent. Facial diplegia is a constant feature of the condition. Clubfeet and relaxation (paralysis) of the diaphragm and its shift into the thoracic cage are frequently encountered (Zellweger & Ionasescu, 1973). Serum creatine kinase and electromyography are normal. Myotonic discharges in the electromyogram, clinical signs of myotonia, such as delayed relaxation of the grip, and percussion myotonia appear only after several months. Muscle biopsy is usually normal, but in some instances it shows unspecific myopathy. The typical lesions of myotonic dystrophy such as triangular fibers, annular fibers, varying fiber size, type I fiber atrophy, and multiple central nuclei may appear only later. The atonic phase of EOmyD lasts for several months or years. Eventually the patients become more alert, yet psychomotor development is delayed, and mental retardation and dysarthria are more pronounced than in cases of classical myD. Articulation defects are somewhat similar to those seen in many P-W patients.

The diagnosis of EOmyD is difficult. EOmyD is not distinguishable from other forms of infantile hypotonia with cerebral depression. The correct diagnosis can be made by examining the mother for evidence of myD. By simply shaking hands with her, delayed relaxation of the fist may be noticed. However, not all mothers of an EOmyD child show myotonia. In such cases the examiner may search for other signs of this multisystem disease, e.g., abnormalities of the eyes such as iridescent dust in the lens, cataracts, decreased intraocular pressure, abnormal electroretinography, and abnormalities of the immunoglobulin metabolism. It has been shown that EOmyD occurs only in children who inherit the mutant gene from their mother. Children who inherit the normal gene from the mother and children who inherit the mutant gene from the father do not develop EOmyD. In other words, EOmyD is the result of a combination of the mutant gene and an intrauterine environment created by a mother who carries the gene for myD. MyD represents one of the most frequent dystrophies; EOmyD is not rare either, its incidence being at least as high as that of spinal muscular atrophy.

Essential Hypotonia Finally a condition should be mentioned that is quite frequent and commonly runs in families, namely essential (EH) or benign congenital hypotonia (Walton, 1956; Zellweger, 1946a). The hypotonia is less severe than that in P-W syndrome, and the strength of the alpha-innervated muscle is good. Discrepancy between decrease of tone and good strength of muscle is characteristic for supranuclear hypotonia in general and EH in particular. The tendon reflexes are positive, although they are obtained only if the muscles are fully relaxed. Hyperlaxity of the joints is often associated with EH. Dysmorphic stigmata, such as clinodactyly, and epicanthus, are more frequent than in controls. The milestones of motor development are reached at a slow pace, yet intellectual development is normal. It should not be overlooked, however, that muscular hypotonia is often the prevailing symptom in infants who after some years show evidence of mental retardation. Careful scrutiny of hypotonic children for mental alertness and intellectual responsiveness is, therefore, of paramount importance. Elevated serum creatine kinase, abnormal electromyogram, and hypogonadism are not features of EH. The prognosis for EH is good. It usually disappears during the early school years. If, however, considerable hypotonia persists, the diagnosis EH becomes doubtful and further tests should be performed in order not to miss the diagnosis of a more serious neuromuscular disease, notably a benign congenital myopathy.

TREATMENT OF THE FIRST PHASE OF P-W SYNDROME

The treatment of P-W syndrome, notably the control of hyperphagia and prevention of excessive weight gain in the second phase, is difficult or even disappointing. This is particularly so for those patients with P-W syndrome who not only eat when food is in sight, but who are constantly plagued by a painful feeling of hunger and who therefore eat incessantly. Therapy for the second phase has been discussed elsewhere (Soper, Mason, Printen, & Zellweger, Chapter 9, this volume; Zellweger & Soper, 1979), and its management is covered in other parts of this book (Holm, Chapter 20; Pipe, Chapter 7; Sulzbacher, Crnic, & Snow, Chapter 11). This discussion is therefore limited to the treatment of the first phase of P-W syndrome, which includes physiotherapy, temperature control, and behavior modification with respect to feeding.

It is well known that immobilized muscles atrophy. Muscles of the inactive young P-W infant are prone to undergo atrophy from disuse. Thus, passive exercises of all extremities and frequent changes of position, in the crib as well as outside it, several times daily are indicated. Physiotherapy should also be given on weekends. If such exercises are continued regularly, it is hoped that the child will actively participate after the cerebral depression phase subsides. The P-W child without physiotherapy is notoriously inactive. Institution of a vigorous physiotherapy program before obesity appears may keep the child in an active condition (see also Carman, Chapter 24, this volume).

The body temperature has a tendency to drop to subnormal values during the early days of the first phase. Later, constitutional hyperthermia is not infrequent. Efforts to maintain the temperature within the normal range should be undertaken in every case.

Most important is the establishment of correct feeding habits which should start during the first phase, when the child is still anorectic. There is a special reason for this. As already mentioned, feeding the P-W child during the first phase is a cause of constant worry and unending frustration for the mother or whoever is concerned with feeding. In spite of major efforts, food intake and weight gain are poor. When, finally, after weeks and months, the infant begins to show appetite, the mother is happy. The more the infant takes, the happier the mother is and the more she will praise the child. Thus, a pattern is established whereby the child learns that eating earns praise, and eating more earns more praise. Now comes the constitutional hyperphagia of the second phase of P-W syndrome, which is initially supported by the praising mother. What is more enjoyable for a hyperphagic child than to be praised for the excessive food intake he or she demands? This establishes a feeding pattern that is almost impossible to reverse. Thus, it seems logical to prevent the development of this pattern by the institution of a feeding program during the first anorectic phase.

The program consists of the following components. Feeding should be at regular hours and always in the same place in the house or apartment. Bib and table mat should be a special bright color, which is only used and seen by the child during feeding. A special acoustic stimulus, e.g., a bell, may ring, but only at the beginning of the meal. In that way the creation of a Pavlovian reflex is attempted. The child should have no similar stimuli except during feeding times. The caloric intake must be regulated by the nutritionist and should be kept to the minimum necessary to ensure adequate weight increase. No praise should be given for eating, although other activities of the child should be praised. Love and praise may be given at any other time except during meals. To perform such a behavior modification program correctly, the whole family has to be informed and be willing to cooperate. No presents in the form of food should enter the house. Parents and grandparents and others can give any present to the child except food. Frequent meetings between physician, nutritionist, other professionals, and the families are needed to keep the parents alert and the program going. So far four P-W children with intelligent and cooperative parents are enrolled in this program at the Children's Hospital of the University of Iowa. Results have been satisfactory, but a much longer follow-up is needed for a final evaluation of the early onset behavior modification program.

SUMMARY

There are two phases in P-W syndrome. The first phase is characterized by severe cerebral depression, muscular hypotonia or atonia, and areflexia. During the second phase hyperphagia and obesity develop. Small stature, hypogonadism, and, often, mental subnormality are further features.

Various diseases of the lower motor unit, spinal cord lesions, and hypotonias of cerebral origin have been considered by emphasizing criteria distinctive from P-W syndrome.

Treatment of the first phase includes passive physiotherapy, control of body temperature, and institution of early behavior modification with respect to feeding practices. Treatment of the second phase is discussed elsewhere in this volume.

REFERENCES

Afifi, A.K., & Zellweger, H. Pathology of muscular hypotonia in the Prader-Willi syndrome: Light and electron microscopic study. *Journal of the Neurological Sciences,* 1969, *9,* 49-61.
Askanas, V., & Engel, K.W. Diseased human muscle in tissue culture. L.P. Rowland (Ed.), *Pathogenesis of human muscular dystrophies: Proceedings of the Fifth International Scientific Conference of the Muscular Dystrophy Association.* Amsterdam: Excerpta Medica, 1977.
Brooke, M. *A clinician's view of neuromuscular diseases.* Baltimore: Williams & Wilkins Co., 1978.
Dunn, H.G., Ford, D.K., Auersperg, N., & Miller, J.R. Benign congenital hypotonia with chromosomal anomaly. *Pediatrics,* 1961, *28,* 578-591.
Engel, K.W. H_2O syndrome. In *Current concepts of myopathies.* Philadelphia: J.B. Lippincott Co., 1965.
Ford, F.R. *Diseases of the nervous system in infancy, childhood and adolescence.* Springfield, Ill.: Charles C Thomas, 3rd ed., 1952; 4th ed., 1960.
Ionasescu, V., Zellweger, H., & Braga, S. Myasthenia gravis. In P. Schweier & H.G. Wolf (Eds.), *Pharmakotherapie im Kindesalter.* Munich: Hans Marseille Verlag, 1977.
Jenab, M., Lade, K.T., Chiga, M., & Diehl, K.M. Cardiorespiratory syndrome of obesity in a child. *Pediatrics,* 1959, *24,* 23-30.
Prader, A., Labhart, A., & Willi, H. Ein Syndrom von Adipositas, Kleinwuchs, Kryptorchismus, and Oligophrenie nach myatonieartigem Zustand im Neugeborenenalter. [A syndrome of obesity, short stature, cryptorchidism, and oligophrenia, with amyotonia in the newborn period.] *Schweizersche Medizinische Wochenschrift,* 1956, *86,* 1260-1261.
Schochet, S.S., Zellweger, H., Ionasescu, V., & McCormick, W.F. Centronuclear myopathy: Disease entity or syndrome? *Journal of the Neurological Sciences,* 1972, *16,* 215-228.
Walton, J.N. Amyotonia congenita: A follow-up study. *Lancet,* 1956, *1,* 1023-1025.

Zellweger, H. Ueber geburtstraumatische Rückenmarkslaesionen. *Helvetica Paediatrica Acta*, 1945, *1*, 13-30.
Zellweger, H. Die essentielle Muskelhypotonie bei degenerativen Kindern. *Helvetica Paediatrica Acta*, 1946, *1*, 495-504. (a)
Zellweger, H. Über verschiedene Formen von Muskelhypotonie im Kindesalter. *Helvetica Paediatrica Acta*, 1946, *1*, 427-488. (b)
Zellweger, H. The genetic heterogeneity of spinal muscular atrophy (SMA). *Birth Defects: Original Article Series*, 1971, *7* (2), 82-89.
Zellweger, H. Cerebro-hepato-renal or Zellweger syndrome. In D. Bergsma (Ed.), *Birth defect compendium* (2nd ed.) New York: National Foundation-March of Dimes, 1979.
Zellweger, H., & Ionasescu, V. Early onset myotonic dystrophy in infants. *American Journal of Diseases of Children*, 1973, *125*, 601-604.
Zellweger, H., & Schneider, H.J. Syndrome of hypotonia-hypomentia-hypogonadism-obesity (HHHO) or Prader-Willi syndrome. *American Journal of Diseases of Children*, 1968, *115*, 588-598.
Zellweger, H., Schneider, H., & Schuldt, D.R. A new genetic variant of spinal muscular atrophy. *Neurology*, 1969, *19*, 865-869.
Zellweger, H., Schochet, S., Pavone, L., & Bodensteiner, J. Malattia di Charcot-Marie-Tooth ad insorgenza precoce. Presentazione di una famiglia. *Pediatria*, 1971, *79*, 199-214.
Zellweger, H., Smith, J.W., & Cusminsky, M. Muscular hypotonia in infancy: Diagnosis and differentiation. *Revue Canadienne de Biologie*, 1962, *21*, 599-612.
Zellweger, H., & Soper, R.T. The Prader-Willi syndrome. *Médicine & Hygiène*, 1979, *37*, 3338-3345.

chapter 6

CLINICAL EXPERIENCE WITH 23 CASES OF PRADER-WILLI SYNDROME

Henry G. Dunn, W. Jun Tze,
Robert M. Alisharan, and Michael Schulzer

> In this chapter Drs. Dunn, Tze, Alisharan, and Schulzer discuss 23 cases of Prader-Willi syndrome, including six atypical variants for whom they think the diagnosis may be questionable. They include information about etiology and differential diagnosis of the syndrome.—*Eds.*

Five years after the original description of the Prader-Willi (P-W) syndrome (Prader, Labhart, & Willi, 1956), one of the present writers participated in a report concerning a boy with closely similar features who had a chromosomal abnormality later identified as XYY (Dunn, Ford, Auersperg, & Miller, 1961). This patient was included in a subsequent article that reviewed published reports and nine personal cases (Dunn, 1968). The mean parental ages at the birth of these nine patients were abnormally high (as in Down syndrome), but this finding was not confirmed on analysis of cases seen by some other observers. Delay in dentition and in closure of the anterior fontanelle, marked dental caries often superimposed on defective enamel, a somewhat characteristic facies, and strabismus were commonly encountered. The prepuce was often phimotic. The dermatoglyphic pattern showed no consistent striking aberration, but a low average total ridge count. The weight tended to be at least 1 SD below the mean during the first year and only became significantly high (+2 SD for height-age) at a mean age of over 3 years, while growth in height did not accelerate. Behavioral development appeared to slow down during the preschool years, whereas the initial hypotonia improved. Electroencephalograms (EEG) did not show any gross paroxysmal activity, but at times revealed dysrhythmic patterns. Nerve conduction studies and electromyography (EMG) were generally within normal limits. Apart from the case with the XYY chromosome abnormality, two of the seven other cases had minor chromosomal aberrations, such as elongated Y chromosomes.

In the present communication, 23 cases of P-W syndrome examined by one or both senior authors in the years 1958 to 1979 are reviewed. These cases were mostly derived from consultations with physicians in British Columbia, Canada; four cases involved inpatients at Woodlands, the main provincial residential school for the retarded. The diagnostic criteria for the syndrome established by Prader and his associates, i.e., *marked* hypotonia in early infancy, *subsequent* onset of obesity, mental retardation, cryptorchidism and hypoplastic scrotum in males, small stature, and acromicria have been closely followed. The characteristic facies with high, often narrow forehead and initially pleasant features, fair or auburn hair and blue eyes in many instances, and the associated stigmata, like early dental caries, strabismus, transverse palm creases, clinodactyly, and partial syndactyly were also helpful in the diagnosis. However, six cases best described as atypical have also been included:

Case no. 12 (male)—not significantly obese, testes small but descended

Case no. 13 (female)—no amyotonia at birth, full-scale Wechsler Intelligence Scale for Children (WISC) IQ 85 at 8½ years, spike-wave discharges on EEG

Case no. 20 (female)—not significantly obese, full-scale WISC IQ 76 at 7 years 4 months, plantar responses extensor

Case no. 21 (female)—neonatal hypocalcemia, only transiently obese

Case no. 22 (male)—not significantly obese, no acromicria

Case no. 23 (male)—not significantly obese, generalized seizures, head circumference more than 4 SD below the mean, testes small but descended.

These atypical "variants" were analyzed separately in some respects, and are discussed further below. With their inclusion, the total number of cases is 23, 15 males and 8 females. The ages at which they were examined ranged from 6 days to 22 years, and most of them were seen repeatedly. Except for one Oriental boy, they were all Caucasians.

RESULTS AND COMMENTS

In the series reported here family history revealed that the disease never occurred in siblings and that the parents were never consanguineous. The mean number of earlier pregnancies for the mothers at the birth of these children was four. Twenty-two mothers with adequate documentation had had a total of 15 miscarriages. The average age of the parents at the time of the affected child's birth was 28.3 years for the mother and 30.9 years for the father. If the six atypical cases are excluded, the mean maternal age was 29.5 and the mean paternal age 32.6 years.

The data concerning parental age and parity were subjected to statistical analysis. Table 6.1 lists the 23 cases, providing the year of birth and contrasting the maternal and paternal ages and parity with the corresponding means in the general population during the particular year of the patient's birth.

Maternal Age

1. Total sample: mean deviation = average (mother's age minus mean population age) = 1.915, SD = 6.749, $n = 23$.

    $t_{22} = 1.361$, $0.05 < p < 0.10$, one-sided

    Thus, the mean maternal age is higher than that of the general population, but the difference fails to reach statistical significance.
2. "Pure" sample of P-W syndrome only: mean deviation = 2.714, SD = 7.027, $n = 17$.

    $t_{16} = 1.592$, $0.05 < p < 0.10$
3. Variants of syndrome only: mean deviation = -0.350, SD = 5.841, $n = 6$.

    $t_5 = -0.146$, p not significant

    Thus, in the pure sample the t value is slightly higher than in the whole group, but the difference from the general population is still not significant. On the other hand, the mean maternal age in the sample of variants does not differ from that of the general population at any level of significance.

Paternal Age

1. Total sample: mean deviation = average (father's age minus mean population age) = 0.879, SD = 5.88, $n = 21$.

    $t_{20} = 0.685$, $p \sim 0.25$, no significant difference
2. Pure P-W syndrome subsample: mean deviation = 2.254, SD = 6.072, $n = 15$.

    $t_{14} = 1.437$, $0.05 < p < 0.10$, no significant difference
3. Variants of syndrome only: mean deviation = -2.558, SD = 3.903, $n = 6$.

    $t_5 = -1.605$, p not significant

    Thus, the mean paternal age is also higher than that of the general population but not significantly. Again, the difference nearly reaches significance in the pure subsample of the syndrome.

Table 6.1. Parental ages and maternal parity in P-W syndrome

Case no.	Year of birth	Maternal age	Population mean maternal age[a]	Paternal age	Population mean paternal age[b]	Parity	Population mean parity[c]
1	1944	29	27.4	33	32.2	4	2.4
2	1951	39	27.4	43	31.4	3	2.5
3	1951	27	27.4	27	31.4	5	2.5
4	1956	26	27.2	31	31.4	6	2.7
5	1956	34	27.2	38	31.4	6	2.7
6	1958	40	27.0	?	30.6	7	2.7
7	1958	34	27.0	31	30.6	3	2.7
8	1959	24	27.0	31	30.6	3	2.8
9	1959	18	27.0	?(adopted)	30.6	?	—
10	1960	38	26.9	39	30.5	3	2.8
11	1960	42	26.9	45	30.5	6	2.8
V 12	1962	24	26.7	28	30.4	3	2.9
V 13	1965	22	26.1	22	30.1	2	2.7
14	1967	31	25.6	31	29.6	3	2.4
15	1968	21	25.4	26	29.4	4	2.4
16	1968	25	25.4	31	29.4	2	2.4
17	1970	23	25.1	26	29.0	2	2.4
18	1970	24	25.1	35	29.0	2	2.2
19	1970	21	25.1	22	29.0	2	2.2
V 20	1970	21	25.1	30	29.0	2	2.2
V 21	1973	26	25.1	26	28.7	1	2.0

| V 22 | 1973 | 36 | 25.1 | 31 | 28.7 | 2 | 2.0 |
| V 23 | 1974 | 22 | 25.1 | 23 | 28.6 | 2 | 1.9 |

[a] In calculating population mean maternal ages, Provincial Board of Health (1946) data in British Columbia were used for 1944. Department of Health and Welfare 1953, 1957 statistics were used for 1951 and 1956 (live births by ages of parents). A listing of mean maternal ages of live births in British Columbia in alternate years 1958-1974 was used, with *linear* interpolation, for the remaining years.

[b] In calculating population mean paternal ages, Provincial Board of Health (1946) data were used for 1944. The data in Vital Statistics for 1956 (Department of Health and Welfare, 1957) are given in 5-year ranges for father's age. Extrapolation was used from the *1951* table (Department of Health and Welfare, 1953) in calculating mean father's age *within* each 5-year group. These values were then used with the 1956 data to obtain a mean paternal age for 1956. A listing of mean paternal ages in alternate years 1958-1974 was used, again with *linear* interpolation for intermediate years, for the remaining years in the sample.

[c] Provincial data on parity were used for the years 1951-1974 (Department of Health and Welfare, 1953-1960; Department of Health Services and Hospital Insurance, 1961-1972; Department of Health, 1975-1976). For the year 1944, provincial figures were obtained from Canadian statistics (Dominion Bureau of Statistics, 1946).

V = variant.

Parity

Table 6.1 also contrasts maternal parity in this study with that in the general population of British Columbia (Department of Health and Welfare, 1953-1960; Department of Health Services and Hospital Insurance, 1960-1972; Department of Health, 1975-1976).

1. Total sample: $n = 22$. Mean deviation = average (parity minus mean population parity) = 0.8534, SD = 1.5104, $t_{21} = 2.6503$, $0.005 < p < 0.01$. There is less than a 1% significance level, suggesting that the mean parity of the sample is higher than that of the general population.
2. Pure subsample: $n = 16$. Mean deviation = average (parity minus mean population parity) = 1.2816, SD = 1.5517, $t_{15} = 3.30$, $0.0005 < p < 0.005$. There is an even higher significance ($p < 0.005$) to suggest that parity in the pure subsample is higher than in the general population.
3. Variant subsample: $n = 6$. Mean deviation = average (parity minus population parity) = -0.2824, SD = 0.4554, $t_5 = 1.5512$, p not significant. Thus, there is a marked contrast between the highly significant excess of parity in the pure syndrome and the relatively *low* parity of mothers of the variants which was not different from that of the general population.

Fetal Movements

The fetal movements in these pregnancies were described by the mothers as being weak in eight cases and normal in seven, and were inadequately documented in eight.

Birth History

Breech presentation occurred in five and cesarean section in three out of 20 children, for whom details of delivery are available. The average length of gestation was 39.7 weeks in the series; if the variants are excluded, the mean gestation period was exactly 40 weeks. The mean birth weight was 2,679 grams (5 lb 14½ oz), i.e., below 3,000 grams, as noted by Prader and his colleagues. Only seven of the 23 patients had a birth weight above 3,000 grams; interestingly, three of these were among the six considered atypical for other reasons. Of the 21 patients whose birth history was known in detail, 15 had been reported as showing asphyxia; of the six who had not been considered asphyxiated, three were among the six considered atypical in other respects. Twenty-one of the 23 patients had feeding difficulties in early infancy.

Development

The mean age at which the children were able to remain sitting freely was 11.9 months (18 cases). The average age when they learned to walk freely was 24.3 months (20 cases). Thus, findings of this study confirm the original observation by Prader and Willi (1963) that most of the patients learn to sit at 1 year and to walk at 2 years. Patients said the first word with meaning at an average age of 22.8 months (20 cases). The weight became significantly excessive (more than 2 SD above mean for height-age) at a mean age of 35.7 months in 18 cases, i.e., at 3 years.

Physical Findings

The height of the patients was below North American means in all cases, and at the latest examination it was more than 2 SD below the mean (according to the standards of Simmons, 1944) in 19 of the 23 cases. Figures 6.1 and 6.2 show that the patients tend to grow along the lower limit of the normal range of height curves and to terminate their growth somewhat early, perhaps because of early fusion of epiphyses.

The children were usually significantly obese after the age of 3 years, but the degree of obesity depended on the diet. This aspect is discussed elsewhere (Pipes, Chapter 7, this volume).

The head circumference was normal (± 2 SD for age) in 18 of the 23 cases. Of the five abnormal cases, three had a significantly small and two a significantly big head; of the three cases with a small head, two were variants.

Some of the other physical findings are listed in Table 6.2. *All* the patients considered to have "classical" P-W syndrome had a small stature ($-$ >1 SD for age), significant obesity, and acromicria, and all the boys in this category had undescended testes. The children with the classical P-W syndrome, with only one or two exceptions, had asphyxia neonatorum, marked hypotonia at birth ("amyotonia congenita"), subsequent mental retardation (global IQ <70), and a normal head circumference. Several of these features were found less constantly in the variants.

The presence of frequent minor stigmata was observed previously (Dunn, 1968). Thus, an arched palate was noted in 12 of the 23 patients, transverse (simian) palm creases were found in both hands in three cases and in one hand in four other cases, and Brushfield spots were detected on the irides in seven of the 23 patients.

Dermatoglyphic Patterns

Laurance (1967) reported palm and fingerprint patterns in six boys with P-W syndrome. Two of the six boys had an *atd* angle higher than 57° by comparison with 10% of the normal population. Five of the six boys had a

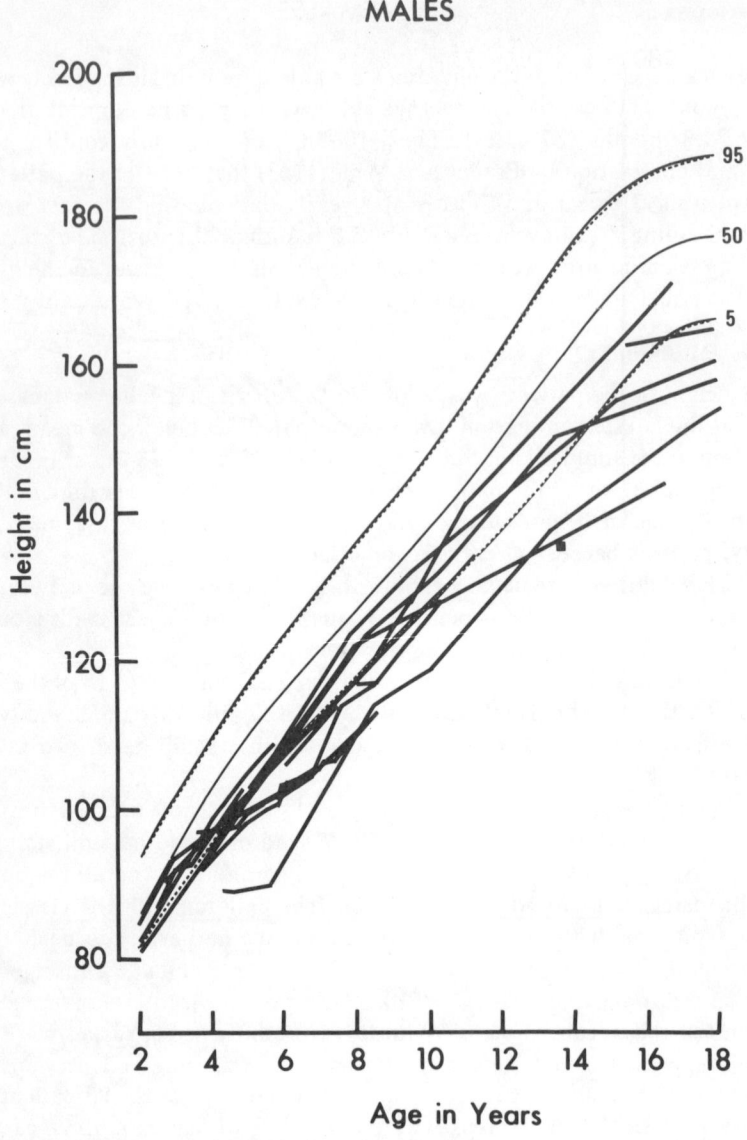

Figure 6.1. Linear growth in 15 P-W syndrome males.

hypothenar loop pattern, whereas 15% of the general population were said to have this pattern.

Cohen and Gorlin (1969) found 7 whorls on the digits of one patient and 10 whorls on the fingers of another.

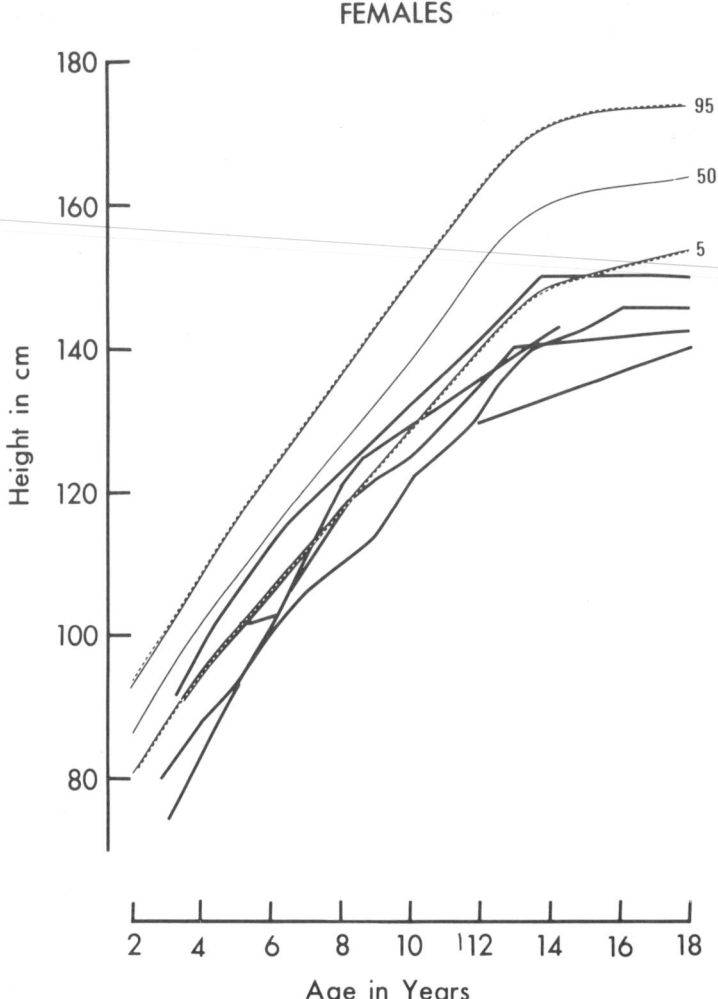

Figure 6.2. Linear growth in eight P-W syndrome females.

In the nine cases previously published (Dunn 1968), an *atd* angle above 57° was only found in one hand of one patient and there was no excess of whorls, while hypothenar loop patterns were noted in six hands of five out of the nine patients. A notable finding in those nine cases was that the mean total ridge count of 112.8 was low as compared to a Canadian population mean of 133.9 ± 1.6 (J.R. Miller, personal communication).

Holt (1975) analyzed the fingerprints, palm prints, and soleprints of

Table 6.2. Frequency of some clinical features in Prader-Willi (P-W) syndrome

	Proportion of cases		
		Classical P-W syndrome	Variants
Decreased fetal movements	56% (10/18)	7/13	3/5
Birth weight < 3000 grams	70% (16/23)	13/17	3/6
Asphyxia neonatorum	71% (15/21)	12/15	3/6
Amyotonia congenita	82% (18/22)	14/16	4/6
Small stature (− >1 SD)	96% (22/23)	17/17	5/6
Very small stature (− >2 SD)	83% (19/23)	14/17	5/6
Acromicria	91% (21/23)	17/17	4/6
Cryptorchidism (males)	87% (13/15)	12/12	1/3
Significant obesity (weight) + >2 SD for height-age)	78% (18/23)	17/17	1/6
Mental retardation (latest global IQ < 70)	87% (20/23)	16/17	4/6
Normal head circumference (mean ± 2 SD for CA[a])	78% (18/23)	14/17	4/6
Strabismus	74% (17/23)	13/17	4/6
Early caries, enamel hypoplasia	80% (16/20)	12/15	4/5

[a]CA = chronological age.

13 patients. She concluded that the dermatoglyphics differed little, if at all, from those of the normal population. The pattern intensity on the hands, and particularly the feet, appeared low.

Among the present 23 cases, 13 have had their dermatoglyphics analyzed by Drs. James R. Miller and Barbara McGillivray. Hypothenar loop patterns have been noted in seven hands of the 13 patients (radial in six hands, ulnar in one). Since hypothenar radial loops are found in 24% of the general population (J.R. Miller, personal communication), this appears to be well within the normal range.

The mean ridge count of the 13 patients is 122.9 and thus closer to the normal Canadian mean of 133.9 ± 1.6 than that recorded previously; if two variant cases are excluded, the mean ridge count of 11 patients is 117.7. If only the eight *males* are considered who have classical P-W syndrome, the mean ridge count is still only 113.1 (normal Canadian male average, 140.8 ± 2.1).

Mental Development

It was noted previously (Dunn, 1968) that the developmental quotients (DQ) and global intelligence quotients (IQ) of children with P-W syndrome tend to fall during the preschool years. Vischer and associates (quoted by Hall & Smith, 1972) stated that among their younger patients some were found to have a normal IQ, only to fall below normal as they became older. The findings in 20 patients of the present group are plotted in Figure 6.3. In 16 patients, serial measurements were obtained. The general downward trend is evident, particularly in the first 6 to 10 years, and ultimately the IQ ranged from about 30 to 70.

Behavior Problems

Hall and Smith (1972) commented that serious personality problems occurred in most patients by adolescence and adulthood. The present study includes 17 patients beyond 10 years of age, eight of whom had emotional disorders ranging from temper outbursts to psychotic behavior and intermittent "rages" reminiscent of those produced by hypothalamic lesions in cats.

Neurological Findings

In addition to the mental retardation and labile emotional state, it was noted that 17 of the 23 patients had strabismus, and some residual hypotonia was present in all cases. One variant case (no. 23) had generalized seizures, and his EEG was abnormal with symmetrical spike-wave discharges; another patient (no. 19) had febrile convulsions at $3\frac{1}{2}$ years, but was then free of seizures at 5 years when his EEG showed only a mild dysrhythmia; a third child had attacks of dizziness or syncope but no proven seizures and had a mildly dysrhythmic EEG. The remaining 20 never had fits. The EEG of 15 patients had been recorded; epileptiform discharges were only found in 2 variant cases; in the remaining 13, six records were considered mildly abnormal, i.e., dysrhythmic or of low voltage, while the remaining seven tracings were interpreted as normal. Nerve conduction studies performed in 10 cases were normal except in one diabetic male of $16\frac{1}{2}$ years (case no. 6) who had a conduction velocity of 45 m/sec in the motor fibers of the median and only 37 m/sec in the motor fibers of the lateral popliteal nerve, perhaps indicating early diabetic neuropathy.

Bone Age

In a previous study (Dunn 1968), it was noted that bone age, determined by x-ray of hand and wrist, was significantly delayed in all *boys* below the

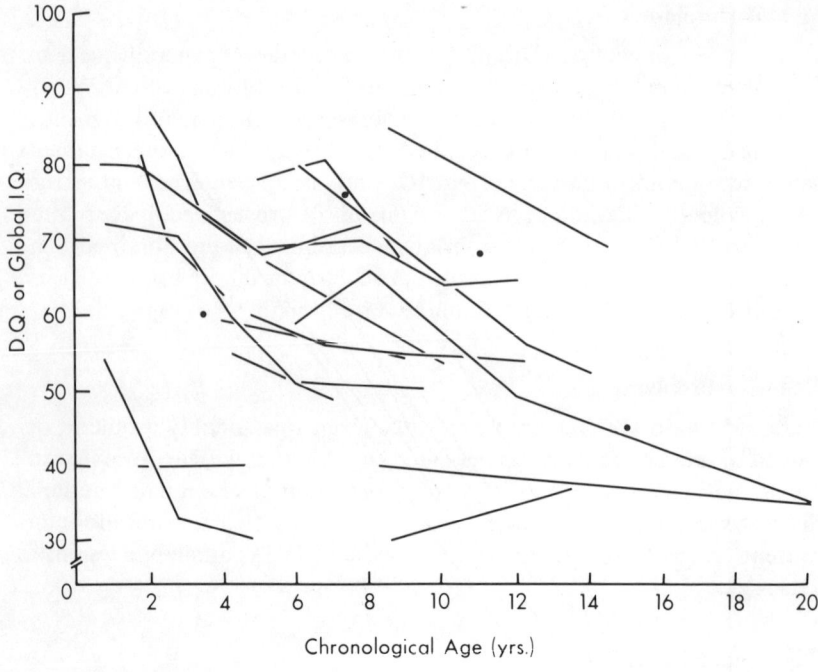

Figure 6.3. Mental development in P-W syndrome. Note the tendency to a gradual fall, particularly in the first 6 to 10 years.

age of 4 years, but subsequently bone maturation tended to "catch up." Figure 6.4 again shows this trend in 15 boys; Figure 6.5 does not indicate it as clearly in girls. (The advance in bone age, like obesity, is not usually associated with increased growth.) As the bone age advances, the epiphyses fuse and the ultimate stature tends to be small (see Figures 6.1 and 6.2) (see also Nugent & Holm, Chapter 21, this volume).

The luteinizing hormone-releasing hormone (LH-RH) stimulation test was performed on 15 patients. There was the expected abnormal "blunted" response, consistent with hypothalamic hypofunction, in nine (60%) patients. Interestingly, among the five variants selected on clinical grounds, only one had such an abnormal response, whereas eight out of 10 patients with the classical P-W syndrome exhibited the expected abnormality (see also Tze, Dunn, & Rothstein, Chapter 22, this volume).

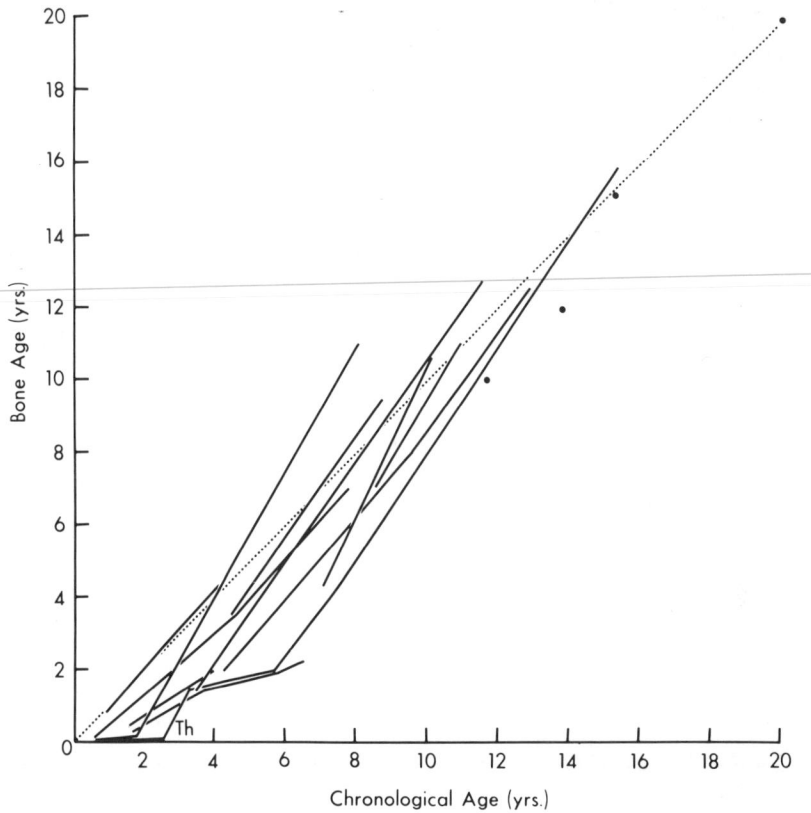

Figure 6.4. Relationship of bone age to chronological age in P-W syndrome in males. Note the trend to catch up (and even advance) after an initial delay. Th = thyroid therapy.

DISCUSSION

The question of parental ages and maternal parity in P-W syndrome remains open. The mean maternal age of 28.3 years in these 23 cases (29.5 years if the variants were excluded) and of 29.6 years in the 32 cases reported from the state of Washington by Hall and Smith (1972) certainly appears high in comparison to general population figures in British Columbia. The difference fails to reach statistical significance in the present study but might, of course, do so with a larger number of patients. The

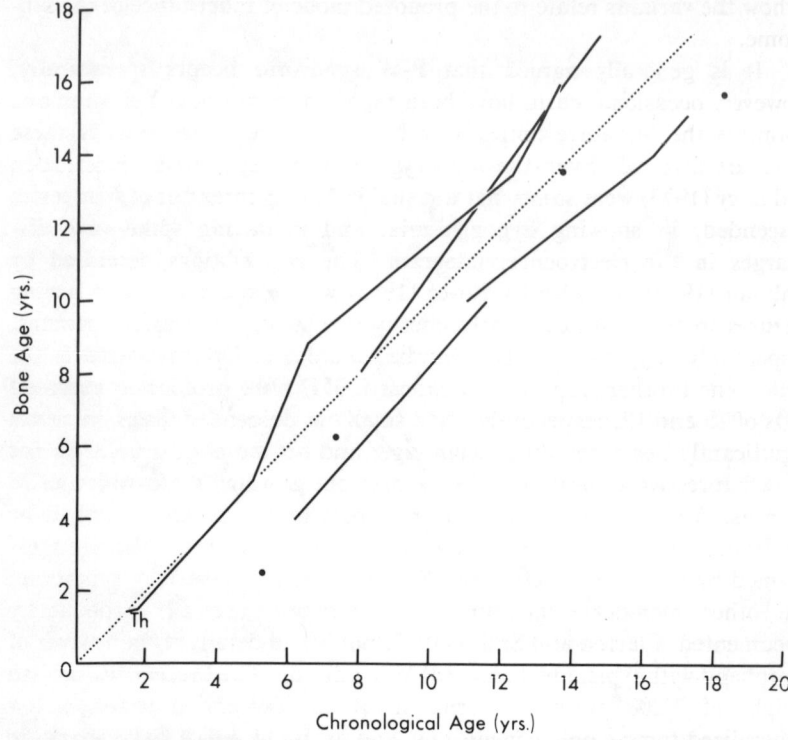

Figure 6.5. Relationship of bone age to chronological age in P-W syndrome in females. Th = thyroid therapy.

mean paternal age of 30.9 years in the 21 cases in whom it was known (32.6 years if the variants were excluded) and of 29.7 years in the series of Hall and Smith appears relatively less elevated in comparison to our general population figures. The mean maternal parity figures in our study show the most impressive difference from the general population because they are significantly higher at the 1% level in our total sample and at $p < 0.005$ in the classical cases, whereas mean parity in the six variants is not significantly different from that in the general population and, if anything, slightly lower.

The fact that the variants differed from the more classical cases of the syndrome in these respects is of interest, because they were labeled on the basis of other criteria, namely, the differences from the clinical picture originally described by Prader and his associates. This raises the question of how the variants relate to the proposed mode of inheritance of the syndrome.

It is generally agreed that P-W syndrome occurs sporadically. However, occasional cases have been reported in siblings. Yet when one examines the literature critically, it becomes evident that most of these cases are atypical. Even the monozygotic twins reported by Brissenden and Levy (1973) were somewhat unusual in having three out of four testes descended, in showing hypoglycemia, and in having spike-wave discharges in the electroencephalogram. The two siblings described by Gabilan (1962) and also by Royer (1963) were more atypical in having seizures in the first year, early obesity (beginning at 8 and 6 months, respectively), hypersensitivity to insulin, and descended small testes in the male. The brothers reported by Jancar (1971) were profoundly retarded (IQs of 15 and 12, respectively), had small but descended testes, were not significantly heavy for their height-age, and on the photographs do not show impressive acromicria. The younger one also had a convulsion at 30 months. Among the five affected members of the family described by DeFraites, Thurmon, and Farhadian (1975), only three had been examined by the authors. One boy (X-5) appeared to have P-W syndrome; the other members, including three females, are all inadequately documented. Clarren and Smith (1977) published details of the brother of a proband with typical features of P-W syndrome. The brother had a birth weight of 3,200 grams at term, small but descended testes, a few generalized tonic-clonic convulsions, and an IQ of only 13 at 8 years; he never learned to walk or talk. The authors admit that the brother was "more profoundly affected than the patients usually described," but one may question whether the diagnosis of P-W syndrome should be made at all. The same question applies to the cousin of a patient with P-W syndrome described by Hall and Smith (1972). The cousin had a birth weight of 3,856 grams (8½ lb), gained weight rapidly at the unusually early age of 2 months, and had normal stature and intelligence at 22 years of age.

Clarren and Smith (1977), also noting a history of increased frequency of spontaneous late miscarriage (17%) by mothers of affected offspring, suggest that P-W syndrome represents a defect of greater variety than has been appreciated in the past, and calculate an occurrence rate of 1.6% in siblings of probands. It seems risky to widen the spectrum in this manner when there is no single pathognomonic feature in the syndrome to prove the diagnosis. It appears that the syndrome *as originally described* occurs only as a sporadic event, and unless more familial aggregation is demonstrated it remains possible that the condition is due to a recurrent autosomal dominant mutation (J.R. Miller, personal communication quoted by Dunn, 1968). If we include all the variants, the mode of inheritance is likely to be obscured, for it is known that other hypothalamic syndromes may be inherited as autosomal recessive traits, e.g., the Laurence-Moon-Biedl and the Alström (1959) syndromes, which show some similar features. Two of the authors (W.J.T., H.G.D.) have participated in the description of another syndrome of congenital monochromatism, cataracts, and sensorineural deafness in two obese sisters with diabetes mellitus (Jan, Tze, Johnston, & Dunn, 1976). A similar syndrome was reported earlier by Weiss (1932). The Cohen syndrome with its additional abnormalities (Carey & Hall, 1978; Cohen, Hall, Smith, Graham, & Lampert, 1973) and other familial "hypothalamic" syndromes (Lynch, Kaplan, Henn, & Krush, 1966; MacMillan, Kim, & Weisskopf, 1972; Parkin, 1973; Weinstein, Kliman, & Scully, 1969) should also be differentiated. Recently Urban, Rogers, and Meyer (1979) published a description of a familial condition resembling P-W syndrome in which two affected brothers with mental retardation, short stature, obesity, and genital anomalies had contractures of the hands, generalized osteoporosis, and frequent fractures. Another new familial syndrome characterized by hypogonadotropic hypogonadism, mental retardation, short stature, and obesity, without acromicria and with gynecomastia and small head size has been reported as X-linked recessive (Vasquez, Hurst, & Sotos, 1979). These syndromes should remain distinct until their pathogenesis and genetic characteristics are better understood; meanwhile, the variants of P-W syndrome should be viewed with caution and analyzed separately.

This distinct analysis of variants will affect calculations concerning the frequency of the various features in the syndrome, as shown by analysis of the clinical aspects, parental ages, and parity in this study. For instance, it is generally agreed that the mature stature of the patients is usually significantly small as seen in the series reported here (Hall & Smith, 1972; Wannarachue, Ruvalcaba, & Kelley, 1975). Hall and Smith (1972) found that this growth deficiency need not be constant, but cases of normal stature should be checked with care to see whether they are variants in other respects. With regard to the dermatoglyphics, no abnormal patterns have been demonstrated to occur with increased frequency, but the question whether the mean ridge count is reduced remains open and should be investigated in larger samples, again distinguishing classical cases from variants.

SUMMARY

The cases of twenty-three patients with Prader-Willi syndrome seen during the years 1958–1979 have been reviewed. They were divided into 17 classical cases and six atypical variants. Fifteen were males and eight were females. Twenty-two were Caucasians, and one was a Canadian of Chinese ancestry.

At the time of the child's birth the mean maternal age was 28.3 years and the mean paternal age was 30.9 years. If the six atypical cases were excluded, the mean maternal age was 29.5 and the mean paternal age 32.6 years. The mean maternal age was numerically higher than that of the general population, but the difference failed to reach statistical significance even when only pure cases of the syndrome were considered; among the variants the mean maternal age did not differ from that of the general population. The mean paternal age was not significantly higher than that of the general population, even in the pure subsample, and was relatively less elevated than the maternal age. The mean age of the fathers of variants did not differ from that of the general population.

The mean maternal parity was higher than that of the general population at the 1% significance level, and in the pure sample mean parity exceeded that of the general population at the level of $p < 0.005$, whereas the parity of mothers of the variants was numerically (although not significantly) *low* in comparison to that of the general population.

Breech presentation occurred in five and cesarean section in three out of 20 children for whom details of delivery were available. The average length of gestation was 39.7 weeks; if the variants were excluded, the mean length of gestation was exactly 40 weeks. The mean birth weight was 2,679 grams. Neonatal asphyxia occurred in 71%, profound hypotonia in 82%, and feeding difficulties in 91% of the patients.

The patients were able to remain sitting at a mean age of nearly 1 year, to say the first word with meaning at nearly 2 years, and to walk freely at approximately 2 years; they became significantly obese ($+ >2$ SD for height-age) at a mean of 3 years. The height was below North American means in all cases; the patients grew along the lower limit of the normal range and achieved significantly small stature. The head circumference was usually within normal limits.

The dermatoglyphic patterns were unremarkable except for a slightly low mean ridge count, particularly in cases of pure P-W syndrome.

Plotting of DQs and global IQs shows a downward trend, particularly in the first 6 to 10 years, with an ultimate IQ range of approximately 30 to 70.

Behavior problems ranging from temper outbursts to rages and psychotic states occurred in at least eight out of 17 patients after the age of 10 years.

Seventeen of 23 patients had strabismus. Epilepsy with generalized seizures occurred in one variant and febrile convulsions in another patient. The remaining 21 were free of seizures. Electroencephalograms were recorded in 15 patients; two variant cases had epileptiform discharges, six records were mildly abnormal (dysrhythmic or of low voltage), and the remaining seven tracings were normal. Nerve conduction studies in 10 cases were normal except for mild slowing in the motor fibers of the median and lateral popliteal nerves of a boy of 16½ years with maturity-onset type of diabetes mellitus.

The radiological bone age tended to be delayed in the first decade and then to catch up with increased chronological age.

LH-RH stimulation produced an abnormally blunted response in nine of 15 patients, consistent with hypothalamic hypofunction. This expected response was found in eight of 10 patients with the classical syndrome but in only one of five variants.

The findings have been discussed and the literature concerning the genetics of this and other presumed hypothalamic syndromes has been reviewed. It is concluded that P-W syndrome as originally described might be due to an autosomal dominant mutation and should be differentiated from variants in which other modes of inheritance may be operative. Further evaluation of clinical, cytogenetic, and biochemical criteria for the classical syndrome is needed.

ACKNOWLEDGMENTS

The authors wish to express their thanks to Drs. James R. Miller and Barbara C. McGillivray, of the Department of Medical Genetics, University of British Columbia, for helpful advice and interpretation of dermatoglyphic patterns; to Mr. D.H.G. Renwick, of the Division of Vital Statistics of the Ministry of Health, Province of British Columbia, for assistance in supplying vital statistics; to Mrs. Betty Whitehead, Mrs. Carolyn Graves, R.N., and Mrs. Doreen Yasui for clerical assistance; and to the Department of Biomedical Communications, University of British Columbia, for help with the figures.

REFERENCES

Alström, C.H., Hallgren, B., Nilsson, L.B., & Asander, H. Retinal degeneration combined with obesity, diabetes mellitus and neurogenous deafness. *Acta Psychiatrica et Neurologica Scandinavica,* 1959, *34,* suppl. 129.

Brissenden, J.E., & Levy, E.P. Prader-Willi syndrome in infant monozygotic twins. *American Journal of Diseases of Children,* 1973, *126,* 110-112.

Carey, J.C., & Hall, B.D. Confirmation of the Cohen syndrome. *The Journal of Pediatrics,* 1978, *93,* 239-244.

Clarren, S.K., & Smith, D.W. Prader-Willi syndrome: Variable severity and recurrence risk. *American Journal of Diseases of Children,* 1977, *131,* 798-800.

Cohen, M.M., Jr., & Gorlin, R.J. The Prader-Willi syndrome. *American Journal of Diseases of Children,* 1969, *117,* 213-218.

Cohen, M.M., Hall, B.D., Smith, D.W., Graham, C.B., & Lampert, K.J. A new syndrome with hypotonia, obesity, mental deficiency and facial, oral, ocular and limb abnormalities. *The Journal of Pediatrics,* 1973, *83,* 280-285.

DeFraites, E.B., Thurmon, T.F., & Farhadian, H. Familial Prader-Willi syndrome. *Birth defects: Original article series,* 1975, *11,* 123-126.

Department of Health. *Vital Statistics of the Province of British Columbia for the years 1973-74. 102nd to 103rd Reports.* Victoria: Queen's Printer, 1975-1976.

Department of Health and Welfare. *Vital Statistics of the Province of British Columbia for the years 1951-58. 80th to 87th Reports.* Victoria: Queen's Printer, 1953-1960.

Department of Health Services and Hospital Insurance. *Vital Statistics of the Province of British Columbia for the years 1959-70. 88th to 99th Reports.* Victoria: Queen's Printer, 1960-1972.

Dominion Bureau of Statistics. *Vital Statistics 1944: 24th Annual Report.* Ottawa: King's Printer, 1946.

Dunn, H.G. The Prader-Labhart-Willi syndrome: Review of the literature and report of nine cases. *Acta Paediatrica Scandinavica,* 1968, Suppl. 186, 1-38.

Dunn, H.G., Ford, D.K., Auersperg, N., & Miller, J.R. Benign congenital hypotonia with chromosomal anomaly. *Pediatrics,* 1961, *28,* 578-591.

Gabilan, J.C. Syndrome de Prader, Labhart et Willi. *Journées Pédiatriques,* 1962, *1,* 179-185.

Hall, B.D., & Smith, D.W. Prader-Willi syndrome. *The Journal of Pediatrics,* 1972, *81,* 286-293.

Holt, S.B. Dermatoglyphics in Prader-Willi syndrome. *Journal of Mental Deficiency Research,* 1975, *19,* 245-258.

Jan, J.E., Tze, W.J., Johnston, A.C., & Dunn, H.G. Familial congenital monochromatism, cataracts and sensorineural deafness. *American Journal of Diseases of Children,* 1976, *130,* 1349-1350.

Jancar, J. Prader-Willi syndrome (hypotonia, obesity, hypogonadism, growth and mental retardation). *Journal of Mental Deficiency Research,* 1971, *15,* 20-29.

Laurance, B.M. Hypotonia, mental retardation, obesity and cryptorchidism associated with dwarfism and diabetes in children. *Archives of Disease in Childhood,* 1967, *52,* 126-139.

Lynch, H.T., Kaplan, A.R., Henn, M.J., & Krush, A.J. Familial coexistence of diabetes mellitus, hyperlipemia, short stature, and hypogonadism. *American Journal of the Medical Sciences,* 1966, *252,* 323-330.

MacMillan, D.R., Kim, C.B., & Weisskopf, B. Syndrome of growth resistance, obesity, and intellectual impairment with precocious puberty but without menarche. *Archives of Disease in Childhood,* 1972, *47,* 119-121.

Parkin, J.M. Syndrome of growth resistance, obesity and intellectual impairment with precocious puberty. *Archives of Disease in Childhood,* 1973, *48,* 86-87.

Prader, A., Labhart, A, & Willi, H. Ein Syndrom von Adipositas, Kleinwuchs, Kryptorchismus und Oligophrenie nach myatonieartigem Zustand im Neugeborenenalter. *Schweizerische Medizinische Wochenschrift,* 1956, *86,* 1260-1261.

Prader, A., & Willi, H. Das Syndrom von Imbezillität, Adipositas, Muskelhypotonie, Hypogenitalismus, Hypogonadismus und Diabetes mellitus mit "Myatonie"-Anamnese. *Second International Congress on Mental Retardation,* Vienna, *1961.* (Part I, 353-357) Basel and New York: S. Karger, 1963.

Provincial Board of Health. *Vital Statistics of the Province of British Columbia for the year 1944. 73rd Report.* Victoria: King's Printer, 1946.

Royer, P. Le diabète sucré dans le syndrome de Willi-Prader. *J. Ann. Diabet. Hôtel-Dieu,* 1963, *4,* 91-99.

Simmons, K. *Growth and development. Monographs of the Society for Research in Child Development,* Vol. IX, No. 1. Washington, D.C.: National Research Council, 1944.

Urban, M.D., Rogers, J.G., & Meyer, W.J., III. Familial syndrome of mental retardation, short stature, contractures of the hands, and genital anomalies. *The Journal of Pediatrics,* 1979, *94,* 52-55.

Vasquez, S.B., Hurst, D.L., & Sotos, J.F. X-linked hypogonadism, gynecomastia, mental retardation, short stature, and obesity—a new syndrome. *The Journal of Pediatrics,* 1979, *94,* 56-60.

Wannarachue, N., Ruvalcaba, R.H.A., & Kelley, V.C. Hypogonadism in Prader-Willi syndrome. *American Journal of Mental Deficiency,* 1975, *79,* 592-603.

Weinstein, R.L., Kliman, B., & Scully, R.E. Familial syndrome of primary testicular insufficiency with normal virilization, blindness, deafness, and metabolic abnormalities. *New England Journal of Medicine,* 1969, *281,* 969-977.

Weiss, E. Cerebral adiposity with nerve deafness, mental deficiency and genital dystrophy: A variant of the Laurence-Biedl syndrome. *American Journal of the Medical Sciences,* 1932, *183,* 268-272.

part II

OBESITY MANAGEMENT

chapter 7

NUTRITIONAL MANAGEMENT OF CHILDREN WITH PRADER-WILLI SYNDROME

Peggy L. Pipes

> This chapter describes the nutritional intervention program at the University of Washington for children with Prader-Willi syndrome. Individually planned low calorie diets and environmental control of access to food has resulted in success when begun at an early age. —*Eds.*

Hyperphagia, food-seeking behaviors, and obesity are problems common to all individuals with Prader-Willi (P-W) syndrome. A number of different approaches to weight reduction and later maintenance of weight loss have been described. In every case stringent environmental controls have been necessary both at home and in other settings. When these have not been implemented the result has been failure. Dietary treatment methods reported in the literature include an individualized low calorie balanced diet (Pipes & Holm, 1973), a protein-sparing modified fast (Bistrian, Blackburn, & Stanbury, 1977), a 1,000 kcal ketogenic diet (Nelson, Hayles, Novak, Margie, & Vernet, 1970), and other hypocaloric regimens (Coplin, Hine, & Gormican, 1976). Other approaches to weight control include the use of anorectic drugs (Zellweger, 1969), increasing physical exercise (Carman, Chapter 24, this volume), behavior therapy (Hirsch & Altman, Chapter 15, this volume; Marshall, Wallace, Elder, Burke, Oliver, & Blackmon, Chapter 14, this volume) and gastric bypass surgery (Soper, Mason, Printen, & Zellweger, 1975, Chapter 9, this volume). This chapter is limited to a discussion of the author's experience in dietary management of P-W syndrome prefaced by a brief discussion of diet approaches not covered in other chapters of this volume.

DIET PROGRAMS DESCRIBED BY OTHERS

Bistrian, Blackburn, and Stanbury (1977) reported success in achieving weight loss in four adolescents and young adults with P-W syndrome 12 to 24 years of age in a metabolic unit with a protein-sparing modified fast consisting of 1.5 g of meat protein per kg of ideal body weight. Vitamin, mineral, and fluid supplements meeting daily requirements were included. One patient continued to lose weight as an outpatient. Two others did not lose as rapidly as outpatients and ultimately regained weight, although they insisted they had complied with the protein-sparing regimen. The fourth patient, a 12-year-old male, did not adhere to the protein-sparing regimen as an outpatient and immediately regained the weight lost. The protein-sparing modified fast produced ketonuria within 24 to 72 hours, which allows for a convenient check of diet compliance. This diet is reported to result in absence of hunger.

Nelson and his colleagues (1970) reported that three patients, 4 to 14 years of age, lost 12% of their body weight in 3 months on a 1,000 kcal ketogenic diet. All mothers noted a decrease in their children's appetites. This diet is further described in the following chapter (Nelson, Huse, Holman, Kimbrough, Wahner, Callaway, & Hayles, Chapter 8). The problems and complications associated with it are also discussed and are similar to those encountered in the protein-sparing diet.

Attempts to reduce and maintain weight with a conventional low calorie diet have been mentioned in a few case reports. In every case severe caloric restriction was necessary. Evans (1964) effected an initial weight loss to 116 pounds in a 16-year-old male. By the age of 21 he had regained 26 pounds despite a diet of starch-reduced wheat flakes, crisp bread, meat, eggs, cheese, green vegetables and salads, apples, and oranges. An 8-year-old also lost 22 pounds during hospitalization on a 300 kcal diet after dieting at home had proved ineffective. Laurance (1967) reported lack of success in effecting weight loss on an 800 kcal diet in a 2½-year-old female who later, at 8 years, lost 13 kg on the same diet. Jancar (1971) and Juul and DuPont (1967) reported weight loss in P-W adults on weight-reducing diets only after institutionalization or hospitalization.

NUTRITIONAL MANAGEMENT PROGRAM

Early intervention with diet therapy that was effective and that resulted in appropriate loss and maintenance of weight in growth channel has been described previously (Pipes & Holm, 1973). The diet plan was individualized for each child. The parents were provided with gram weight scales and requested to record all food offered and returned for 60 to 90 consecutive days. The amount of additional food taken was estimated as accurately as possible and recorded. During this period the children were weighed on beam balance scales at least every 2 weeks.

The energy value of food consumed was calculated from these records. To this the energy cost of weight lost or gained was added or subtracted, using a conversion figure of 7.7 kcal/g of weight change. The child's energy need per centimeter of height was estimated from these data and a diet plan was designed to effect a weight loss or weight maintenance in growth channel, depending on the child's needs.

Data collected on preschool and school-age children with P-W syndrome indicated that 8.5 kcal/kg is a reasonable energy intake to effect a slow weight loss and that 10 to 11 kcal/cm of height will maintain appropriate weight in growth channel. In every case but one it was necessary to reduce energy intake below that consumed by normal children of the same age.

If mothers were unable or unwilling to weigh and record the food intake, reductions in the child's current food intake were based on weight gained during a certain time period. For example, parents of a child who gained an unwanted 500 g during 30 days would be requested to reduce the child's energy intake by 130 kcal/day ($7.7 \times 500/30 = 128$), which was necessary to prevent further weight gain. An additional reduction in caloric intake was added if it became necessary to effect weight loss.

The diet recommendation utilized an exchange system originally designed to simplify diet calculations for diabetics (*Exchange lists for meal planning*, Note 1). It can be used successfully in most calorie-controlled diets. Exchanges are lists of similar foods in portion sizes that have approximately equivalent amounts of protein, fat, carbohydrates, and energy. Therefore, foods within each list can be exchanged or substituted for other foods in the same list. There are six major lists: milk, vegetable, fruit, bread, fat, and meat exchanges. Portion sizes are appropriate for adults, but modification of the exchanges is adopted for use with young children.

Children with P-W syndrome have many behavioral characteristics that make adherence to such a rigidly controlled low energy diet difficult. Food must be locked up or otherwise made unavailable (Holm & Pipes, 1976). Parents need support and guidance to carry out this nutritional management program. In addition, everyone who offers food to the child, including teachers, the extended family, and respite caregivers must support the diet program, which often necessitates extensive educational efforts.

Results of Nutritional Management

Although the difficulties in maintaining dietary control increase as the children become older, prevention of obesity has been possible in the majority of cases. Some of the children in our program are shown in Figure 7.1. In 1976 reasonable success was reported in 12 of 14 children with P-W syndrome, ranging in age from 2 years, 3 months (2;3) to 11 years, 3 months (11;3), using an interdisciplinary approach to an individualized nutrition management program (Holm & Pipes, 1976). Since that report the num-

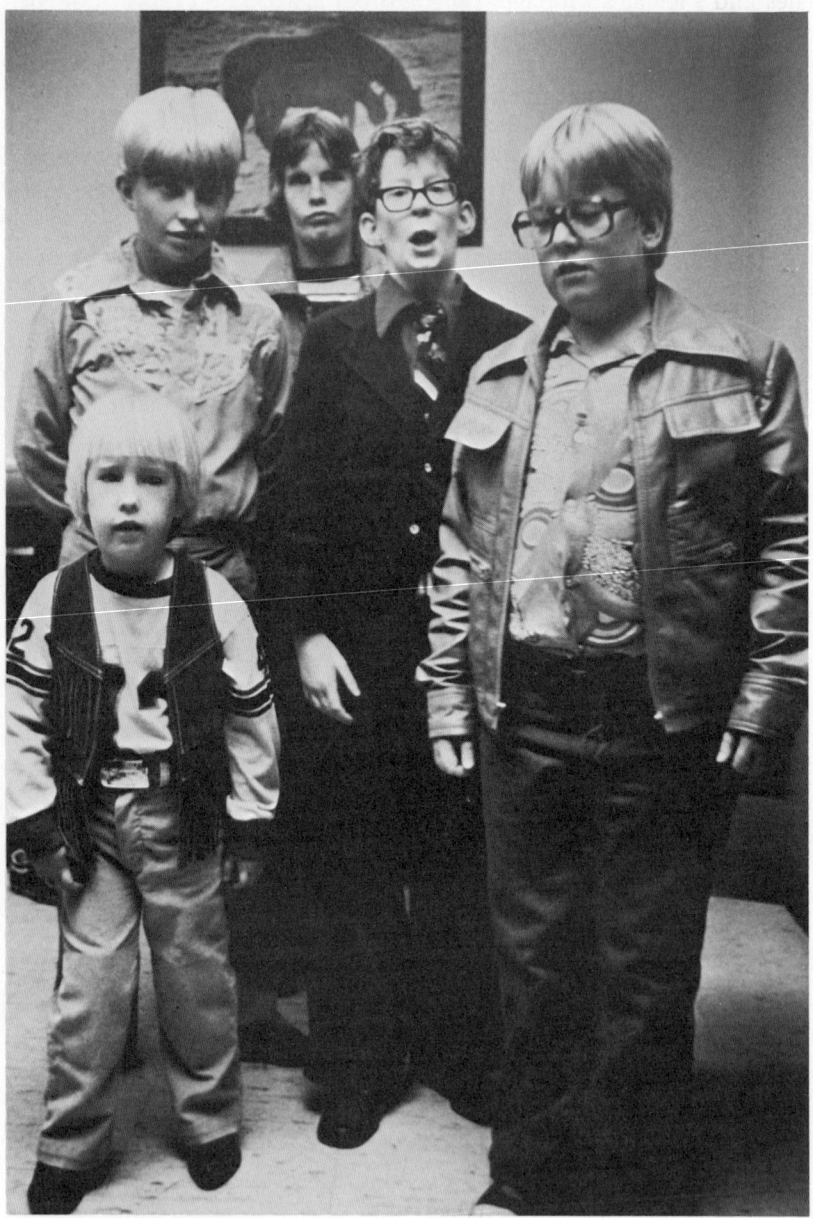

Figure 7.1. P-W syndrome boys who are involved in the University of Washington P-W Syndrome Clinic nutritional management program.

ber of children that have been followed up closely has increased to 24, 15 males and 9 females with ages ranging from 3;9 to 21;8 (Table 7.1). An additional five boys and two girls have been seen only occasionally while being followed up by private physicians in their local communities. Six of this group are preschoolers and their families have been able to effect weight control.

Four of the children seen initially for periods of 1 to 3 years have dropped out of the program. One, by teacher's report, remains at normal

Table 7.1. Weight control

Case	Sex	Age at initial contact	Number of years followed up	Result of weight control
1	M	1;2	8;6	U[a]
2	M	1;6	9;1	S[b]
3	M	1;10	9;1	S
4	F	2;2	3;7	S
5	F	2;9	1	S
6	F	3;6	7;1	S
7	M	4;2	8;2	S
8	F	4;4	1	S
9	M	5;10	4;3	S
10	M	6	2	S
11	M	6;2	5;5	S
12	M	6;9	7	S
13	F	8;10	2	U
14	M	9;2	4;4	U
15	M	10	5	S
16	M	10	5	U
17	M	10;6	6	S
18	F	10;11	3	U
19	M	11	7	S
20	F	11;11	8;9	U
21	M	13;2	2;4	S
22	F	14;3	4	U
23	M	15;10	3;2	S
24	F	17;3	2	S

[a] U = unsuccessful.
[b] S = successful.

weight, while the current weights of the other three are unknown. Two of the original patients are deceased; one with a slender physique was accidentally drowned, the other was grotesquely obese and died in his sleep from an undetermined cause.

As can be seen in Table 7.1, 11 of 12 children who came to the clinic before 7 years of age have continued to be reasonably successful in preventing obesity for 9;1. Twelve youngsters were first seen after age 8 and were for the most part grossly obese initially. Five of the older seven males lost weight and have maintained weight in growth channel. Three of these are living in group homes. Of the five older females, only one has achieved success with weight management (case no. 24). This girl's mother had learned to control the food available to her daughter prior to the diagnosis of P-W syndrome. One 9-year-old girl (case no. 13) has neither gained nor lost weight. The other three older females (case nos. 18, 20, and 22) initially lost some weight, but regained it and have continued to gain.

Weight control programs have not been effective in three males. Case no. 16 initially lost 12.5 kg and maintained his weight in growth channel for 3 years. He had always been a difficult child, but behavior problems with food intensified as he approached adolescence. He used temper tantrums to force his mother not to involve the school in the program for weight control. Money earned from neighbors for odd jobs was spent on food and he persuaded his schoolmates to give him their unwanted lunch food.

Another boy (case no. 14) never lost weight because the diet plan was not implemented and environmental controls on food availability were never put into effect. His parents at times housed a variety of needy adults in their home, who gave him food to keep him quiet. At other times the family has been dependent on donated food and therefore has had no choice in food selection.

The third boy for whom weight control has been ineffective (case no. 1) has been known to the clinic since he was 14 months of age. He lives in a one-parent household. His young mother works and he is fed by a number of different babysitters and relatives who do not support the diet program. His mother understands the diet and is concerned about his weight, but has been unable to organize the needed environmental constraints on her son's food intake.

The oldest successful youngster (case no. 24) has never been grossly obese because control of food availability was begun early, even though she had not been diagnosed before entering the program. The oldest obese child who lost weight and has maintained weight control was 15 years, 10 months at the time services were first provided. Thus, long-lasting weight loss instituted in adolescents is possible, but early age entrance into a weight control program seems an important factor in determining success.

Figure 7.2 shows that in spite of some cases in which treatment has been judged to be ineffective by clinical standards, the results of this study compare very favorably with those for untreated P-W syndrome children. The figure depicts weight data on 22 boys and 13 girls who have been seen in the University of Washington P-W Syndrome Clinic. Most of the weight plots represent many observations on individual children followed up over time, but some show one or just a few weights on a single child. The connected plots in Figure 7.2A show the weight curve of case no. 19 (Figures 7.3 and 7.4). The connected plots in Figure 2B show the weights of case nos. 18 and 20, respectively. With occasional exceptions, most of which were pre-intervention weights, the weights of the patient population are below the regression line for untreated P-W patients and in the normal range for age.

Observations

The need for severe caloric restriction to effect weight reduction in P-W syndrome was reported earlier (Pipes & Holm, 1973). A number of other clinicians have made similar observations. However, the range of kilocalories per centimeter appropriate for individual children varies. One of the patients in this study, a 15-year-old male, maintains his weight in growth channel while consuming more calories than Beal's 10th percentile (Beal, 1970). Thus, the diet has to be individualized.

During weight loss most families have followed the exchange system weight reduction regimen previously described. However, they have usually found portion control of family menu items coupled with calorie counting easier and equally effective during weight maintenance. Parents and siblings have stayed alert to the possibility of food foraging. When it has occurred adjustments are made in portion sizes or choice of food items offered at mealtime. At times, restriction of energy intake at regular meals has been so great that the adequacy of a child's intake of vitamins and trace minerals has been of concern. As a preventive measure a multiple vitamin supplement that includes trace minerals has been prescribed for all children.

Weight control for children with P-W syndrome requires control both of dietary intake and behavior. When parents lack motivation or ability to make food unavailable and cannot supervise their child at mealtime, the result is unsuccessful weight control. Lack of support of the dietary program by babysitters and members of the extended family compounds the problem, as illustrated in one of our cases. Schools add another dimension. One common problem stems from classmates tempting the P-W

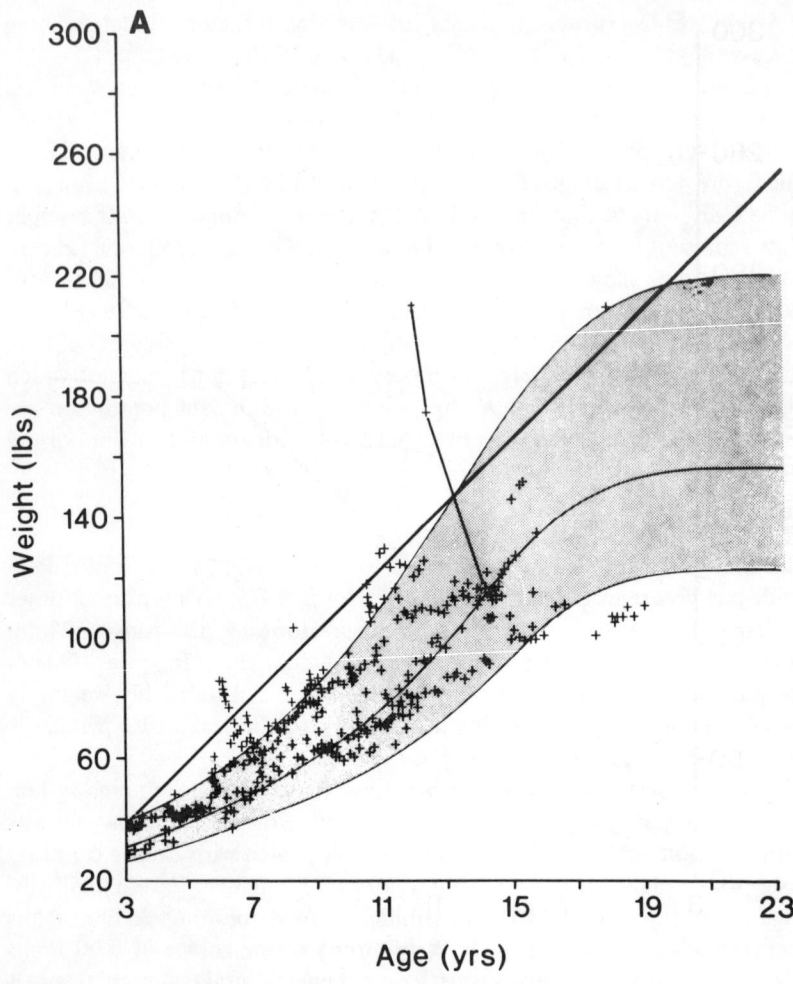

Figure 7.2. Longitudinal weight data of University of Washington P-W Syndrome Clinic patients compared to the regression line of untreated P-W children and the 5th, 50th, and 95th percentiles for the general population. *A*, 22 boys; *B*, 13 girls.

child with food. Easy access to food causes difficulties; as the children grow older, school lunchrooms are less closely monitored and vending machines become available. Accessibility to money for food buying increases. Tantrums and behavior problems related to food seem to become more severe in adolescence.

Regardless of the age of the individual with P-W syndrome, there seems to be a relationship between general attitude and impulsive food

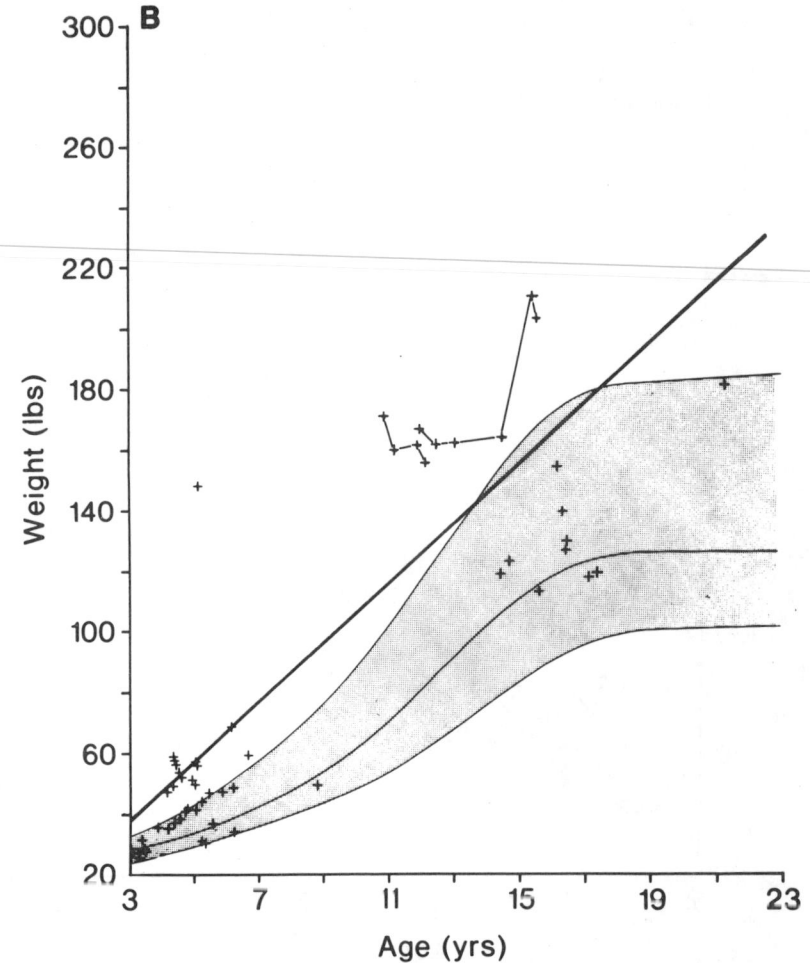

behavior. Many parents say that holidays are particularly difficult. Impulsive and manipulative behavior occurs when sweets and other holiday foods are in the house. Foraging for food is the biggest problem when children are not busy, when they feel that they need extra attention, or when they see someone else eating.

Several parents have commented on the effect they feel refined sugar has on the children's behavior. One mother writes that when "she eats regular sugar she becomes nasty, more stubborn and uncontrollable" (E. Reiss, personal communication). Another states that after holiday seasons with access to much sugar "she becomes motorically hyperactive.

100 Pipes

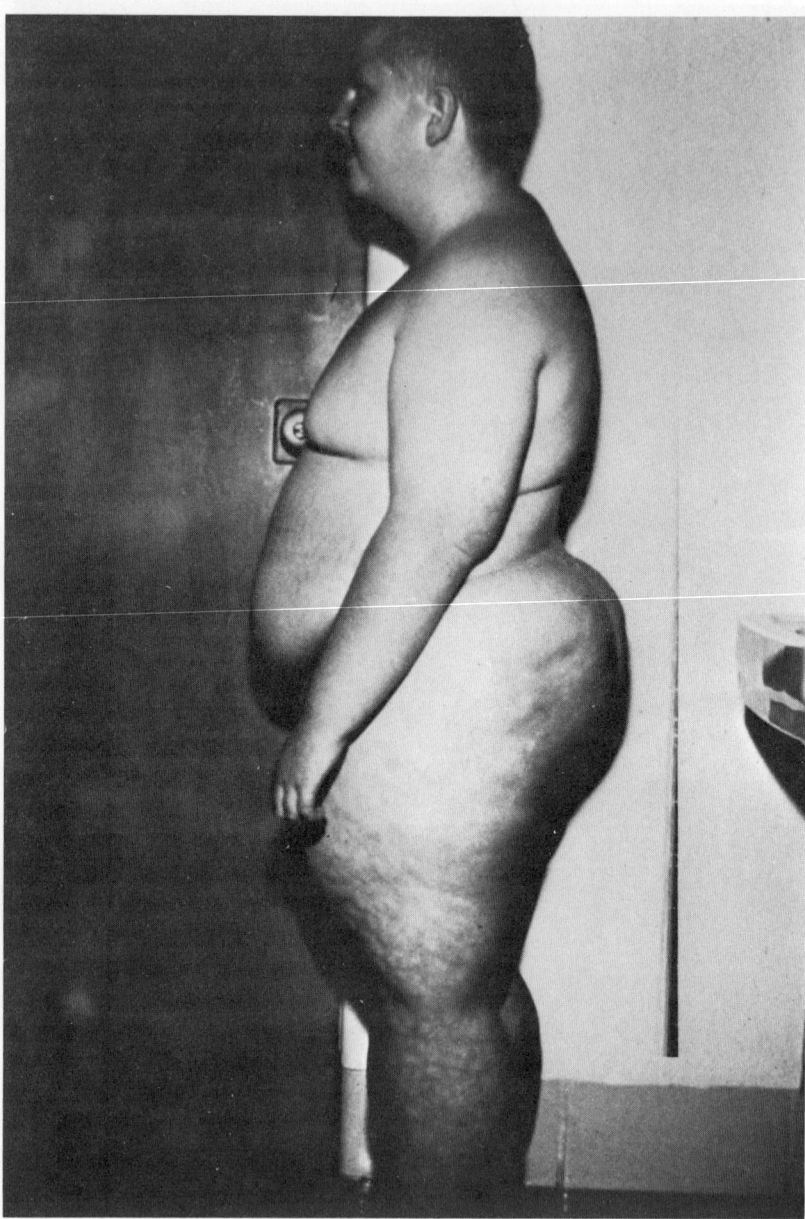

Figure 7.3. A P-W patient before nutritional intervention.

Nutritional Management of Children 101

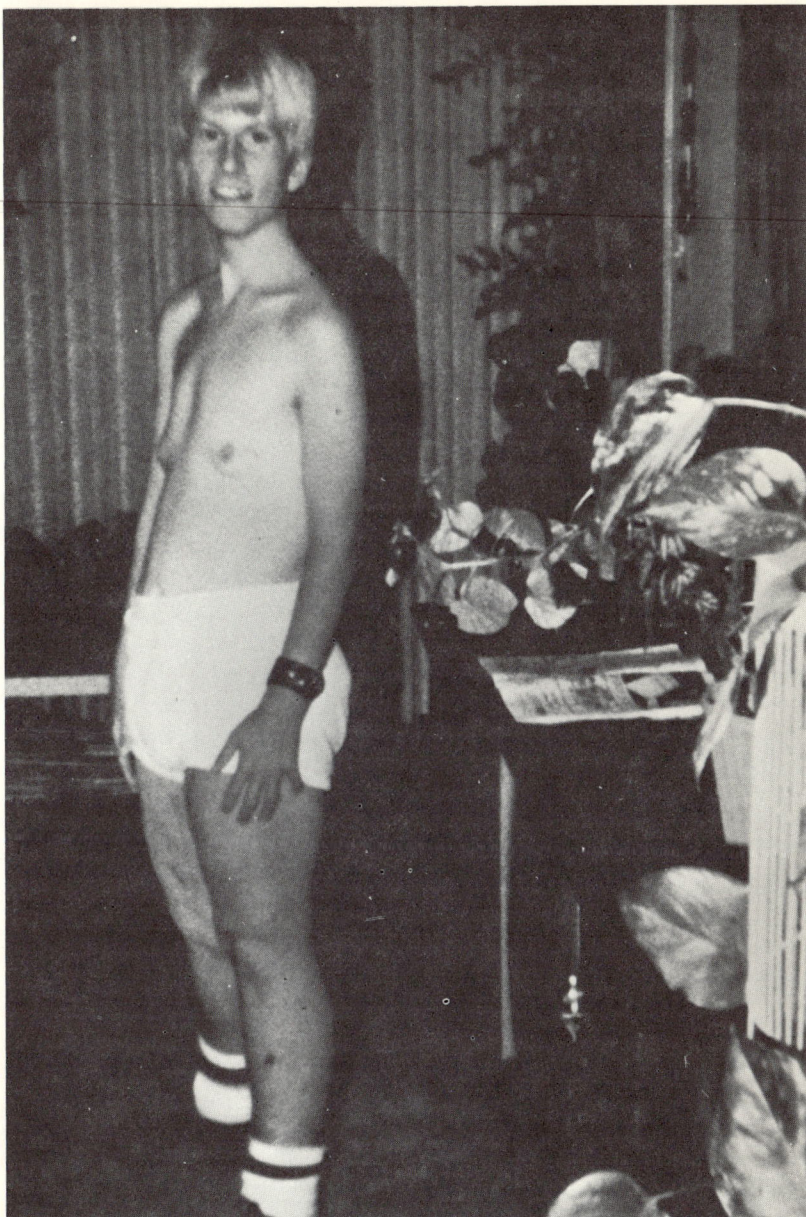

Figure 7.4. The patient shown in Figure 7.3 after nutritional intervention.

The behavior continues for weeks after the holiday season before she settles down."

Our experience strongly indicates that early intervention for control of obesity offers the greatest hope for children affected with P-W syndrome. If the diagnosis is made in early childhood, the child, family, and everybody in the environment learns to accept the fact that the child has a disorder that needs special treatment (a low calorie diet). Some parents refer to P-W syndrome as a "metabolic condition like diabetes" and teach their afflicted offspring to use similar terminology. If parents understand the condition, food-related behavior can be dealt with unemotionally as it develops, and conflicts around food and eating are minimized. The earlier in the child's life that this understanding occurs, the more likely it seems that the result will be a rational approach to a difficult problem.

SUMMARY

Prevention of the grotesque and ultimately fatal obesity in P-W syndrome patients is possible if dietary therapy and environmental controls of food availability are begun when the children are young. Successful programs require the full cooperation of everyone who supervises the child. Individually planned low calorie diets and environmental controls will probably be needed throughout the lifetime of affected persons. Weight control programs can be implemented in adolescents and young adults with P-W syndrome, but are less likely to be successful. Families need continuing contact and support from clinic personnel and from other families who face similar problems.

REFERENCE NOTE

1. *Exchange lists for meal planning.* New York: American Diabetes Association, and Chicago: The American Dietetic Association, 1976. (This publication may be purchased from: The American Dietetic Association, 430 North Michigan Avenue, Chicago, Illinois 60611.)

REFERENCES

Beal, V.A. Nutritional intake. In R.W. McCammon (Ed.), *Human growth and development.* Springfield, Ill.: Charles C Thomas, 1970.

Bistrian, B.R., Blackburn, G.L., & Stanbury, J.B. Metabolic aspects of a protein-sparing modified fast in the dietary management of Prader-Willi obesity. *The New England Journal of Medicine,* 1977, *296,* 774–779.

Coplin, S.S., Hine, J., & Gormican A. Out-patient dietary management in the Prader-Willi syndrome. *Journal of the American Dietetic Association,* 1976, *68,* 330–334.

Evans, P.R. Hypogenital dystrophy with diabetic tendency. *Guy's Hospital Reports*, 1964, *113*, 207-222.

Holm, V.A., & Pipes, P.L. Food and children with Prader-Willi syndrome. *American Journal of Diseases of Children*, 1976, *130*, 1063-1067.

Jancar, J. Prader-Willi syndrome (hypotonia, obesity, hypogonadism, growth and mental retardation). *Journal of Mental Deficiency Research*, 1971, *15*, 20-29.

Juul, J., & Dupont, A. Prader-Willi syndrome. *Journal of Mental Deficiency Research*, 1967, *11*, 12-22.

Laurance, B.M. Hypotonia, mental retardation, obesity, and cryptorchidism associated with dwarfism and diabetes in children. *Archives of Disease in Childhood*, 1967, *42*, 126-139.

Nelson, R.A., Hayles, A.B., Novak, L.P., Margie, J.D., & Vernet, J. Ketogenic diet and Prader-Willi syndrome. *American Journal of Clinical Nutrition*, 1970, *23*, 667. Abstract.

Pipes, P.L., & Holm, V.A. Weight control of children with Prader-Willi syndrome. *Journal of the American Dietetic Association*, 1973, *62*, 520-524.

Soper, R.T., Mason, E.E., Printen, K.J., & Zellweger, H. Gastric bypass for morbid obesity in children and adolescents. *Journal of Pediatric Surgery*, 1975, *10*, 51-58.

Zellweger, H. The HHHO or Prader-Willi syndrome. *Birth Defects: Original Article Series*, 1969, *5*(2), 15-17.

chapter 8

NUTRITION, METABOLISM, BODY COMPOSITION, AND RESPONSE TO THE KETOGENIC DIET IN PRADER-WILLI SYNDROME

Ralph A. Nelson, Diane M. Huse,
Ralph T. Holman, Barbara O. Kimbrough,
Heinz W. Wahner, C. Wayne Callaway,
and Aldine B. Hayles

> In this chapter the authors describe their efforts to determine more accurately the nature of Prader-Willi syndrome obesity and to find a method of therapy. They found that Prader-Willi syndrome subjects differed somewhat from controls in their metabolic processes, in body composition, and in the nature of their adipose tissue. Their research led to the experimental use of the ketogenic diet to control obesity. This was initially successful but had less satisfactory long term results.—Eds.

The clinical study was begun with the aim of defining better nutritional management of the complex Prader Willi (P W) syndrome. In order to accomplish this, a number of studies were performed over a period of several years. Body composition and substrate utilization, the use of a ketogenic diet to produce weight loss, adipose tissue composition, and hyperphagia were studied.

An early hypothesis stated that in the postabsorptive state children with P-W syndrome exhibited an inhibition of release of fat from adipose tissue for energy needs and, since energy was required, a stimulus to eat resulted. At the time, there were no data relating the extreme obesity of these children to their use of carbohydrate, fat, and protein for metabolic

---

This investigation was supported in part by Public Health Service Grant AM 04524 from the National Institutes of Health, by the Hormel Foundation, and by the Northwest Area Foundation, St. Paul, Minnesota.

This chapter was presented in part at the meeting of the Federation of American Societies of Experimental Biology in Anaheim, California, 1976.

processes and the way in which these factors might be related to hyperphagia.

BODY COMPOSITION AND SUBSTRATE UTILIZATION FOR BASAL AND EXERCISE METABOLISM

The first studies involved body composition and substrate utilization for basal and exercise metabolism. The 11 P-W syndrome children studied (mean ± standard error) were 9 ± 1 years old, 126 ± 6 cm in height, and weighed 56 ± 9 kg. Populations used for comparison purposes were 13 children whose only problem was exogenous obesity (12 ± 2 years old, 151 ± 8 cm tall, 90 ± 14 kg of body weight) and 12 children in good health and at ideal body weight (8 ± 1 years old, 129 ± 7 cm tall, and 28 ± 4 kg of body weight).

Body composition was assessed in P-W syndrome and normal obese children by determination of total body water using the non-radioactive isotope D_2O. Total body potassium was determined in the Mayo Clinic whole body counter. Anthropometric measurements of the skeleton and skin folds were also made. From these data, lean body mass and total body fat were calculated according to the method described previously (Nelson, Hayles, & Wahner, 1973).

Substrate utilization was calculated by measuring oxygen consumption and carbon dioxide production at rest and during mild step exercise for P-W syndrome, normal obese, and normal weight children while fasting. Haldane analysis of the expired air was performed and respiratory quotients were determined. A 24-hour collection of urine was simultaneously made and total nitrogen was determined. With these data the utilization of carbohydrate, protein, and fat were calculated by indirect calorimetry (Nelson, Hayles, & Wahner, 1973).

Body composition studies revealed that the P-W group had more adipose tissue than the obese group, 52% and 45%, respectively (Table 8.1.). In some of the children with P-W syndrome, more than 60% of their body weight was adipose tissue, representing the highest value, in the authors' experience, for obese subjects.

On the other hand, respiratory quotients were quite similar in all three groups for basal metabolism (Table 8.1). Since the respiratory quotient is a function of metabolic use of carbohydrate, fat, and protein, these substrates were used in similar fashion in all three groups (P-W, normal obese, and ideal weight children). The much greater quantity of adipose tissue reserves in the P-W and normal obese children did not appear to be a factor in determining the quantity of fat used. In each group, an average of between 53% and 57% of total calories for basal metabolism came from adipose tissue deposits.

Table 8.1. Body composition and basal and exercise metabolism before and after 12 months of ketogenic diet in Prader-Willi syndrome children

	Prader-Willi group			Normal groups	
	Before	12 months later		Obese	Ideal weight[a]
Basal metabolism					
Respiratory quotients	0.81 ± 0.01 (9)[b]	0.76 ± 0.01 (10)		0.80 ± 0.02 (12)	0.81 ± 0.01 (12)
Utilization (g/hr)					
Carbohydrate	4.4 ± 1	1.9 ± 5		5.1 ± 1	4.2 ± 1
Fat	3.6 ± 1	3.9 ± 4		5 ± 1	3.2 ± 0.4
% Calories from fat	53 ± 5	73 ± 4		57 ± 5	53 ± 4
Protein	2.6 ± 0.3	1.7 ± 0.4		3.3 ± 0.3	2.3 ± 0.2
Total kcal/hr	60	50		79	55
Exercise metabolism					
Respiratory quotients	0.80 ± 0.02 (4)	0.70 ± 0.02 (9)		0.84 ± 0.02	0.73 ± 0.02
Utilization (g/hr)					
Carbohydrate	14.4 ± 4	3.1 ± 2		45.4 ± 13	4.6 ± 2
Fat	11.8 ± 2	12 ± 2		19.2 ± 3	12.2 ± 2
% Total calories from fat	63 ± 6	86 ± 3		53 ± 8	80 ± 4
Total kcal/hr	174	127		368	137
Body composition					
Lean body mass (kg)	31.4 ± 5 (7)	22.9 ± 3 (8)		52.5 ± 4 (10)	22
Total body fat (kg)	33.4 ± 6	21.3 ± 6		42.2 ± 6	4
% Total body fat	52	42		45	15

[a]Body composition estimated.
[b]Values in parentheses indicate number of subjects.

However, groups differed in their use of fat and carbohydrate during exercise. It should be noted that only four P-W children were exercised early in the studies because it was difficult to get them to step up and down a step for 5 minutes. Initially, some exercised only 2 minutes and a steady state was not realized. (In the authors' experience, 3 to 5 minutes of mild exercise is necessary to produce a steady state of oxygen consumption and carbon dioxide production.)

During mild step exercise the respiratory quotients decreased in normal weight children, remained about the same in the P-W group, but increased in normal obese children. These differing responses showed that normal weight children used the most fat as substrate for exercise metabolism (80% of total) and that normal obese children used the most carbohydrate (47% of total). Curiously, P-W children appeared midway between the two groups, using about 63% from fat and 37% from carbohydrate.

The response of normal weight children to mild exercise was as predicted for well trained individuals, that is, increased contribution from fat as energy substrate. The response of the normal obese group was also as expected because of the increased use of carbohydrate resulting from much more stressful exercise (lifting of a heavy frame by untrained individuals).

The response of P-W children could not be readily explained. Although the data obtained showed that fat, indeed, was used as substrate for basal and exercise metabolism, the responses of P-W children were somewhat different and could not be easily explained from known physiological data. Inhibition of fat release from adipose tissue possibly might be present, but to a lesser degree than hypothesized. It was decided, therefore, to conduct a clinical trial of a diet high in fat and compare it with a diet high in carbohydrate of equal caloric content. It was reasoned that a metabolic derangement might exist in one or both of the pathways (fat absorption, storage, and release, or carbohydrate absorption, conversion to fat, storage, and release). Accordingly, three children were given a diet prescription for a ketogenic diet and followed up closely for the succeeding 3 months. However, the children's response to the ketogenic diet was so gratifying to the parents that they did not wish to try the high carbohydrate diet.

Since the aim of the investigators was to find the best means of therapy and since the usual calorie-controlled weight reduction diet had been a failure in these children, it was decided to adopt the ketogenic diet in treating obesity in P-W children.

LONG TERM RESULTS OF A KETOGENIC DIET

A calorie-controlled ketogenic diet to produce weight loss was prescribed for P-W children (Committee on Dietetics of the Mayo Clinic, 1971). The ketogenic to antiketogenic ratio was 2.7:1; the subjects were fed 2.7 g of fat for every 1 g of carbohydrate and protein combined. Adherence to the diet prescription was assessed by 7-day diet diaries that were completed by the parents. Total nitrogen was determined in timed overnight 24-hour urine collections. The total 24-hour excretion of nitrogen in urine should be within ±2 g of calculated nitrogen intake for accuracy of diary information (Huse, Nelson, Briones, & Hodgson, 1974). This indirect but objective measure of diet reliability holds for timed overnight collections when corrected to 24-hour totals.

During the 1- to 6-year follow-up of these patients indirect calorimetry, body composition, and 24-hour urine collections were analyzed for total nitrogen, uric acid, and total and free ketones, and 7-day diaries were kept at least once each year. Blood samples taken while fasting were analyzed for glucose, cholesterol, and triglycerides. All determinations were made by the Mayo Clinic Department of Laboratory Medicine.

Retrospective data of height and weight for the P-W group were obtained from their medical records and from parents. This information provided control data for growth and development in the untreated state, since the parents uniformly indicated their inability to inhibit excessive food intake by the children.

Prior to starting the ketogenic diet, hematocrit, hemoglobin, white blood cell counts, serum potassium, calcium, and phosphorus were normal. Mean serum cholesterol and triglycerides were also normal—182 and 82 mg/dl, respectively. During the first year of therapy the diet prescription compared favorably with actual food intake as judged from 7-day food diaries kept by parents. Children ate approximately 14 g of carbohydrate, 102 g of fat, and 26 g of protein each day. The mean diet prescription was 1,078 kcal/day, about 8.6 kcal/cm of height, similar to the caloric intake in growing children experiencing weight loss according to Pipes and Holm (1973). Protein supplied at least 1.0 g/kg of body weight, calculated on the basis of predicted ideal body weight. Daily replacement of vitamins, calcium, and iron was prescribed. Food was not used as a reward. There was no penalty for dietary excesses above the prescription. No special arrangements were made in schools or other institutions that P-W children attended without parental supervision. Adherence to the diet for the first 12 months was good.

In the five P-W children on whom body composition studies were made before and after being placed on the ketogenic diet, lean body mass decreased from 28.6 to 24.0 kg and total body fat decreased from 28.8 to 23.6 after 1 year of therapy. Lean body mass loss was thought to represent the loss in body water that occurs when a ketogenic diet is followed.

Long term body weights prior to and in response to the diet are shown in Figure 8.1. The regression line represents the line of best fit for gain in body weight based on readings when the children were eating normally. The increase in total body weight with age was somewhat greater in boys than in girls. The slopes of the lines in body sexes were much greater than the curve for the 84th percentile for normal developing children of similar ages. Between ages 8 and 12, P-W children have the prospect of gaining between 20 and 30 kg in body weight if not treated.

All children lost weight during the first 12 months of following the calorie-reduced ketogenic diet. All of the older children except one began to eat foods not in the diet prescription and their body weights began to increase to fit the predicted weight curve for untreated P-W children. However, all P-W children age 6 or less not only lost weight but eventually placed between the 16th and 84th percentiles of normals. Some maintained these positions for 6 years of therapy only to rebound with rapid weight gain when they went off the diet. (These responses after 6 years are not on the graph.) One young patient went off the diet after 30 months of favorable progress and quickly gained weight to a point where she exceeded the curve for untreated P-W children.

Figure 8.2 compares the four boys who followed the ketogenic diet for the longest period of time (responders) with the two boys and two girls who did not stay on the diet (non-responders). In the non-responding group, total body fat increased significantly from 35% to 60% of body weight during the 5 years of observation. Lean body mass increased slightly in the non-responders. The change that occurred in one younger girl who at first responded but became a non-responder when she went off the diet is depicted below the general curve for non-responders. The curve was very similar to that for the older, non-responding children.

In the responders, lean body mass increased at a rate similar to that of the non-responders. Apparently, the ketogenic diet did not inhibit growth of lean body mass. Body fat increased slightly in the responding group. The primary effect of the diet appeared to be inhibition of excessive fat accumulation. The ratio of fat to lean body mass remained constant as the children slowly grew in height; this placed them within the normal distribution of children for height and weight (Figure 8.1)

P-W children were shorter than normal. No change in height development was noted as a result of the ketogenic diet prescription. It was similar to that of children who did not stay on the diet and to published reports about other P-W children.

Indirect calorimetry studies after 1 year on the diet showed that the utilization of fat changed considerably. Contribution to basal metabolism increased from 53% to 73% and from 63% to 86% in exercise metabolism (Table 8.1)

This is a response to be expected in normal individuals who eat high fat diets. In P-W children a similar reaction occurred. Apparently, when

Nutrition, Metabolism, Body Composition, and the Ketogenic Diet

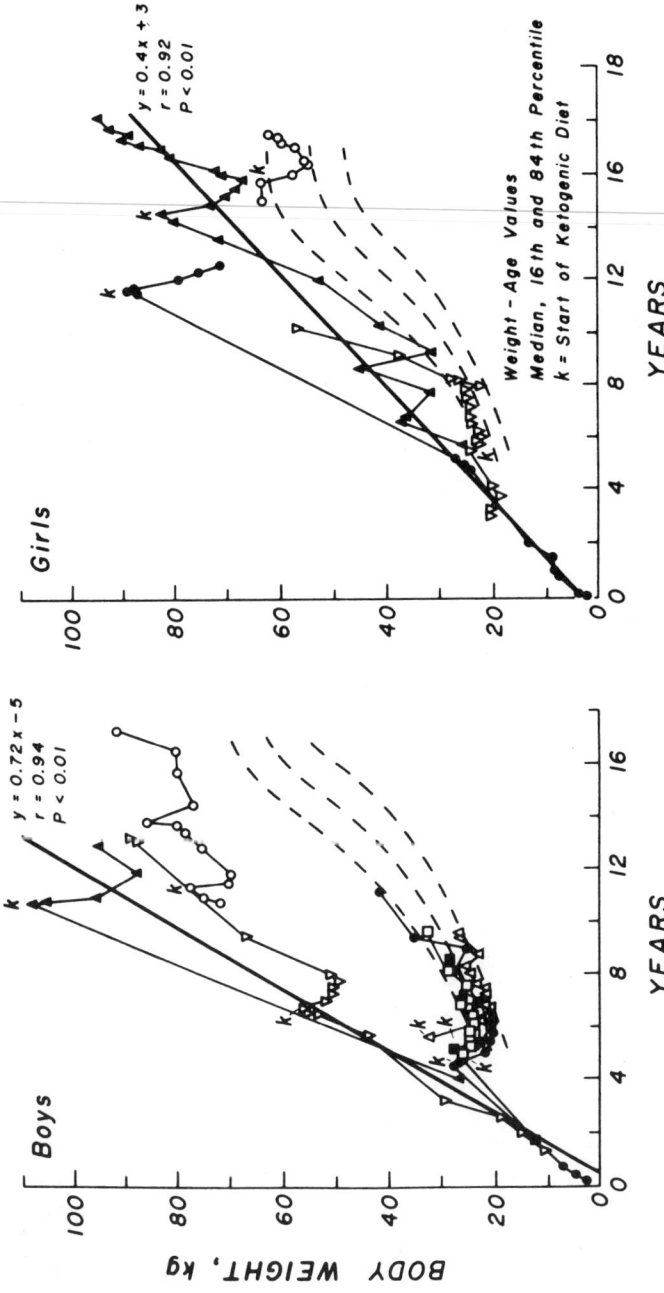

Figure 8.1. Changes in body weight of P-W children during time before and after treatment with the ketogenic diet.

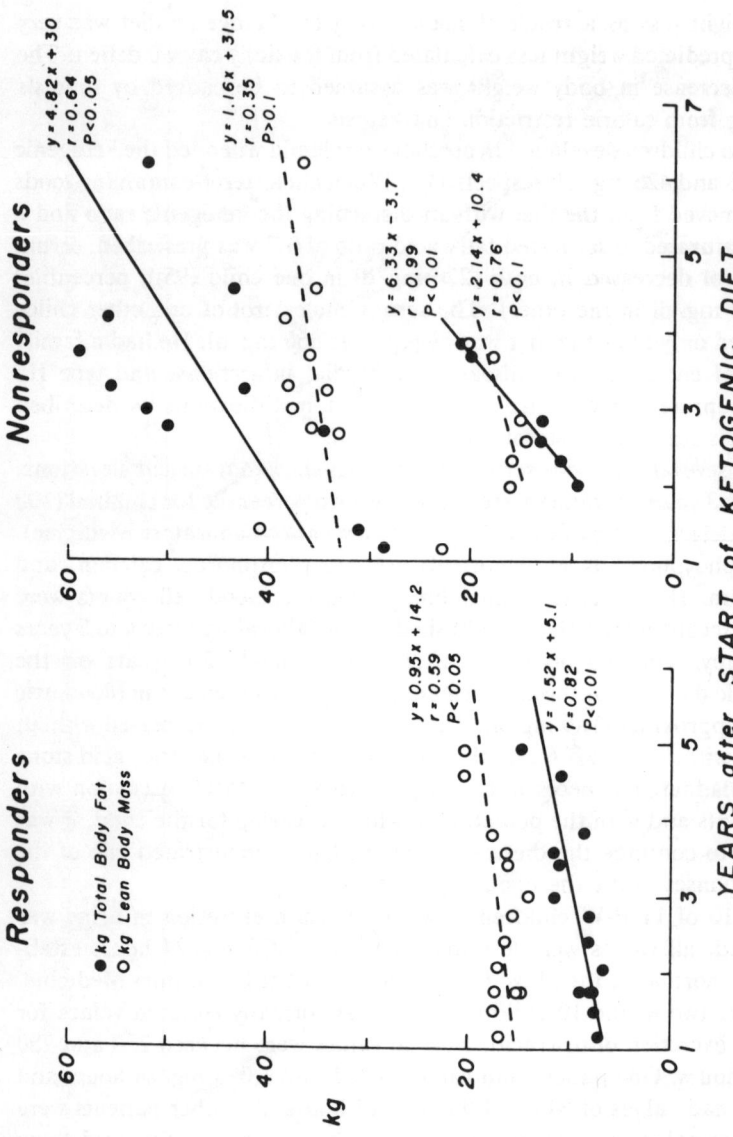

Figure 8.2. Changes in body composition of P-W children who adhered (responders) and who did not adhere (non-responders) to the ketogenic diet. The bottom curve on the non-responding portion represents data from one subject.

dietary fat was fed in large amounts, circumventing carbohydrate to fat conversion, it was absorbed, deposited, and released normally from adipose tissue. Parents also noted that hyperphagia seemed easier to control.

Weight loss as a result of maintaining the ketogenic diet was very close to predicted weight loss calculated from the daily calorie deficit. The initial decrease in body weight was assumed to be caused by diuresis resulting from calorie restriction and ketosis.

Two children developed hypercholesterolemia when fed the ketogenic diet (375 and 425 mg/dl, respectively). When cholesterol-containing foods were removed from the diet without disturbing the ketogenic ratio and a polyunsaturated to saturated fatty acid ratio of 0.7 was prescribed, serum cholesterol decreased in both (220 mg/dl in one child (95th percentile) and 290 mg/dl in the other). The serum cholesterol of one other child, measured only after the diet was begun, was 560 mg/dl. He had a family history of coronary heart disease, myocardial infarctions, and type IIa hyperlipoproteinemia. After 5 years of diet modifications as described above, his serum cholesterol was 238 mg/dl.

On several occasions serum triglycerides showed transient elevations, but after 3 years all values were below the 95th percentile for children (100 mg/dl, determined by Mayo Clinic Department of Laboratory Medicine). Serum phospholipids were normal, as were phosphorus, calcium, and potassium. Hematocrit, hemoglobin, and white blood cell counts were normal according to values established by the laboratory after 4 to 5 years of therapy. On two occasions after approximately 2½ years on the ketogenic diet, two of the children demonstrated an increase in blood uric acid to approximately 9 mg/dl. These values, however, decreased without therapy within the next 6 months. One child developed a uric acid stone in the bladder that necessitated surgical removal. After discussion with the parents and with the pediatrician who was caring for the child, it was decided to continue the diet. This patient had demonstrated one of the best responses to the therapeutic program.

In 10 of 11 P-W children in whom calcium excretion in urine was measured, all values were less than the 250 to 275 mg/24 hours established as normal by the Mayo Clinic Department of Laboratory Medicine. However, two of the 10 children showed abnormally elevated values for 24-hour excretion of uric acid. Normal values were between 250 and 750 mg/24 hours. One patient had values of 951 and 1,073 mg/24 hours and another had values of 844 and 980 mg/24 hours. All other patients were within normal ranges, including the child who developed a uric acid stone in his bladder. Values for this patient varied between 250 and 513 mg/24 hours, recorded on five separate occasions. During therapy, total ketone excretion in urine ranged from 128 to 2,782 mg/24 hours.

Our earlier experience (Nelson, Hayles, Novak, Margie, & Vernet, 1970) and that of others (Bistrian, Blackburn, & Stanbury, 1977) showing that the ketogenic diet has potential to control the massive gain in body fat was not confirmed by the long range studies. The most obvious reason was inability of patients to comply. The ketogenic diet only "buys time" before massive obesity develops. All the children studied became massively obese after leaving parental control. However, all parents of younger children preferred the ketogenic diet because it was effective in producing weight loss and helped control hyperphagia. All P-W children when considered for diet therapy should receive the usual calorie-restricted diet that contains all essential nutrients for growth and development. If this fails, the ketogenic diet will buy time but some other form of therapy must be found.

The ketogenic diet was tried for several normal obese children who had not responded to the conventional weight reduction program. It was found that it did not control appetite and it offered no particular benefits for this population. This point should be stressed in light of current interest by the lay public in low carbohydrate diets for weight reduction. In the authors' opinion such diets have potential for producing atherosclerosis and gout in normal individuals and should not be prescribed, although these writers and the parents of P-W children were willing to accept these risks. The ketogenic diet has had a long history of use for the treatment of children with convulsive disorders. In the experience of Keith (1963) children on the ketogenic diet did lose weight. However, over a period of weeks weight stabilizes or actually increases. Many of the children who achieved ketosis complained of not receiving enough food. The diet, therefore, should not be considered as one that inhibits appetite in healthy individuals.

ADIPOSE TISSUE COMPOSITION

After almost 4 years of experience using the ketogenic diet, it was decided to determine whether the structure of fat in adipose tissue of P-W children was different from that of normal adipose tissue. Palpation of adipose tissue deposits revealed softer texture in P-W children.

Under local anesthesia nine biopsy specimens of 2 to 5 g of subcutaneous adipose tissue were obtained from abdominal fat of P-W children. Total lipid was extracted from approximately 1 g of tissue and its fatty acid composition was measured by gas-liquid chromatography. These analyses were performed at the Hormel Institute. Thin layer chromatography of the extract revealed that it was more than 98% triglyceride (Hofstetter, Sen, & Holman, 1965). For comparison, adipose tissue was obtained from nine normal weight subjects at surgery. Seven biopsies were from abdominal fat and two were obtained after operations for elbow and for hip disease. Eight of the nine subjects varied in age from 2½ years to 11 years. The subject with hip disease was 62 years old. In the test for significance, the comparison between P-W and normal means was made using the higher standard deviation of the two.

The analysis of adipose tissue triglycerides from P-W children revealed significantly smaller percentages (12:0 and 18:0) of the saturated fatty acids but a noticeable elevation in long-chained polyunsaturated fatty acids (PUFA) (Table 8.2). The content of fatty acids with double bonds at carbon atoms positions Δ 2 to 7 was three times that found in the normal samples. These long-chained fatty acids (double bonds in carbon atom positions Δ 2 to 7), which were found in excess in P-W adipose triglycerides, are metabolic products from the linoleic and linolenic acids found in PUFA oils commonly used in foods. Therefore, the diet consumed by the children prior to the fat biopsy was analyzed for inclusion of such foods. Three of the subjects were biopsied while they were consuming diets ad libitum containing usual quantities of carbohydrates. Three biopsies were taken from children on the ketogenic diet, but the PUFA/saturated fatty acids ratio was between 0.1 and 0.2 with very low linoleic or other polyunsaturated fatty acid content. The elevated PUFA content of adipose tissue was, therefore, probably not directly of dietary origin.

Although metabolic data showed that children with P-W syndrome can release and use fat in the postabsorptive state in basal and exercise metabolism, and although hyperphagia appeared to be most likely caused by altered hypothalamic control of appetite, the results of fat biopsies in P-W children did suggest an abnormality in their body fat composition. There is a noticeable elevation on long-chained PUFA in triglycerides. The content of fatty acids having double bonds in carbon atom positions Δ 2 to 7 in adipose triglycerides was three times greater than in adipose tissue from normal individuals. The content of long-chained PUFA in adipose triglycerides is usually low. Elevated contents indicate altered fatty acid or lipid metabolism. These high PUFA levels may inhibit not only the hydrolysis of the triglycerides in which they are contained, but hydrolysis of other stored triglycerides with the more common fatty acids as well.

Lipases are generally considered to hydrolyze all fatty acids without regard for their structures. Pancreatic lipase was previously considered to have specificity for positions 1 and 3 of a triglyceride, but no specificity with respect to fatty acid structure. Bottino, Vandenburg, and Reiser (1967) found that fish oils containing high proportions of PUFA resisted hydrolysis by pancreatic lipase. Esters of 3-enoic acids from plant sources

Table 8.2. Fatty acid patterns of human adipose tissue in two populations

Fatty acids(s)		Experimental (n = 9)		Normal (n = 10)[a]	
		Mean	SD	Mean	SD
12:0	—[a]	0.57	0.54	1.24	0.59
14:0		3.83	1.51	5.17	1.44
14:1	—[b]	1.73	1.05	1.02	0.42
16:0		17.46	3.82	19.33	3.13
16:1W7[c]	—[a]	8.40	1.68	6.79	1.98
16.2	—[b]	0.98	1.43	0.50	0.09
18:0	—[a]	5.60	2.62	9.06	3.82
18:1W9		38.06	10.36	39.30	5.77
18:2W6		13.97	2.48	13.73	4.37
18:3W6	—[b]	0.47	0.76	0.00	0.00
18:3W3	—[b]	3.54	2.57	1.52	0.52
20:2W9		0.84	0.36	0.65	0.54
20:2W6	—[b]	0.61	0.58	0.23	0.16
20:3W9		0.02	0.03	0.11	0.31
20:3W6	—[b]	0.52	0.39	0.18	0.08
20:4W6	—[b]	1.23	1.13	0.29	0.13
20:4W3	—[b]	0.15	0.14	0.03	0.05
20:5W3	—[a]	0.20	0.16	0.06	0.10
22:4W6	—[b]	0.61	0.52	0.06	0.08
22:4W3	—[b]	0.01	0.03	0.00	0.00
22:5W6	—[b]	0.31	0.40	0.00	0.00
22:5W3	—[b]	0.25	0.18	0.06	0.08
22:6W3	—[b]	0.22	0.31	0.04	0.07

[a] Indicates average difference greater than 1 standard deviation.
[b] Indicates average difference greater than 2 standard deviations.
[c] W indicates the carbon position of the first double bond.

also resist pancreatic lipase action (Kleiman, Earle, Tallent, & Wolff, 1970). One of the authors (RTH) has made a study of hydrolysis of triglycerides, each containing a single *cis* positional isomer of oleic acid by pancreatic lipase, and found that fatty acids having double bonds in carbon atom positions Δ 2 to 7 resist its action (Heimermann, Holman, Gordon, Krowalyshyn, & Jenson, 1973). If the triglyceride lipase of adipose tissue behaves similarly in its ability to hydrolyze triglycerides with fatty acids having double bonds in positions Δ 2 to 7, retention of PUFA in adipose triglycerides and the accumulation of total triglycerides of P-W children could be explained. Just a few percent of PUFA could have profound effects upon lipolysis of other triglycerides because, being more polar than common fatty acids, a relatively high concentration of PUFA would occur at the interface of the fat droplet. Lipase action is at that interface, and if triglycerides containing PUFA cannot be hydrolyzed by lipase, this could effectively prevent most release of fat from the fat depot for energy purposes. Despite the great quantity of fat stores in P-W children, only 55% of the energy used in basal metabolism was derived from fat, compared with 57% in obese children and 71% in obese adults (Nelson, Anderson, Gastineau, Hayles, & Stamnes, 1973).

The recent demonstration of marked elevation of adipose tissue lipoprotein lipase in P-W children (Schwartz, Brunzell, & Bierman, Chapter 10, this volume) could be the consequence of resistance of polyunsaturated adipose triglycerides to lipolysis. Furthermore, increased quantity of PUFA could be the reason for softness of fatty tissue in these children.

The contribution of dietary carbohydrate in fatty acid biosynthesis remains unclear. Certainly, the almost total absence of dietary carbohydrate and the excessive fat content of the ketogenic diet improved fat utilization in basal and exercise metabolism.

HYPERPHAGIA

The final portion of the study involved documentation of hyperphagia. Some parents denied its existence. If the hypothesis relating fatty acid structures to ease of hydrolysis of adipose tissue triglycerides has merit, hyperphagia should be present in those who have increased quantities of polyunsaturated fatty acids with double bonds between carbon atom positions $\Delta 2$ to 7. Accordingly, three P-W children with these changes in their fatty acid composition were studied for existence of hyperphagia.

In order to quantitate the degree of hyperphagia found, it was necessary to admit the three children to the Clinical Research Center (CRC) for 33, 26, and 19 days, respectively. The study was approved by the Human Studies Committee of the Mayo Clinic and parental consent was obtained in all cases. The children, ages 19, 13, and 11 years, were studied under two dietary conditions. In the first phase the children selected their own food and ate three meals and three snacks daily. They were instructed to eat only in the CRC dining room and told they could eat whenever they wished if they simply asked the dietitian.

Daily caloric intake was calculated by weighing the food offered and subtracting the weight of food refused. Calculated intake was divided into grams of protein, fat, and carbohydrate. Body weight was measured daily after voiding and before breakfast.

In the second phase the children also planned their own menus but were served substitutes for bread, peanut butter, and cookies that were high in dietary fiber (DF). The DF foods were developed by General Mills, Inc., and Wonder Bread Baking Co. The DF ingredients were on the FDA list of foods generally recognized as safe and consisted of approximately one-fourth cellulose and lignin and three-fourths arabinogalacta, galactomannans, acidic polysaccharides, and xylan hemicellulose.

Twenty-four-hour urine collections were analyzed for total nitrogen, uric acid, calcium, and magnesium. Blood samples taken during fasting were analyzed for glucose, cholesterol, and triglycerides. Determinations were done by the Mayo Clinic Department of Laboratory Medicine.

Hyperphagia was found in all P-W children admitted to the CRC. Associated with it was weight gain under ad libitum conditions (Table 8.3). When children were allowed to select their food and snacks for 5 to 8 days, the excess calorie intake varied between 961 and 1,895 kcal. The diets contained 10% to 20% protein, 50% carbohydrate, and 30% to 40% fat of total kilocalories eaten. This is slightly higher in carbohydrate than the usual percentage found in the American diet. For the next 5 to 8 days the three foods high in DF were added to the diet and incorporated wherever possible into the menus planned by the children. The average amount of DF consumed was 38 g/day (the usual amount is approximately 4 to 8 g/day). While eating the foods high in DF the children continued to eat excessively and to gain weight. Although weight gain tended to be somewhat less, only in one case did the intake of available food decrease significantly. In the other two children it did not increase at all,

Table 8.3. Daily nutrient intake under ad libitum conditions in three patients with Prader-Willi syndrome

Patient	Dietary fiber	Kilocalories		No. of days	Weight gain (kg)
		Available	Excess consumed		
1	5[a]	3,696	1,895	8	2.2
	41[b]	3,298	1,498	8	0.8
2	3[a]	3,125	1,225	5	1.5
	38[b]	3,125	1,225	5	0.5
3	4[a]	2,898	1,098	5	1.6
	34[b]	2,761	961	5	0.6

[a]Crude fiber estimate.
[b]Crude fiber estimate + known additions of pure dietary fiber.

and all subjects complained of hunger while consuming 3,000 kcal/day of the high DF diet. The appetite of one subject could best be described as ravenous; on three occasions he was found seeking food outside the CRC. The data showed that hyperphagia persisted despite use of foods high in DF and low in caloric density.

SUMMARY

The natural progression of the untreated state of most patients with P-W syndrome is one of continuing weight gain with increasing age. The gain in weight is primarily in adipose tissue, not lean body mass. The extreme obesity appears directly related to hyperphagia. It is proposed here that hyperphagia be considered a part of the syndrome rather than an associated finding. Furthermore, hyperphagia is present in P-W children who have increased quantities of polyunsaturated fatty acids with double bonds between carbon atom positions Δ 2 to 7 in triglycerides of adipose tissue. This finding supports the hypothesis that fatty acid structure is related in some fashion to hyperphagia. Also, the original hypothesis that there may be inhibition of fat release in response to energy demands and that this is related, in some manner, to hyperphagia has some support from the experimental data collected thus far.

REFERENCES

Bristrian, B.R., Blackburn, G.L., & Stanbury, J.B. Metabolic aspects of a protein-sparing modified fast in the dietary management of Prader-Willi obesity. *The New England Journal of Medicine*, 1977, *296*, 774-779.

Bottino, N.A., Vandenburg, G.A., & Reiser, R. Resistance of certain long-chain polyunsaturated fatty acids of marine oils to pancreatic lipase hydrolysis. *Lipids*, 1967, *2*, 489-493.

Committee on Dietetics of the Mayo Clinic. *Mayo clinic diet manual* (4th ed.). Philadelphia: W.B. Saunders Co., 1971.

Heimermann, W.H., Holman, R.T., Gordon, D.T., Krowalyshyn, D.E., & Jenson, R.G. Effect of double bond position in octadecenoates upon hydrolysis by pancreatic lipase. *Lipids*, 1973, *8*, 45-46.

Hofstetter, H.H., Sen, M., & Holman, R.T. Characterization of unsaturated fatty acids by gas-liquid chromatography. *Journal of the American Oil Chemists Society*, 1965, *42*, 537-540.

Huse, D.M., Nelson, R.A., Briones, E.R., & Hodgson, P.A. Urinary nitrogen excretion as an objective measure of dietary intake. *American Journal of Clinical Nutrition*, 1974, *27*, 771-773.

Keith, H.M. *Convulsive disorders in children with reference to treatment with ketogenic diet*. Boston: Little, Brown & Co., 1963.

Kleiman, R., Earle, F.R., Tallent, W.H., & Wolff, I.A. Retarded hydrolysis by pancreatic lipase of seed oils with *trans*-3 unsaturation. *Lipids*, 1970, *5*, 513-518.

Nelson, R.A., Hayles, A.B., Novak, L.P., Margie, J.D., & Vernet, J. Ketogenic diet in the Prader-Willi syndrome. *American Journal of Clinical Nutrition,* 1970, *23,* 667.

Nelson, R.A., Anderson, L.F., Gastineau, C.F., Hayles, A.B., & Stamnes C.L. Physiology and natural history of obesity. *Journal of the American Medical Association,* 1973, *223,* 627-639.

Nelson, R.A., Hayles, A.B., & Wahner, H.W. Exercise and urinary nitrogen excretion in two chronically malnourished subjects. *Mayo Clinic Proceedings,* 1973, *48,* 549-555.

Pipes, P.L., & Holm, V.A. Weight control of children with Prader-Willi syndrome. *Journal of the American Dietetic Association,* 1973, *62,* 520-524.

chapter 9
SURGICAL TREATMENT OF MORBID OBESITY IN PRADER-WILLI SYNDROME

Robert T. Soper, Edward E. Mason,
Kenneth J. Printen, and Hans Zellweger

> This chapter discusses the surgical treatment of obesity and its role in treating Prader-Willi syndrome patients. The authors report moderate success in gastric bypass and gastroplasty operations on 11 Prader-Willi syndrome children and adolescents.—*Eds.*

In this chapter, attempts at surgical control of morbid obesity in both adults and children are briefly reviewed, and the experience with 11 children suffering from Prader-Willi syndrome who were subjected to gastric bypass or gastroplasty in treatment of their morbid obesity is discussed in some detail. An attempt is made to establish the place of surgical therapy in managing the morbid obesity of P-W syndrome. This, with its complications, is the most disabling component of P-W syndrome from the therapeutic angle.

Paradoxically, in early infancy P-W syndrome is characterized by hypotonia and failure to thrive nutritionally. However, a different pattern emerges, leading to rapid and sustained weight gain, which usually produces obesity of Pickwickian dimensions during the latter half of the first decade of life. Most P-W children appear to be persistently hungry, constantly asking for food and foraging in the refrigerator, pantry, and garbage can in search of something edible. They have been known to consume dog food, K-Y jelly, and other inappropriate substances. However, a few P-W children eat only when food is available, seeming to lack the intense hunger drive when they are out of contact with food (Hoefnagel, Costello, & Hatoum, 1967).

The fat is typically deposited on the trunk, buttocks, and proximal extremities. Diabetes mellitus, probably simply a complication of the obesity, develops in as many as one-third of P-W adolescents (Zellweger & Schneider, 1968), although a lower incidence has been found in some other series of patients (Holm, Chapter 3, this volume). As the obesity worsens during the second decade of life, the children become more sedentary and may develop recurrent and progressive respiratory problems characterized by hypercapnia, hypoxemia, and right-sided heart failure. This appears to be little different from the Pickwickian respiratory problems suffered by normally intelligent but morbidly obese adults; it is probably related to the huge fat mass compressing the lung, inhibiting intercostal and respiratory diaphragm function and leading to CO_2 retention, acidosis, constriction of the pulmonary arterioles, and pulmonary hypertension. A shortened life expectancy is characteristic of P-W syndrome; the oldest known afflicted individual with this syndrome died at the age of 43 (Bier, 1970).

Since the obesity is etiologically related to the most dangerous complications of the syndrome (diabetes mellitus and respiratory acidosis), weight control is necessary to improve life quality and expectancy. However, dietary therapy has had only limited success in treating P-W obesity (Coplin, Hine, & Gormican, 1976; Dunn, 1968; Evans, 1964; Hall & Smith, 1972; Jenab, Lade, Chiga, & Diehl, 1959; Laurance, 1967; Zellweger & Schneider, 1968), faring little better than dietary control of the obese older patient of normal intelligence (Drenick & Johnson, 1978; Merritt, 1978; Stunkard & McLaren-Hume, 1959). Painstaking efforts by interested and motivated parents, dietitians, and physicians can control weight in some P-W children by carefully supervised dietary management (Bistrian, Blackburn, & Stanbury, 1977; Holm & Pipes, 1976; Pipes & Holm, 1973), including calorie restriction, behavior modification, and protein-sparing diets.

In view of the devastating psychological and physiological effects of morbid obesity and the high relapse rate with dietary management, surgical procedures have been developed for its control. The most popular operation bypasses 90% of the small intestine (Payne, DeWind, Schwab, & Kern, 1973; Schwartz, Varco, & Buchwald, 1973; Scott, Sandstead, Brill, Burko, & Younger, 1971), and has been used in a handful of adolescents (Randolph, Weintraub, & Rigg, 1974; White, Cheek, & Haller, 1974) and in one child with P-W syndrome (Randolph et al., 1974). Small intestinal bypass controls morbid obesity by producing a short bowel syndrome, with reduced absorption of fats and carbohydrates. Weight loss is effected because of rapid transit of ingested material through the shortened small intestine, reflected by diarrhea. Food intake is not limited, except for those patients who become anorexic from severe diarrhea. Postoperative weight loss is excellent in most patients treated by small intestinal bypass, but it may be accompanied by dehydration, electrolyte imbalance, protein malnutrition, cirrhosis, renal and gallbladder stones, polyarthritis, pancreatitis, and other metabolic and psychiatric side effects (Alden, 1977; Sorrell, Knight, & Burcher, 1975; Winkelman, 1974). These adverse metabolic effects of jejunoileal bypass have been confirmed and studied in the rat (Grosfeld, Cooney, Csicsko, and Madura, 1976; Grosfeld, Harris, Csicsko, Cooney, & Madura, 1977; Madura, Csicsko, Cooney, & Grosfeld, 1975). Especially disturbing are the adverse effects of jejunoileal bypass on growth and development in the rat (Grosfeld et al., 1976).

In contrast, Mason and others bypass all but a measured 50-ml volume of the stomach to effect weight loss (Alden, 1977; Mason & Ito, 1969; Printen & Mason, 1973). Gastric bypass reduces weight by curbing intake; the small residual gastric pouch distends to produce a feeling of satiety with only small amounts of food. The small stoma size delays passage of food out of the proximal gastric pouch, and, ideally, prolongs satiety for several hours. Postoperative weight loss often is not as spectacular as after jejunoileal bypass, but gastric bypass is free of the metabolic complications and side effects provoked by diarrhea in the intestinal bypass (Alden, 1977; Buckwalter, 1977; Griffen, Young, & Stevenson, 1977). During the past 11 years, 800 morbidly obese patients have been subjected to gastric bypass and gastroplasty at the University of Iowa, with acceptable morbidity and mortality and with satisfactory weight reduction in the majority (Mason, 1979; Mason & Printen, 1978; Mason, Printen, Blommers, & Scott, 1978).

In this chapter, the authors' experience with gastric bypass operations in morbidly obese P-W syndrome children (Soper, Mason, Printen, & Zellweger, 1975) is updated, summarizing the data from 11 of these patients.

MATERIALS AND METHODS

Eleven children (seven boys and four girls) with P-W syndrome who ranged in age from 8 to 19 years (mean age of 13 years) were subjected to bypass of 90% of their stomach in an attempt to control morbid obesity. These children had resisted all attempts at weight control initiated by their referring physicians. Because of the natural history of continuing morbid obesity in P-W syndrome, the twice-ideal weight requirement for operation developed by Printen and Mason (1973) was waived.

Ten of the 11 patients underwent gastric bypass, whereas one was treated by gastroplasty. Both of these operations, developed by Mason, have been previously reported in detail (Mason & Ito, 1969; Printen & Mason, 1973) and are diagrammatically represented in Figure 9.1.

Gastric bypass excludes 90% of the distal stomach, gastrointestinal continuity being reestablished by gastrojejunostomy either to a short retrocolic jejunal loop or, as is being done more recently, to a longer jejunal loop brought in front of the colon. The critical features of this procedure are: 1) a small proximal gastric pouch (50 ml) which eliminates the stom-

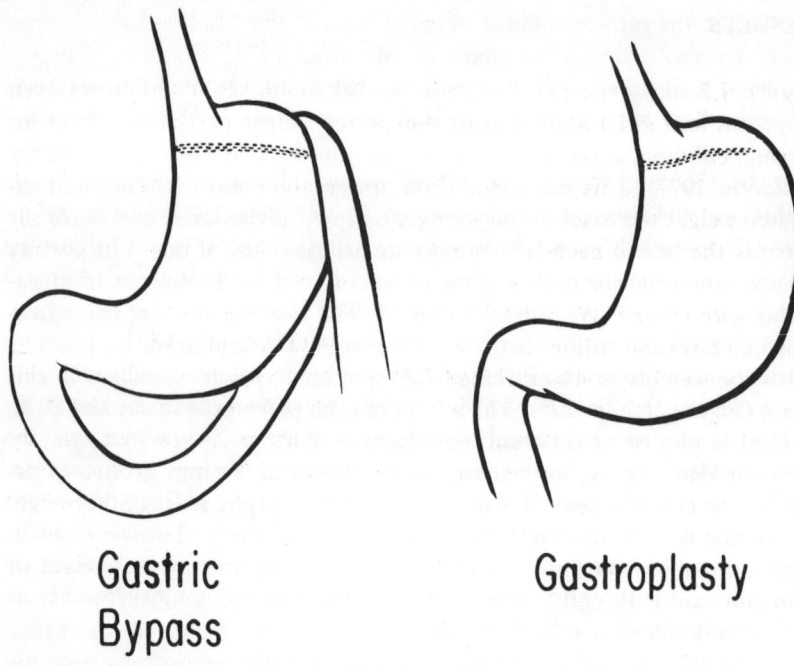

Figure 9.1. Diagrams of gastric bypass and gastroplasty operations.

ach's reservoir function, and 2) a narrow (1.2 cm) gastroenterostomy stoma to delay gastric emptying and prolong satiety. Gastroplasty consists of taking a large tuck in the stomach, leaving a 9-mm non-distensible channel along the greater curvature for continuity between the upper and lower gastric pouches. As originally described by Printen and Mason (1973), gastroplasty was less effective in producing weight loss than gastric bypass, but recently (Gomez, 1980; Pace, Martin, Tetrick, Fabri, & Carey, 1979) slightly different surgical modifications have been introduced which make gastroplasty an acceptable alternative to gastric bypass.

Operating time has decreased from 310 minutes prior to 1969 to 220 minutes in 1975 (Soper et al.) and has been further reduced to about 100 minutes with special retractors, instruments, and stapling devices to obviate laborious hand suturing. Transfusions are rarely required. Concurrent procedures (five liver biopsies, two appendectomies, one tubal ligation, and one splenectomy) were performed as indicated by operative findings. Mean postoperative hospital stay was 15 days in these 11 patients, although one patient with a wound infection remained in the hospital considerably longer.

RESULTS

Figure 9.2 shows the postoperative weights for the P-W children (seven boys and four girls) plotted against expected weight percentile curves for normal children, adolescents, and young adults (*NCHS growth curves for children*, 1977). This method of data presentation takes into account expected weight increases of the younger patients as they grow and faithfully records the fate of each individual patient. However, it does not portray trends very well, nor does it allow us to compare easily this group of patients with other P-W patients. Nevertheless, one can see that the operation can favorably influence the weight curve of P-W children.

The weights of 44 untreated P-W patients appear elsewhere in this book (Figure 21.2, p. 275). The weight of each patient (24 males and 20 females) is plotted at different ages from 3 years to 23 years of age, the straight lines representing the regression lines of the two groups of patients; the curved lines in the lower parts of the graphs are the 50th weight percentile for normal males and females, respectively. This provides us with untreated P-W children who will serve as controls against which we can compare P-W children treated by gastric bypass.

Figure 9.3 plots the weights for age of the seven P-W males and four P-W females treated by gastric bypass against this regression curve for untreated P-W controls as well as against a backdrop of the 50th percentile for normal children. Again, although individual patients do indeed vary in their results, it is clear from these data that gastric bypass provides certain patients with a very favorable result as compared with the untreated controls. Treatment failures are also evident.

Figure 9.4 shows the postoperative average absolute weight changes in the 11 P-W children. All were followed up for 1 year after surgery, their average weight dropping from 85 kg to 73 kg, an absolute average weight loss of 12 kg. Ten of the patients have been followed up for 3 years and have, on an average, almost regained their preoperative weights. The seven patients followed up for 5 years are just back to their preoperative weight levels. Although not dramatic or ideal, these results again compare favorably with the regression line in the untreated P-W children. Children who were still growing at the time of operation continued to grow in height at a normal rate for those with this syndrome.

Figure 9.5 depicts the post-gastric bypass results in the 11 P-W children when the weights are transformed into the percentage of what the ideal weight should be for the age of the patient. Ideal weight for the growing child was defined as the 50th percentile of expected weight for age shown on growth charts, and for the older adolescents it was defined by Metropolitan Life Insurance Co. actuarial tables. For each patient at each postoperative age the following formula was used:

$$\% \text{ ideal body weight} = \frac{\text{actual body weight}}{\text{ideal body weight}} \times 100.$$

This index is especially useful for comparing postoperative weights of young children who are still growing. At the end of the first postoperative year, the weight of the 11 surgically treated P-W children decreased from an average 230% of ideal weight down to 177% of ideal body weight. The 10 children who were followed up for 3 years after operation increased up to approximately 180% of ideal body weight and the seven who had been followed up for 5 years are down to nearly 170% of their ideal weight. Again, these are not ideal results, but the downward trend in percentage of ideal weight is significant and sustained. Serial electrolytes and liver

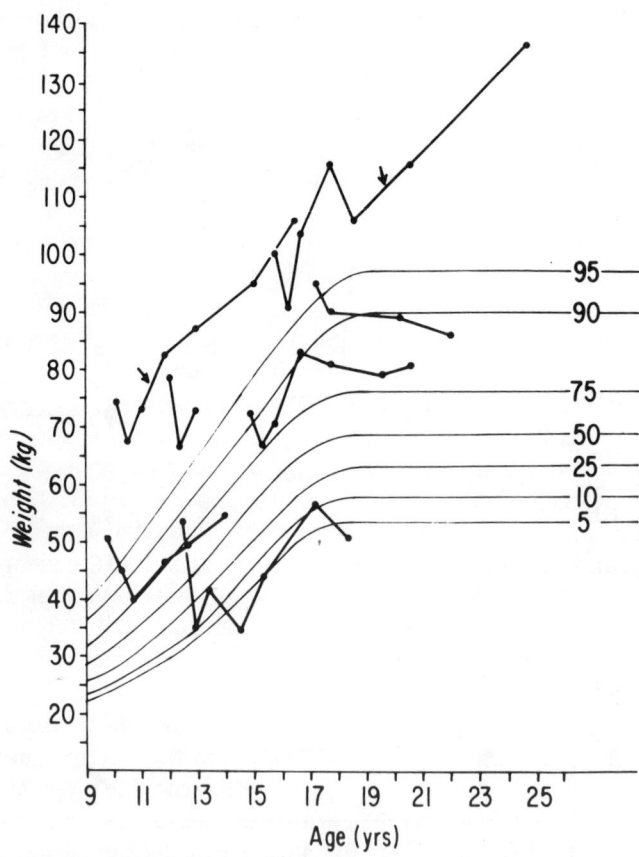

Figure 9.2. Post-gastric bypass weight curves of Prader-Willi children plotted on NCHS percentile growth charts for age. A, 7 boys; B, 4 girls. Each arrow (←) indicates an operative revision; each cross (†) signifies one death.

function studies performed during the follow up have not shown any significant deviation from normal.

The rates of morbidity and mortality were acceptable. One child developed a wound infection soon after the operation, which prolonged his postoperative hospital stay. There was one late death that occurred 50 months after surgery, the cause of death being listed as acute congestive heart failure (case no. 11, Figure 3B). This patient declined the surgical revision of her operation which had been strongly recommended, and her unchecked weight gain led to her death. This operative failure was due to repeated ingestion of food throughout the waking hours; with time, the proximal pouch and stoma gradually became distended, allowing her to eat larger quantities of food at progressively shorter intervals. The proposed revision would have been directed toward reestablishing a small gastric pouch and small stomal opening to again effectively inhibit intake.

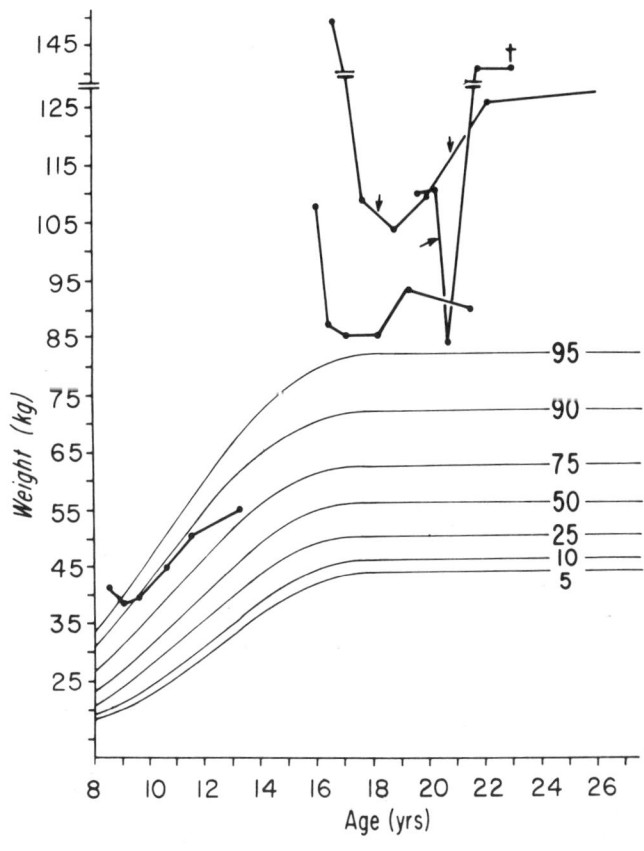

Figure 9.2. B

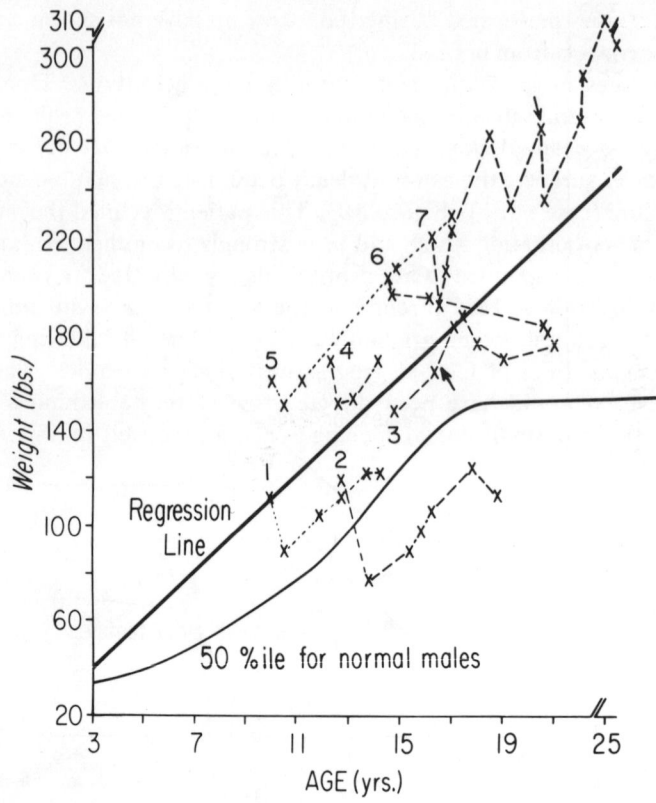

Figure 9.3. Weights of 11 Prader-Willi children treated by gastric bypass superimposed on the regression lines of untreated controls (see Figure 21.2) as well as the 50th percentile weights for age of normal children. A, 7 males; B, 4 females.

Although representing a failure of surgical treatment, this death is not directly related to the operation.

DISCUSSION

Morbid obesity has been implicated in sudden death of unknown cause, hypertension, diabetes, and coronary artery disease (Kannel, Troy, & McNamara, 1967; Keys, Aravanis, Blackburn, Van Buchem, Buzina, Djordjevic, Fidanza, Karvonen, Menotti, Puddu, & Taylor, 1972). The short life expectancy of the P-W child is likely due to morbid obesity leading to diabetes and pulmonary complications, and is perhaps the most compelling argument for surgical control of obesity.

Arguments against surgical treatment of morbid obesity in the young include the fact that it may impair normal growth and development

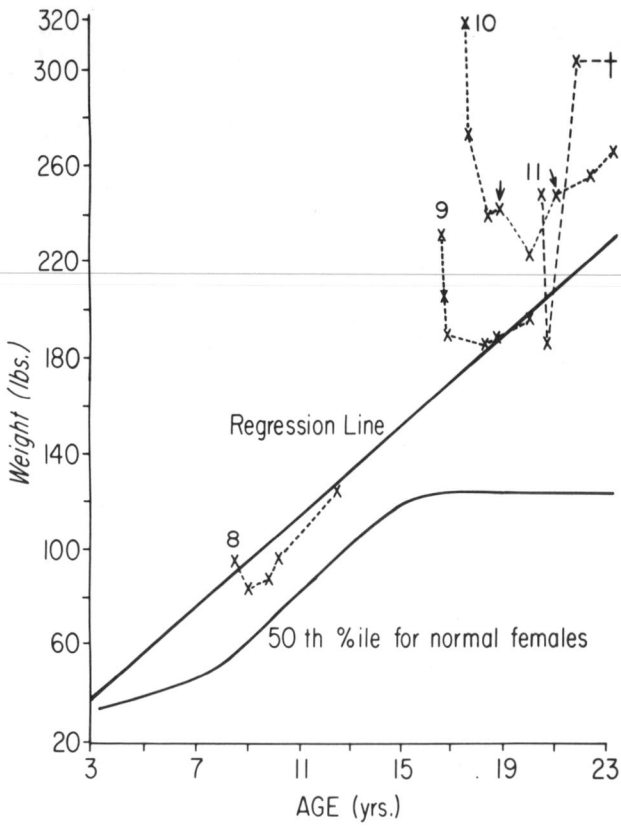

Figure 9.3. B

and that with the normal pubertal changes in body function, attitude, and interest, the operation may not be necessary. However, non-surgical control of morbid obesity has met with only limited success (Drenick & Johnson, 1978; Merritt, 1978; Stunkard & McLaren-Hume, 1979). It is especially difficult when dealing with a group of mentally subnormal children with P-W syndrome (see the regression lines for untreated P-W children in Figure 21.2). Certainly, if an operation is safe enough and morbid obesity severe enough, a major operative procedure to control the obesity is justified.

Surgeons have been actively involved in treating morbid obesity for only the past 25 years. In 1954 Kremen, Linner, and Nelson reported that extensive small bowel bypass with preservation of the ileocecal valve was effective in producing weight loss in a single patient. Later, various modifications of intestinal bypass were perfected with differing degrees of

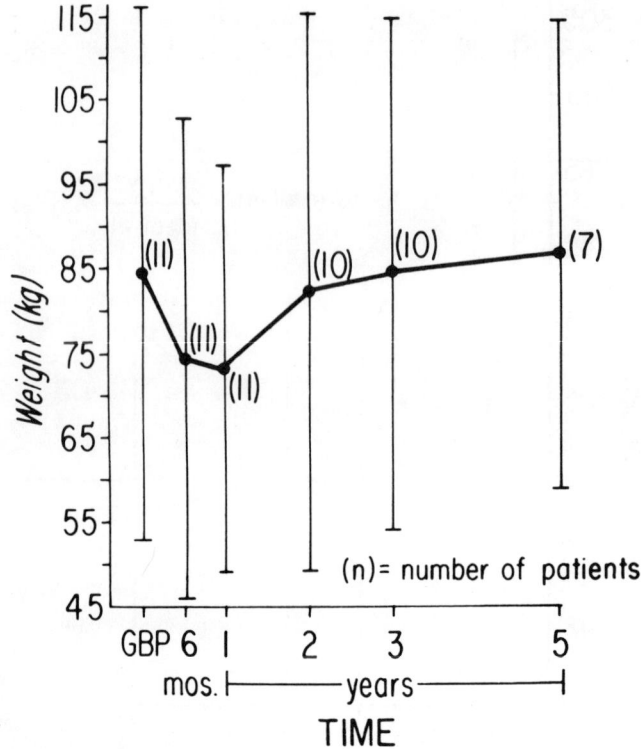

Figure 9.4. Average absolute post-gastric bypass (GBP) body weight changes in 11 Prader-Willi children.

success. Payne and his colleagues (1973) and Scott and his colleagues (1971) developed two of the more popular small bowel bypass operations for morbid obesity. Although these operations produce significant and sometimes dramatic weight loss, they are capable of causing dire metabolic complications which include acute and chronic liver failure, potassium and calcium abnormalities, gallstones, renal stones, peripheral neuropathies, pancreatitis, migratory arthritis, and anemia (Alden, 1977; Sorrell et al., 1975; Winkelman, 1974). These metabolic complications have led some surgeons to curtail the use of intestinal bypass for morbid obesity (Buckwalter, 1977; Griffen et al., 1977).

Gastric bypass was developed at the University of Iowa more than a decade ago (Mason & Ito, 1969) in an attempt to induce respectable weight loss without the metabolic complications and side effects of intestinal bypass. Some of the patients in the present study have required revisions of their gastric bypass to improve weight loss. Table 9.1 shows the

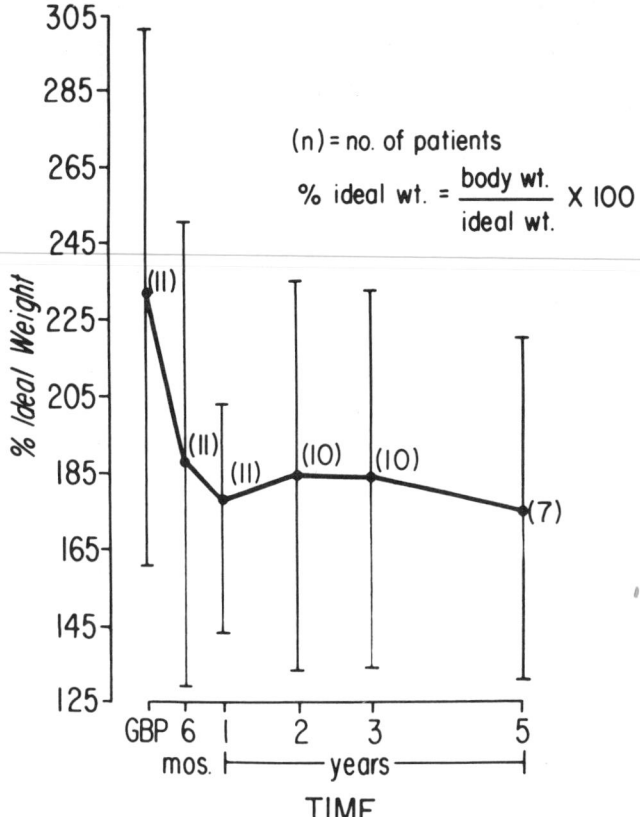

Figure 9.5. Percentage of ideal body weight following gastric bypass (GBP) in 11 Prader-Willi children.

subsequent operations that the 11 P-W children underwent. Five had revision of their gastric bypass, the revisions aimed at reducing the size of the gastric pouch and narrowing the size of the stoma through which it empties. One gastroplasty operation was converted to a gastric bypass operation. The other operations were directed to non-related surgical problems.

The authors have been concerned about long term physiological changes caused by gastric bypass in growing children. However, lengthy follow-up documents normal linear growth with none of the hepatic or other metabolic complications that might threaten growth and development (Mason, 1979; Mason et al., 1978; Mason & Printen, 1978) and that are reported experimentally for intestinal bypass (Grosfeld et al., 1976; Grosfeld et al., 1977; Madura et al., 1975). Because gastric bypass ex-

Table 9.1. Gastric bypass in 11 Prader-Willi children: subsequent operations

Revision	5
Conversion	1
Cholecystectomy	2
Appendectomy	2
Inguinal hernia repair	2
Resect Meckel's diverticulum	1

cludes the gastric antrum from food, there has been some concern about the operation's potential for encouraging stomal or acid-peptic ulceration. These concerns have been laid to rest, because in the authors' total experience with gastric bypass the incidence of marginal or peptic ulcer is only 2% (Mason, 1979). The acid pH of the antrum following gastric bypass suppresses excess gastrin and acid secretion, which accounts for this absence of ulceration.

Anemia has seldom been a problem after gastric bypass, probably as a result of a certain amount of backwash of food into the duodenum to provide adequate stimulus for producing intrinsic factor. Because ingested food passes through the duodenum with gastroplasty, one need not worry about anemia after this operation. Mild dumping is occasionally seen early after gastric bypass; this usually does not persist, probably because of the delay in gastric emptying occasioned by the small gastroenterostomy stoma. One of the P-W children in this study had periodic diarrhea due to dumping; this is a socially troublesome condition that could require surgical correction.

Postprandial vomiting can be a problem, especially early in the convalescence of mentally abnormal patients such as P-W children. Since gastric bypass provides an extremely small reservoir with a tiny outlet, the patient (and parents) must be taught to alter their feeding habits so that there is better mastication of smaller amounts of food. Dietary counseling is an important part of postoperative care, and is instituted while in the hospital. A liquid diet is recommended for the initial 6 weeks following gastroplasty, and a soft diet is advised for 6 weeks following gastric bypass. By this time most patients tolerate a general diet, provided they chew it well and avoid overeating. They usually learn to stop eating before distress occurs, a Pavlovian type of education.

Wound infections have occurred in about 10% of the patients and were the most consistent postoperative hazard. Infections are often followed by incisional hernias as late complications, which in turn require surgical repair.

Weight loss after gastric bypass amounts to a gradual loss of approximately 1 kg/month in P-W children. Weight loss tends to plateau after a certain period of time, with no reliable predictors to forecast the degree of weight loss in any individual patient. In general, the heavier the patient is preoperatively, the more weight will be lost postoperatively. Males usually fare better than females. This gradual weight loss is well tolerated, as evidenced by the lack of hepatic and other metabolic complications, and by continued normal linear growth. This safety factor is especially important in adolescents with their potential for growth and long life expectancy, and is vital in a mentally subnormal P-W child. Since the P-W child normally prefers to eat very large quantities of food, the diarrhea after intestinal bypass would be a very serious complication. This problem is obviated by gastric bypass or gastroplasty, which simply limit intake to reduce weight. Normal weight is not usually attained, but the increase in weight expected in untreated P-W children is not usually seen after successful gastric bypass.

In the authors' judgment, gastric bypass and gastroplasty have a place in managing P-W children with voracious appetites. Ongoing technical improvements are being made in both these operations to improve results. Controlling the morbid obesity of P-W children simplifies their care, reduces the incidence of diabetes mellitus and pulmonary complications, and is likely to improve the quality and length of their lives.

ACKNOWLEDGMENTS

The authors are immensely grateful to David H. Scott and Thomas J. Blommers for expediting data collection and collation, and to Patricia Piper for manuscript preparation.

REFERENCES

Alden, J.F. Gastric and jejunoileal bypass: A comparison in the treatment of morbid obesity. *Archives of Surgery,* 1977, *112,* 799-806.
Bier, D.M. The Prader-Willi syndrome. *California Medicine,* 1970, *112,* 65-73.
Bistrian, B.R., Blackburn, G.L., & Stanbury, J.B. Metabolic aspects of a protein-sparing modified fast in the dietary management of Prader-Willi obesity. *New England Journal of Medicine,* 1977, *296,* 774-779.
Buckwalter, J.A. A prospective comparison of the jejunoileal and gastric bypass operations for morbid obesity. *World Journal of Surgery,* 1977, *1,* 757-766.
Coplin, S.S., Hine, J., & Gormican, A. Outpatient dietary management in the Prader-Willi syndrome. *Journal of the American Dietetic Association,* 1976, *68,* 330-334.
Drenick, E.J., & Johnson, D. Weight reduction by fasting and semi-starvation in morbid obesity: Long term follow-up. *International Journal of Obesity,* 1978, *2,* 123-132.

Dunn, H.G. The Prader-Labhart-Willi syndrome: Review of the literature and report of nine cases. *Acta Paediatrica Scandinavica,* 1968, Suppl. 186, 1-38.

Evans, P.R. Hypogenital dystrophy with diabetic tendency. *Guy's Hospital Reports,* 1964, *113,* 207-222.

Gomez, C.A. Gastroplasty in the surgical treatment of morbid obesity. *American Journal of Clinical Nutrition,* 1980, **33(2),** 406(suppl.).

Griffen, W.O., Young, V.L., & Stevenson, C.C. A prospective comparison of gastric and jejunoileal bypass procedures for morbid obesity. *Annals of Surgery,* 1977, *186,* 500-509.

Grosfeld, J.L., Cooney, D.R., Csicsko, J.F., & Madura, J.A. Adverse effects of jejunoileal bypass on growth and development. *Surgery,* 1976, *80,* 201-207.

Grosfeld, J.L., Harris, R.A., Csicsko, J.F., Cooney, D.R., & Madura, J.A. Increased hepatic synthesis of cholesterol following jejunoileal bypass. *Surgery,* 1977, *81,* 701-707.

Hall, B.D., & Smith, D.W. Prader-Willi syndrome: A resumé of 32 cases including an instance of affected first cousins, one of whom is of normal stature and intelligence. *The Journal of Pediatrics,* 1972, *81,* 286-293.

Hoefnagel, D., Costello, P.J., & Hatoum, K. Prader-Willi syndrome. *Journal of Mental Deficiency Research,* 1967, *11,* 1-11.

Holm, V.A., & Pipes, P.L. Food and children with Prader-Willi syndrome. *American Journal of Diseases of Children,* 1976, *130,* 1063-1067.

Jenab, M., Lade, R.I., Chiga, M., & Diehl, A.M. Cardiorespiratory syndrome of obesity in a child. *Pediatrics,* 1959, *24,* 23-30.

Kannel, W.B., Troy, B.L., & McNamara, P.M. Relation of body weight to development of coronary heart disease: The Framingham study. *Circulation,* 1967, *35,* 734-744.

Keys, A., Aravanis, C., Blackburn, H., Van Buchem, F.S.P., Buzina, R., Djordjevic, B.S., Fidanza, F., Karvonen, M.J., Menotti, A., Puddu, V., & Taylor, H.L. Coronary heart disease: Overweight and obesity as risk factors. *Annals of Internal Medicine,* 1972, *77,* 15-27.

Kremen, A.J., Linner, J.H., & Nelson, C.H. An experimental evaluation of the nutritional importance of the proximal and distal small intestine. *Annals of Surgery,* 1954, *140,* 439-448.

Laurance, B.M. Hypotonia, mental retardation, obesity, and cryptorchidism associated with dwarfism in children. *Archives of Disease in Childhood,* 1967, *42,* 126-139.

Madura, J.A., Csicsko, J.F., Cooney, D.R., & Grosfeld, J.L. The "fat-rat": A new experimental jejunoileal bypass model. *Journal of Pediatric Surgery,* 1975, *10,* 349-352.

Mason, E.E. Gastric bypass. In L.M. Nyhus (Ed.), *Surgical Annual.* New York: Appleton-Century-Crofts, 1979.

Mason, E.E., & Ito, C. Gastric bypass. *Annals of Surgery,* 1969, *170,* 329-339.

Mason, E.E., & Printen, K.J. Gastric bypass for obesity. In H. Buchwald & R.L. Varco (Eds.), *Metabolic Surgery.* New York: Grune & Stratton, 1978.

Mason, E.E., Printen, K.J., Blommers, T.J., & Scott, D.H. Gastric bypass for obesity after ten years experience. *International Journal of Obesity,* 1978, *2,* 197-206.

Merritt, R.J. Treatment of pediatric and adolescent obesity. *International Journal of Obesity,* 1978, *2,* 207-214.

NCHS growth curves for children: Birth-18 years, United States (DHEW Publication No. (PHS) 78-1650). Hyattsville, Md.: National Center for Health Statistics, 1977.

Pace, W.G., Martin, E.W., Jr., Tetrick, T., Fabri, P.J., & Carey, L.C. Gastric partitioning for morbid obesity. *Annals of Surgery,* 1979, **190**(3) 392-400.
Payne, J.H., DeWind, L., Schwab, C.E., & Kern, W.H. Surgical treatment of morbid obesity. *Archives of Surgery,* 1973, *106,* 432-437.
Pipes, P.L., & Holm, V.A. Weight control of children with Prader-Willi syndrome. *Journal of the American Dietetic Association,* 1973, *62,* 520-524.
Printen, K.J., & Mason, E.E. Gastric surgery for relief of morbid obesity. *Archives of Surgery,* 1973, *106,* 428-431.
Randolph, J.G., Weintraub, W.H., & Rigg, A. Jejunoileal bypass for morbid obesity in adolescents. *Journal of Pediatric Surgery,* 1974, *9,* 341-345.
Schwartz, M., Varco, R., & Buchwald, H. Preoperative preparation, operative technique, and postoperative care of patients undergoing jejunoileal bypass for massive exogenous obesity. *Journal of Surgical Research,* 1973, *14,* 147-150.
Scott, H.W., Jr., Sandstead, H.H., Brill, A.B., Burko, H., & Younger, R.K. Experience with a new technique of intestinal bypass in the treatment of morbid obesity. *Annals of Surgery,* 1971, *174,* 560-572.
Soper, R.T., Mason, E.E., Printen, K.J., & Zellweger, H. Gastric bypass for morbid obesity in children and adolescents. *Journal of Pediatric Surgery,* 1975, *10,* 51-58.
Sorrell, V.F., Knight, D.H., & Burcher, S.K. Pancreatitis following intestinal bypass operations for obesity. *Australian and New Zealand Journal of Surgery,* 1975, *45,* 163-167.
Stunkard, A., & McLaren-Hume, M. The results of treatment of obesity: A review of the literature and report of a series. *Archives of Internal Medicine,* 1959, *103,* 79-85.
White, J.J., Cheek, D., & Haller, J.A., Jr. Small bowel bypass is applicable for adolescents with morbid obesity. *American Surgeon,* 1974, *40,* 704-708.
Winkelman, E.I. Disabling sequellae frequent in bypass surgery for obesity. *Hospital Practice,* 1974, *9,* 41-42.
Zellweger, H., & Schneider, H.J. Syndrome of hypotonia-hypomentia-hypogonadism-obesity (HHHO) or Prader-Willi syndrome. *American Journal of Diseases of Children,* 1968, *115,* 588-598.

chapter 10

ELEVATED ADIPOSE TISSUE LIPOPROTEIN LIPASE IN THE PATHOGENESIS OF OBESITY IN PRADER-WILLI SYNDROME

Robert S. Schwartz, John D. Brunzell, and Edwin L. Bierman

> Drs. Schwartz, Brunzell, and Bierman found that Prader-Willi syndrome patients had a higher level of adipose tissue lipoprotein lipase than a control group. They suggest that this might make triglyceride storage more efficient, thus leading to the obesity typical of this syndrome.—*Eds.*

Adipose tissue lipoprotein lipase (AT-LPL) is the key rate-limiting enzyme responsible for the uptake and storage of triglyceride by the adipocyte (Robinson, 1970). Lipoprotein lipase is produced in the cytoplasm of the adipocyte (Robinson & Wing, 1970), but the functionally active enzyme resides at the capillary endothelium (Blanchette-Mackie & Scow, 1971). At this site, it works by hydrolyzing triglycerides that circulate in the plasma as major components of very low density lipoproteins and chylomicrons (Cunningham & Robinson, 1969). The fatty acids released are taken up into the cytoplasm of the adipocyte where they are reesterified to triglyceride which in turn is stored in the lipid droplet.

Because of its unique position with regard to fat storage, the authors became interested in the possible role AT-LPL might play in human obesity. It was shown previously that a significant positive correlation between

---

This chapter is reprinted from *Transactions of the Association of American Physicians*, Vol. 92, 1979, pp. 89-95, and appears by permission of the Association of American Physicians.

This project was supported by NIH Grants AM 02456 and AM 80-0055. This work was performed at the University Clinical Research Center (RR-37), University of Washington. Computational assistance was provided by CLINFO Computer Systems (RR-37), University of Washington.

percentage of ideal body weight (% IBW) and AT-LPL activity per cell (Pykälistö, Smith, & Brunzell, 1975) exists. It also was shown that the AT-LPL activity in a group of previously obese subjects who were weight-stable at a reduced weight was significantly higher than expected for their % IBW (Schwartz & Brunzell, 1978). This appears to be the first description of a metabolic abnormality associated with obesity that does not normalize with weight loss. It was speculated that this elevation in AT-LPL activity in previously obese subjects might account for the difficulty obese patients have in maintaining their weight loss. Recent studies by Gruen, Hietanen, and Greenwood (1978) have shown that elevated AT-LPL activity is the earliest detectable abnormality in the genetically obese Zucker rat. Elevations in AT-LPL activity were documented at 7 to 14 days of age and preceded any rise in the basal insulin level or significant fat cell hypertrophy. They speculated that the very high AT-LPL activity observed in the pre-obese Zucker rat might predispose to fat cell hypertrophy and subsequent obesity. To test whether a similar causal role for AT-LPL might exist in a human form of congenital obesity, the authors measured AT-LPL activity in Prader-Willi (P-W) syndrome.

METHODS

The present study compares the AT-LPL activity in seven patients with P-W syndrome to that in 19 controls. Both groups were composed of weight-stable males with normal fasting glucose levels. Lipoprotein lipase activity in adipose tissue aspirated from the buttock was measured by the heparin-releasable method (Pykälistö et al., 1975) and expressed as $mU/10^6$ fat cells. Fat cell size was determined from formalin-fixed frozen sections and expressed as μg of triglyceride/cell. Immunoreactive insulin, expressed as $\mu U/ml$ of plasma, was measured by a double antibody technique.

RESULTS

There was no significant difference in mean % IBW between the two groups, and there was considerable overlap of their ranges of % IBW (Table 10.1). Overlap of the ranges was also seen for age and fat cell size, but patients with P-W syndrome, on the average, were younger and had larger fat cells than controls. There was no correlation between age and AT-LPL activity in this study or in the literature. Thus, it appears unlikely that the age differences between the groups could account for the large differences seen in AT-LPL activity. Fat cell size has been positively correlated to AT-LPL activity. To correct for differences in fat cell size, statistical evaluation by the analysis of covariance was performed. This

Table 10.1. Group characteristics

	Prader-Willi	Controls	p
Subjects	7	19	
	Males	Males	
	Weight-stable	Weight-stable	
% IBW			
Range	104-288	85-232	
Mean	183	136	NS[a]
±SD	±72	±37	
Fat cell size (µg TB[b]/cell)			
Range	0.4-1.5	0.2-0.8	
Mean	0.9	0.5	0.027
±SD	±0.3	±0.1	
Age			
Range	14-26	13-48	
Mean	20	29	0.002
±SD	±5	±9	

[a] NS = not significant.
[b] TG = triglyceride.

showed ($p < 0.025$) that differences with respect to fat cell size could not fully account for the significant differences in AT-LPL activity between the two groups.

A significant positive correlation between % IBW and AT-LPL activity expressed per 10^6 cells was found for the 19 control subjects (Figure 10.1). This relationship has been described previously by the authors and by others (Schwartz & Brunzell, 1978). Thus, with increasing degrees of obesity there is an elevation in the AT-LPL activity per cell. Comparable data derived from all patients with P-W syndrome are well above the regression line for normals. Because the differences are so large, AT-LPL activity is expressed on a log scale, so that data both from P-W patients and the controls could fit on the same graph.

Because patients with P-W syndrome are hypotonic and could have a reduced lean body mass, it may be incorrect to compare their % IBW with that of a control group. For this reason fat cell volume can be substituted for % IBW. There is a significant positive correlation between fat cell volume and AT-LPL activity in control subjects and, again, data from patients with P-W syndrome are above the regression line for controls (Figure 10.2). Thus, even accounting for a possible abnormality in body

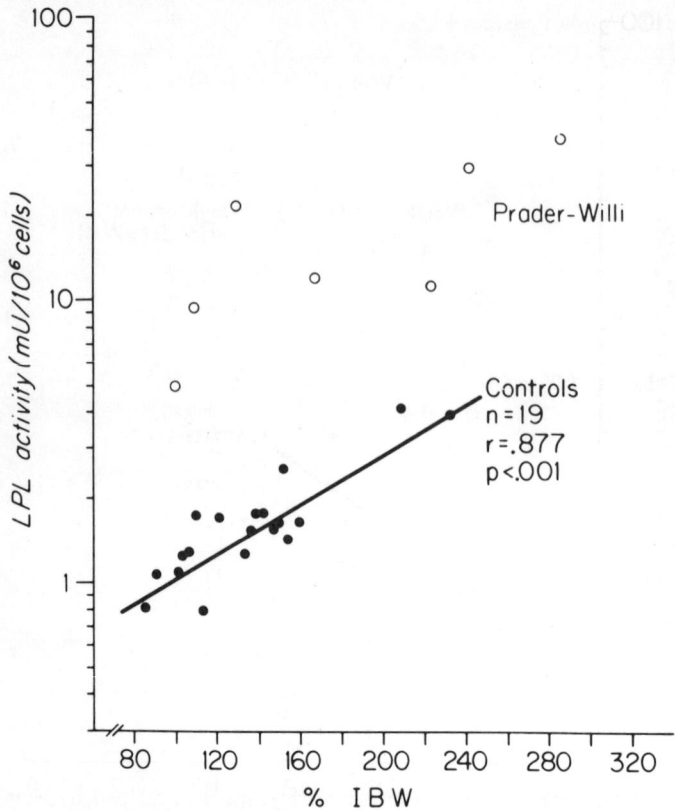

Figure 10.1. Adipose tissue lipoprotein lipase (LPL) activity as a function of percentage of ideal body weight (% IBW).

composition in patients with P-W syndrome, an elevation in the AT-LPL activity per cell compared to a control population is still found.

The mean AT-LPL activity expressed as mU/10^6 cells is 17.4 for patients with P-W syndrome compared to 1.7 for the controls (Table 10.2). This difference is highly significant. It is of interest that the mean basal immunoreactive insulin level in P-W patients is only 20 μU/ml. This is far below the 56 μU/ml that would be expected for their % IBW (Bagdade, Bierman, & Porte, 1967). This relatively low basal insulin level in P-W patients is corroborated by results in several studies in the literature. One example is the study by Parra, Cervantes, and Schultz (1973) in which a mean basal insulin level of 23 μU/ml in patients with P-W syndrome was found compared to 41 μU/ml in weight-matched controls.

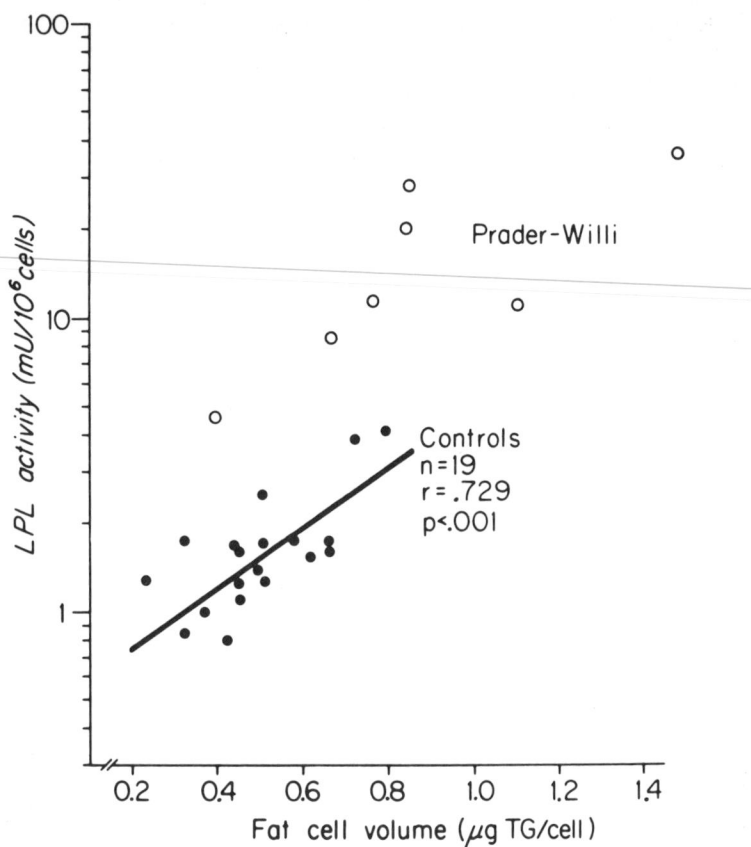

Figure 10.2. Adipose tissue lipoprotein lipase (LPL) activity as a function of fat cell volume.

COMMENT

Results in recent studies (Pykälistö et al., 1975; Schwartz & Brunzell, 1978) have implicated elevated AT-LPL activity as a potentially important predisposing factor for the development of obesity. In the present study the possible role that elevated AT-LPL activity might play in the congenital obesity seen in P-W syndrome was evaluated. Results show that patients with P-W syndrome have a tenfold higher AT-LPL activity when compared to a control group. P-W patients had higher AT-LPL activity per cell for any given fat cell size or % IBW.

Although insulin clearly has been shown to be important in the regulation of AT-LPL activity after feeding (Pykälistö et al., 1975), in the

Table 10.2. Comparison of adipose tissue lipoprotein lipase activity and basal insulin levels in controls and P-W patients

	Prader-Willi	Controls	p
Lipoprotein lipase ($mU/10^6$ cells)	17.4	1.7	< 0.001
Insulin (basal) ($\mu U/ml$)			
This study	20		
Expected for % IBW		56	
Parra et al. (1973)	23	41	< 0.005

present study the extremely high AT-LPL activity in P-W syndrome was not associated with a concomitant elevation in basal insulin level. In contrast, the authors and others have found that the basal insulin levels in non-diabetic P-W patients are lower than expected for their degree of obesity.

Many of the abnormalities seen in P-W syndrome are best explained by a hypothalamic abnormality. Therefore, it is speculated that the elevation seen in AT-LPL activity may also be caused by a primary hypothalamic abnormality. This abnormality might, by an as yet unknown neurohormonal regulation, cause an elevation in the AT-LPL activity at the capillary endothelium site. Since AT-LPL activity is positively correlated to triglyceride uptake and storage (Taskinen & Nikkilä, 1977), elevation of AT-LPL activity might increase the efficiency of triglyceride storage, leading to adipocyte hypertrophy and subsequent obesity. The regulation of this process is most likely independent of the basal insulin level. It is possible that similar but less extensive abnormalities in the regulation of AT-LPL could play a causal role in other more common types of human obesity.

ACKNOWLEDGMENTS

The authors thank Martha Kimura and Steve Hashimoto for their expert technical assistance and Sharon Kemp for skilled secretarial assistance.

REFERENCES

Bagdade, J.D., Bierman, E.L., & Porte, D., Jr. Significance of basal insulin levels in the evaluation of the insulin response to glucose in diabetic and nondiabetic subjects. *Journal of Clinical Investigation*, 1967, *46*, 1549–1557.

Blanchette-Mackie, E.J., & Scow, R.O. Site lipoprotein lipase activity in adipose tissue perfused with chylomicrons: Electron microscope study. *Journal of Cell Biology*, 1971, *51*, 1-25.

Cunningham, V.J., & Robinson, D.S. Clearing factor lipase in adipose tissue. *Biochemical Journal*, 1969, *112*, 203-209.

Gruen, R., Hietanen, E., & Greenwood, M.R.C. Increased adipose tissue lipoprotein lipase activity during the development of the genetically obese rat (fa/fa). *Metabolism*, 1978, *27*, Suppl. 2, 1955-1956.

Parra, A., Cervantes, C., & Schultz, R. Immunoreactive insulin and growth hormone responses in patients with Prader-Willi syndrome. *The Journal of Pediatrics*, 1973, *83*, 587-593.

Pykälistö, O.J., Smith, P.H., & Brunzell, J.D. Determinants of human adipose tissue lipoprotein lipase. *Journal of Clinical Investigation*, 1975, *56*, 1108-1117.

Robinson, D.S. The function of the plasma triglyceride in fatty acid transport. In M. Florkin & E.M. Stotz (Eds.), *Comprehensive biochemistry* (Vol. 18). Amsterdam: Elsevier, 1970.

Robinson, D.A., & Wing, D.R. Regulation of adipose tissue clearing factor lipase activity. In B. Jeanrenaud & D. Hepp (Eds.), *Adipose tissue regulation and metabolic functions*. Stuttgart: Georg Thieme Verlag KG, 1970.

Schwartz, R.S., & Brunzell, J.D. Increased adipose tissue lipoprotein activity in moderately obese men after weight reduction. *Lancet*, 1978, 1, 1230-1231.

Taskinen, M.R., & Nikkilä, E.A. Lipoprotein lipase activity in adipose tissue and in postheparin plasma in human obesity. *Acta Medica Scandinavica*, 1977, *202*, 399-408.

part III

BEHAVIORAL AND SOCIAL ASPECTS

chapter 11
BEHAVIORAL AND COGNITIVE DISABILITIES IN PRADER-WILLI SYNDROME

Stephen Sulzbacher, Keith A. Crnic, and Jeff Snow

> The authors discuss behavioral and cognitive characteristics of Prader-Willi syndrome individuals, with recommendations for treatment. Special considerations for classroom teachers are included. —Eds.

Since 1956, when Prader-Willi (P-W) syndrome was first described, there have been roughly 100 studies of the syndrome published (see the annotated bibliography at the end of this volume). Most of these studies were directed at understanding the diagnosis and etiology of the syndrome, with emphasis on describing the physical characteristics and speculating on possible causes. The few studies suggesting treatment procedures focused mainly on weight control, either through diet or through behavior modification. Since the syndrome also includes significant behavioral and cognitive disabilities, the present study is a discussion of the nature and degree of mental retardation found among some of the 52 patients followed up at the University of Washington Prader-Willi Syndrome Clinic, and an analysis of their behavioral characteristics. In addition, the various treatment tactics employed in modifying some of the behavioral deviations shown by these P-W children are presented.

COGNITIVE DEVELOPMENT

Mental retardation associated with this syndrome is reported to be in the range of >20 IQ to <80 IQ, with most cases between 40 and 60 IQ (Smith, 1976). A case with an IQ of over 100 has been reported by Crnic, Sulzbacher, Snow, and Holm (1980). In that study, there were 10 subjects whose obesity was untreated and who had a mean IQ of 59.9; nine patients who were diagnosed after becoming obese and lost weight under behavioral and nutritional treatment, but whose mean IQ equaled 57.33 after treatment; and a third group of eight children, who were diagnosed in infancy and never became obese, whose mean IQ was 80.25. It was concluded in that report that although IQ declines with age, it also declines with increasing weight. Apparently, dietary and behavior management in the early years were of greatest importance in improving prognosis for intellectual development.

A working hypothesis of many researchers is that P-W syndrome is associated with a hypothalamic defect, a fact that would account for the obvious appetite control difficulties, disorders in gonadal development, and emotional lability most often expressed as unpredictable rage outbursts. The research of Warren and Hunt (Chapter 12, this volume) documents a consistent deficit in short term memory-related tasks that does not improve over time and that could explain the judgment and information-processing deficits in the P-W syndrome girl who has a tested IQ of over 100, but still appears to most casual observers as a mildly retarded person.

Although many P-W syndrome children are mentally retarded on the basis of their tested IQs, their performances are more like those seen in children labeled as learning-disabled, in that there is considerable variability in relative skills and deficits exhibited by each individual. P-W syndrome persons, like the learning-disabled, demonstrate great difficulty in learning some tasks such as arithmetic and significantly less difficulty in learning to read. The emotional lability seen in P-W syndrome children is also more like that seen in learning-disabled than in mentally retarded children. Although educational placement should be decided on an individual basis, most P-W syndrome children seen at the University of Washington Prader-Willi Syndrome Clinic are placed in learning disabilities programs. Outlined below are some of the behavioral interventions that have been found useful at school and home.

TREATMENT TACTICS FOR THE 0- TO 3-YEAR-OLD P-W CHILD

The most important problem in dealing with P-W syndrome children in this age range is assuring adequate nutrition given the general hypotonia and poor suck. Physical therapy is usually indicated (Carman, Chapter 24, this volume; Zellweger, Chapter 5, this volume). From a behavioral standpoint, it is important to encourage mobility wherever possible by arranging toys just outside the child's reach and by helping the child make approximations to pushing or pulling up. P-W syndrome infants and children will need more than the normal amount of encouragement and reinforcement for general motor activity. Since it is during this period that many of the patterns of mother-child interaction are established, it is particularly important that the parents seek professional advice in the subtleties of behavior-shaping that help the child develop the desired behaviors without causing psychological stress. Although it is important to arrange such early childhood learning experiences, it remains of paramount importance that such activities be enjoyable for the child! After the initial battle to get enough food into the child during the early extreme hypotonia, most parents have needed professional reassurance and support in altering their feeding patterns when the child begins to overeat and gain weight toward the end of this developmental period (Zellweger, Chapter 5, this volume).

THE 3- TO 6-YEAR OLD P-W CHILD

Since many P-W syndrome children have language and articulation difficulties (Branson, Chapter 13, this volume) and also have difficulty maintaining social interactions with peers, the single most important behavioral recommendation for P-W syndrome children of this age is enrollment in an organized preschool, Head Start, or an early childhood education program with a behavioral or academic orientation. In order to overcome their deficits, however mild these may be, it is important for P-W syndrome children to receive specific training at the hands of early childhood education specialists. Day care programs and less structured play-oriented preschools will not, in most cases, provide the necessary academic rigor. Appropriate early childhood and language stimulation programs are found in Allen, Holm, and Schiefelbusch (1978) and Rieke, Lynch, and Soltman (1977).

In addition, parents should make extra efforts to arrange for their P-W syndrome children to have as much exposure as possible to other children their age. Whereas encouraging skill acquisition in numbers and letters, prereading, and writing is certainly important, language and social skills should be a first priority at this time in the child's development. Two examples that illustrate successful intervention in improving language and social skills follow.

Case No. 1

After being followed up in the clinic for about 1 year, Joe was enrolled in a language stimulation group when he was 2 years, 10 months old. The program focused on articulation and teaching two-word (verb-object) responses to questions. He learned the latter skill, but continued to need more articulation therapy. As a result, on subsequent intelligence testing when Joe was 3 years, 11 months old, his IQ remained in the borderline range and his language was tested in the normal range. His articulation continued to be poor. He was then enrolled in a special preschool program for P-W children. The target behaviors were improved articulation and improved quality in social interactions with peers and adults. Although it is not possible to say that these interventions "caused" the progress, at 10 years of age Joe's IQ is still 84, his academic progress is satisfactory in a class for disabled learners, and the teachers feel that his language and social skills are adequate.

Case No. 2

A few summers ago a social skills training group was held three times a week at the University of Washington Prader-Willi Syndrome Clinic for six P-W boys, whose ages ranged from 4 years to 8 years. Among those attending was Ted, who was approximately 6 years old at the time and whose inappropriate social behavior consisted of acting as if he were an animal, often a lion, and telling stories about monsters and other imaginary creatures insisting that they were, in fact, real. When asked a question by another member of the group, Ted often responded with a statement that did not relate to the question or he would make an animal sound in response. It was determined that Ted was losing his grasp on reality and that this emotional disturbance was made worse by a television show featuring monsters that he watched avidly and that seemed to figure in his monster fantasies.

It should be noted that Ted's thought disorder may have been an idiosyncratic expression of the central nervous system effects of P-W syndrome, since similar manifestations are rare in other children with the syndrome. It was, however, a central feature of this child's symptom complex. The treatment was essentially what would have been done for another child without the syndrome exhibiting similar behaviors; he was forbidden to watch the particular TV show, and consistent feedback was provided at home and in the social skills group to help Ted distinguish real events from fantasy events. It is important not to discourage fantasy, but to be very sure that the child can distinguish between it and reality, and can move from one thought realm to the other at will. At home, his parents would respond to fantasy statements by saying, "Ted, is what you're telling me real or fantasy? I'll be glad to listen to your story if you'll label it correctly." Similarly, in the therapy group he was asked to label what he wanted to say as real or as fantasy before he began, and when he made animal noises, the others in the group would let him know (prompted by the group leader) whether they wanted to hear such noises. Usually they did not. At first Ted took such feedback badly, and on several occasions he left the group to sit in a corner by himself. However, he did want to be friends with the other boys and, after several sessions, began to control his desires to stay in the fantasy world so that he could relate to his friends. He was also learning that they would interact with him longer if he talked about topics of interest to them. The group leader would give Ted hints such as, "Ask Bill about his pony," which Ted would do to get attention from Bill.

It took over a year before Ted stopped his monster talk, and he still occasionally retreats to his fantasies, but he now seems to be able to return to the "real world" whenever he is asked to do so.

THE 6- TO 12-YEAR-OLD P-W CHILD

Every P-W syndrome child in this study, without exception, has required special education in the elementary school years. However, it has been very difficult to find just the right program for many of these children and to establish their eligibility for special education help. In some cases, the child's IQ score was too high to qualify and the unique characteristics of P-W syndrome did not always fit under any of the various state rules and regulations governing eligibility for special education. Some P-W children in the present study who were followed up had spent a year or so in regular education classes before their academic difficulties and behavioral excesses became sufficiently apparent that special education placement was necessary. Although each individual case differs, it is often socially beneficial for the P-W child to have this exposure to the normal classroom situation. The social benefits can outweigh some lost academic ground. Nevertheless, the authors have found that it is useful to visit schoolteachers and administrators to explain the educational ramifications and to outline the unique features of the P-W syndrome to them. It is important to stress that children with P-W syndrome generally do best with the same academic curriculum and behavior modification procedures commonly employed for children with learning disabilities. The following are specific recommendations for teachers.

Reinforcement

Characteristic of many P-W syndrome children are refusal to do assigned schoolwork, threats of tantrums, and general lack of motivation. In general, social reinforcement procedures and token economies of the sort employed in many special education classrooms are recommended for these children. If these fail, the following alternatives, developed in cooperation with a nutritionist, may be applied.

1. Use the child's lunch as a reinforcer. The lunch may be divided into bite-size portions (ideally, the parent could send the lunch prepared in this way). The child is then instructed that he will get one part of his lunch after he completes each portion of his daily work. For example, he might get a bite of his sandwich after finishing three pages in his Sullivan reader, then another bite after doing four pages of arithmetic, etc. The teacher can arrange to dispense about one-half the lunch in this fashion and let the student have the other one-half during the standard lunch period. If problems are experienced in the afternoon, a small portion of the lunch

can be held back for the end of the day if the student continues to behave himself. If the child does not complete the assigned work, the lunch should be thrown away and a note sent home to the parents to be especially alert for food foraging that afternoon. Obviously, these children will survive quite nicely if they miss a few lunches!

2. Use additional food as a reinforcer. The nutritionist at the University of Washington Prader-Willi Syndrome Clinic has suggested several foods—small slices of celery, carrot, or dill pickle—that children with P-W syndrome may have in unlimited quantities and that may be kept in stock to use as bonus reinforcers in conjunction with the program outlined above. Alternatively, the child may be allowed a "normal" lunch and these foods simply used as additional reinforcers (keeping the parents informed, of course). The children may have as much of these three foods as they wish, but only one thin stick at a time. Sips of dietetic carbonated beverage are another popular reinforcer. These reinforcers might be particularly useful in a classroom where candy-type reinforcers are used with other children, so that the P-W child is reinforced with food of a type he can tolerate. In fact, it is suggested that the entire class would benefit from these reinforcers instead of sweets. One sweet reinforcer, flavored gelatin sticks made with *dietetic* gelatin such as D-Zerta, is recommended. To make these sticks, one-half to one-third the amount of water recommended on the package is used. When the product hardens it is thicker and gummier than normal gelatin, but does not require refrigeration.

Behavioral Problems

The most common behavioral problems reported in the 6- to 12-year-old have been severe but infrequent temper tantrums at school, food stealing at home, and difficulty relating to peer playmates. In general, standard educational practices for the temper tantrums, such as being taken or sent to the principal's office, and/or being sent home, have been recommended but school authorities have been told that regardless of the consequences for the behavior, these behavioral outbursts will persist in P-W children at a rate of three or four times in a school year. It has also been recommended that changes in the home (and where possible, the school) be made so that the temptation of food is not available to the P-W child of this age. However, allowing P-W children some choice in their food is a useful prelude to training them to eventually manage their own dietary regimen.

Social Relationships

Another frequent difficulty of nearly all the P-W children in this study is poor social relationships with peers, parents, and teachers, sometimes said to be related to low self-concept or poor self-esteem. A common denominator in this class of behavior is a lack of certain social skills and a seeming difficulty in picking up social cues from other people. This problem is certainly not unique to children with P-W syndrome, but it seems to be a problem that many children have to some degree (Johnson, 1972). One way to help these children adapt is to provide opportunities to try out social skills in structured social situations. Simple role-playing sessions and guided discussions on selected topics, with children getting feedback on the appropriateness of their comments, are the kinds of experiences that might be helpful and could be conducted in special education classes (Canfield & Wells, 1976; Chase, 1975). It is important, however, that the children actually participate in these experiences, since it appears that they do not seem to profit from lectures on how to behave. Some examples of these exercises are:

1. What to say when you meet a new friend.
2. How do you let someone know that you like them?
3. How do you let someone know that you're angry?
4. Things to do when someone calls you a name.

Another type of activity is assigning a topic for discussion with the children sitting in a circle and giving each child immediate feedback on whether his comments were on-task and appropriate. This teaches children the difference between comments that are silly and immature and those that are of interest to listeners of their age. The important thing in all of these tasks is to allow the children to interact with peers in ways that will enable them to make and keep friends. Such exercises should be continued throughout the elementary grades and junior high school.

In addition to these specific recommendations, it is important to encourage the younger child who encounters difficulties in social relationships to relate to other children as much as possible. For example, when children have "show and tell," they should be instructed to ask questions and make comments after each child does his own "show and tell." When necessary, a child can be directly prompted on what to say, such as, "John, tell Bill you thought he told a good story." Another conversational assignment might be, "Bill, tell John something nice about something he is wearing." "John, tell Bill you're glad he likes your shirt." Even during straight academic instruction, opportunities are available for social learning: "David, ask Jane to give you four blocks and give half of them to Steven." "Steven, did David give you the right number of blocks?" In each of these cases, a social interaction becomes an integral part of what is normally just a response to a teacher request.

Extracurricular Activities

A very important recommendation that has been stressed for all parents of P-W children 6 years to 12 years of age is that the child be enrolled in as many extracurricular organized activities with peers as possible, such as church groups, Girl Scouts or Boy Scouts, organized athletic teams, little league, and Special Olympics. Stamp- or coin-collecting clubs and the arts and crafts activities typically arranged through parks and recreation departments in most municipalities are also recommended. The important features of such activities are that they be supervised by adults, provide for structured social interaction, and lead to correlated activities that the child can continue at home, alone or with his parents. The development of a lifelong hobby can be fostered at this point and lead to continued satisfaction throughout the individual's lifetime.

Physical Education

Careful thought should also be given to the P-W child's physical education classes (Carman, Chapter 24, this volume). Although the chance to get some exercise, recreation, and competitive experience is a reasonable goal for regular education gym classes, participating in group sport activities is often not the best use of the P-W student's time. Since these students are likely to be at least somewhat isolated for most of their lives, it is important that they develop the habit of a personal regimen of daily exercise such as calisthenics or jogging, particularly in light of the obesity problem with which they must cope all of their lives. Teaching these skills may be accomplished either in physical education classes or in the students' home classrooms. It is important that the exercise regimen being taught require no special equipment, since the children should be able to continue the regimen on their own at home, on a daily basis.

A second component of the physical education program for these children should be the programming of social skills such as taking turns, understanding the rules of the game, and working together as a team. One should strive to increase the frequency of peer-appropriate vocal exchanges among the participants in a game. Such opportunities should be encouraged even at the expense of downgrading the actual game performance. For example, the students need to decide among themselves who plays what position in a game. When a student has difficulty with one aspect of the game, another student should help him rather than the teacher. It is also important that the social maturity as well as the physical skill level of a student be considered in deciding which type of sport (amount of competitiveness, team or individual, etc.) would be most satisfying. Considerable time should be spent in discussing the activity and planning strategies. Thus, if a team is preparing for the Special Olympics, individuals should be assigned to find out winning times and discuss them with the group. Relay races are obviously better than individual sprints for fostering peer interaction.

THE 12- TO 17-YEAR-OLD P-W ADOLESCENT

In general, there are fewer options for specialized programs in special education at the junior and senior high school levels. Difficult and significant decisions are required in devising the IEPs (individualized education programs, required by federal law for all special education students) to maximize the child's educational and vocational possibilities. Thought should be given to preparing the P-W child to assume as much responsibility for himself as possible. These preparations should include using savings and checking accounts, using a pocket calculator to keep track of those accounts and as an aid in shopping, and weighing and measuring foods and leaving a ration of food available to consume over a period of several days. A part-time job (preferably *not* in the food service industry!) is most desirable. Being a teacher's helper for kindergarten or first grade or managing a high school athletic team are examples of work experience from which some patients have profited.

The adolescent years are a time when the P-W individual must take increasing responsibility for himself. Parents begin the transition from managers to advisers. Unfortunately, this experiment will not succeed for all, and it will often become apparent that the P-W individual will require a manager for the rest of his life. Others will show some ability to manage their own dietary intake, to accept some responsibility for daily living and part-time jobs, and to apply what they have learned in school to everyday situations.

However, even for those who show tested IQs in the normal range and maintain their weight in proportion to height, significant cognitive deficits prevent them from having a totally independent, self-sufficient life-style, as the following case shows.

Case No. 3

Frank's case illustrates the difficulty of dividing responsibility for important decisions between parents and the increasingly assertive, mildly retarded P-W child. Frank's parents had managed his weight and his behavior effectively through childhood by careful attention to diet and consistent behavior management. Two behavioral techniques especially effective with Frank were contingent reinforcement (administered by varying Frank's weekly allowance) and timeout. Saving money was a particularly strong reinforcer for Frank, who was quite proud of his passbook and kept close track of earned interest. He lost money for temper outbursts, earned extra money for certain chores, and could increase the weekly amount of the allowance by maintaining or losing weight. When he was approximately 13, his temper outbursts increased. Therefore, his father modified a basement washroom into a timeout room. Frank watched his father working on it and was told its intended use (the procedure was not new to Frank since it had been used at school). After the room was built, Frank's behavior improved dramatically and nearly 6 months passed before one of his temper outbursts ever necessitated using the room.

Between Frank's 14th and 15th birthdays, a number of changes occurred: The family moved to another house in a different school district, Frank's scoliosis became worse, his behavior deteriorated, and he began to gain weight. Parental attempts to control his food intake led to more severe and more frequent temper outbursts and his daily behavior became increasingly unpleasant (a very exaggerated version of what is seen in most adolescents). He was ridiculed at school where older children would make him dance for pennies, which he now spent for food instead of saving. He demanded the right to withdraw money from his own savings account to buy food. His parents had been experimenting by allowing Frank a greater voice in choosing his diet and by allowing him to go more places on his own. His "adolescent rebellion" expanded as he became more secretive about his activities while concurrently demanding greater privileges and accepting less advice about his diet. Major confrontations at the dinner table were becoming commonplace and Frank's sister began complaining bitterly that his behavior at school was a source of embarrassment for her. It was around this time that the orthopedist at the University of Washington Prader-Willi Syndrome Clinic discovered that Frank's scoliosis had worsened and recommended a brace, which Frank refused to wear. When the consequences of failure to stop the progressive defect were explained (that he might eventually need surgery to straighten his backbone), he calmly announced, after thinking it over, that he had decided it was not worth it and that he preferred to die rather than undergo the treatment. He had apparently been ruminating about this for some time. He had also made a decision that he did not care if he gained weight.

Unfortunately, the situation described above has no ideal solution. The orthopedic procedures are such that success is possible only with active patient cooperation. Therefore, after many attempts at counseling and cajoling it became apparent that it was futile to continue trying to persuade Frank. However, discussion of the scoliosis problem among clinic staff members and Frank's parents enabled the authors to determine how much parental control was in Frank's best interest and what compromises might be indicated for the psychological health of the rest of the family. The brace was abandoned. Although weight gain was inevitable, restrictions on Frank's food intake and his access to the savings account were significantly relaxed. Predictably, he began to gain weight, but his temper outbursts at home decreased and his general relationships with family members improved. Although he will remain at home for another year or so, his parents have begun to explore group home options for Frank in the future. These decisions were difficult ones for Frank's family and were not the unanimous recommendations of the various professionals at the Prader-Willi Syndrome Clinic. This case is presented to emphasize the importance of sensitive clinical judgment in assisting families with the management of their P-W children.

Running Away

Another serious problem of the P-W adolescent is running away from home, either because of anger or in search of food. These "adventures" can be as brief as a 2-hour jaunt to the local shopping center to ask for handouts or to shoplift, or they can be absences of several days resulting in significant weight gain. There are stopgap measures, such as taking the child's shoes away when he gets home, but the problem really cannot be completely solved by most families. If an older adolescent is running away frequently (more than once a month) alternative living arrangements, such as a group home, which is better equipped to keep the person occupied and has more staff to monitor the adolescent's movements, should be considered. In states where respite care is available, such assistance can help monitor the child's activities while the parents are busy and thus make it possible for the child to remain at home for a few more years. Nevertheless, it is the feeling of the authors not only that active parenthood should be an 18-year commitment for parents of developmentally disabled children, just as it is for parents of normal children, but also that alternative living arrangements are most appropriate for P-W adults. It goes without saying that parents will naturally continue caring and show active involvement with their P-W child, but the actual caring *for* is, in most cases, best transferred to others and, to the degree possible, to P-W individuals themselves.

THE P-W YOUNG ADULT

The experience of the authors with the young adult age group is still limited, but it is believed that a group home/sheltered workshop living arrangement can provide maximum happiness and fulfillment for the P-W individual *and* for the other members of the family. With the treatments outlined in this volume there is unquestionably a far brighter prognosis for P-W persons than institutionalization, which was the most likely outcome as recently as the 1950s and early 1960s.

Whereas group home living appears to be the least restrictive and most rewarding option available for individuals with P-W syndrome, foster homes or nursing homes might be the most appropriate in individual cases. This study includes two P-W individuals who live independently, although one of them is currently doing so against the advice of the authors. He has been experiencing considerable difficulties in interpersonal relationships, does not have a job, and is gaining weight. It is anticipated that he will eventually return to a group home situation. The other person lives in his own apartment and is somewhat obese. He lived for some time in an institution, then moved to a group home for P-W youngsters where they were able to help him make the transition to an apartment. He currently has a job at the same institution in which he formerly lived.

Because of the special diets and restrictions on access to food required for the successful management of most individuals with P-W syndrome, many group homes have found it difficult to serve this population and still maintain a home-like atmosphere (including home-style meals and free access to the kitchen) for their other clients. Nevertheless, some of the patients in this study have been able to lose or maintain weight in such facilities that house other developmentally disabled persons. It is hoped that other group homes can be encouraged to develop programs that will include P-W individuals, enabling these individuals to remain in their home communities near family and friends and to make new friends among other developmentally disabled and normal persons.

At present, it is believed that only one group home exclusively for P-W individuals exists, although several others are being planned in various parts of the country. This original group home, housing five male and three female P-W individuals ranging in age from 13 to 35 years of age, has been described by Thornley (Note 1). She reports that a menu prepared in consultation with a nutritionist provides for family-style meals with daily caloric intake ranging from 1,200 to 1,800 calories. Residents are permitted in the kitchen only under staff supervision. A token reinforcement system is used involving stars on a chart for weight loss, weight maintenance, and "appropriate behavior." During the first 18 months of its operation, five obese individuals lost between 45 and 110 pounds, and two individuals, who were at ideal weight for height, gained slightly (10 and 15 pounds). Some of the individuals in the group home attend public school and others go to a sheltered workshop. Although various recreational opportunities are available on a regular basis, some of the individuals complain that their social contacts are restricted unduly by associating primarily with other P-W persons.

Reports received from several sheltered workshops for developmentally disabled persons confirm that only minimal special consideration need be given to a P-W individual in such a setting: the staff should be alerted to the possibility of food theft and some minimal supervision over its availability is required. It is reported that P-W workers are indistinguishable from their developmentally disabled peers as far as workshop performance and behavior are concerned. One other point to remember in planning adult work opportunities for P-W individuals is that a large percentage of work opportunities for developmentally disabled people are in the food services industry, which is an inappropriate job placement for this population.

CONCLUSION

Although the experiences of the authors are limited thus far, it is increasingly apparent that individuals affected with P-W syndrome can expect to find meaningful and productive lives in school, with their families, and in society. It is equally clear that, in most cases, their diet must be supervised and their cravings for food must be controlled. An approach that has not yet been tried, but that holds some promise, is the peer support group for adults. Model groups that have had some success for obesity management are Weight-Watchers or the kinds of groups associated with Alcoholics Anonymous. It is clearly important that we devise ways of helping P-W individuals establish a sense of personal dignity that comes with increasing freedom to manage their own affairs.

REFERENCE NOTE

1. Thornley, M.L. *Results of a longitudinal intervention program for eight adolescents and adults with Prader-Willi syndrome residing in a controlled living and caloric environment.* Unpublished manuscript, 1979.

REFERENCES

Allen, K.E., Holm, V.A., & Schiefelbusch, R.L. (Eds.). *Early intervention—A team approach.* Baltimore: University Park Press, 1978.
Canfield, J., & Wells, H.C. *100 ways to enhance self-concept in the classroom: A handbook for teachers and parents.* Engelwood Cliffs, N.J.: Prentice-Hall, 1976.
Chase, L. *The other side of the report care: A how-to-do-it program for effective education.* Santa Monica, Calif.: Goodyear, 1975.
Crnic, K.A., Sulzbacher, S., Snow, J., & Holm, V.A. Preventing mental retardation associated with gross obesity in the Prader-Willi syndrome. *Pediatrics,* 1980, *66,* 787-789.
Johnson, D.W. *Reaching out.* Englewood Cliffs, N.J.: Prentice-Hall, 1972.
Rieke, J., Lynch, L., & Soltman, S. *Teaching strategies for language development.* New York: Grune & Stratton, 1977.
Smith, D.W. *Recognizable patterns of human malformation: Genetic, embryologic, and clinical aspects* (2nd ed.). Philadelphia: W.B. Saunders, 1976.

chapter 12
COGNITIVE PROCESSING IN CHILDREN WITH PRADER-WILLI SYNDROME

Judith L. Warren and Earl Hunt

> Drs. Warren and Hunt found that Prader-Willi syndrome children had greater difficulty with short term memory processing than other retarded children with similar IQ scores. The Prader-Willi syndrome group also lost more information from memory over time. The authors believe that further research might discover still more differences between the groups.—*Eds.*

Although there are many causes of mental retardation, it is often assumed that all individuals who have the same intelligence quotient have similar cognitive abilities. Etiological information has rarely been considered as a factor in psychological studies of retarded children. The following studies were undertaken with mildly retarded children who had Prader-Willi (P-W) syndrome. The research investigated the assumption that the causal factors that produced mental retardation were unimportant in determining the precise nature of the cognitive impairment found. The results suggest that there are unique cognitive deficits found in P-W children that are not the same as those seen in other youngsters with comparable IQ scores. These information-processing differences may have some implications for educational treatment of P-W children.

EXPERIMENT 1

These studies employed picture recognition tasks in which subjects were shown a large number of pictures and asked to determine whether or not they have seen a particular picture before. When unique pictures are used as stimuli, the accuracy levels of both normal and retarded persons are quite high (Brown, 1972). Because a very large number of pictures are presented, common verbal strategies such as naming and rehearsal are not particularly useful in aiding recall, and their possible confounding effect on performance is minimized.

Method

Subjects   P-W children were compared with two control groups. The first was a group of undifferentiated retarded children of comparable age and IQ whose retardation was attributable to unknown causes. The second control group was made up of children of normal intelligence whose mental ages (MA) were equivalent to or less than those of the retarded groups. Since the P-W children and the undifferentiated retarded group both spanned a wide age range, the groups were split at the chronological age (CA) of 8 years into an older and a younger group. Subject characteristics are shown in Table 12.1.

Stimulus Materials   Colored pictures were cut from children's books and mounted in the center of black posterboard cards. Two sets of 120 cards were assembled, each composed of 50 duplicate pairs of pictures and 20 single pictures. The pictures were ordered so that the second picture of a pair appeared after a specified number of distractor pictures had intervened. The number of intervening items, or lag, was either 0, 5, 10, 25, or 50. There were 10 tests of each lag and these were distributed as evenly as possible throughout the deck.

Procedure   After a brief pretraining session that ensured that each child understood the task, the first set of pictures was presented to each child individually. The child's task was to determine whether or not each picture had occurred previously in the set. The children returned on the

Table 12.1.   Subject characteristics for experiment 1

Group	MA (years)	CA (years)	IQ
Prader-Willi	6.4	10.1	65.0
($n = 11$)	SD = 1.9	SD = 3.3	SD = 13.8
Younger	4.9	6.2	70.3
($n = 3$)	SD = 0.9	SD = 0.7	SD = 14.2
Older	6.9	11.5	64.3
($n = 8$)	SD = 1.9	SD = 2.7	SD = 13.6
Undifferentiated	7.7	11.7	65.5
($n = 12$)	SD = 2.8	SD = 3.3	SD = 10.0
Younger	4.5	7.4	57.3
($n = 4$)	SD = 0.46	SD = 0.22	SD = 6.2
Older	9.4	13.9	71.4
($n = 8$)	SD = 1.7	SD = 1.1	SD = 9.7
Normal	5.6	5.4	95.9
($n = 13$)	SD = 0.88	SD = 0.61	SD = 11.2

following day and were tested in an identical manner with the second deck of pictures.

Results

Figure 12.1 shows the group differences at each lag combined over the 2 days of testing. The d' statistic is used as the measure of accuracy because it considers both the percentage of "old" pictures the subject correctly identifies as having been previously seen and the percentage of "new" items accurately rejected as being novel. Both the group effect and the lag effect were significant ($p < 0.01$). Lag did not interact with group, and longer lags were more difficult for all those tested. The day

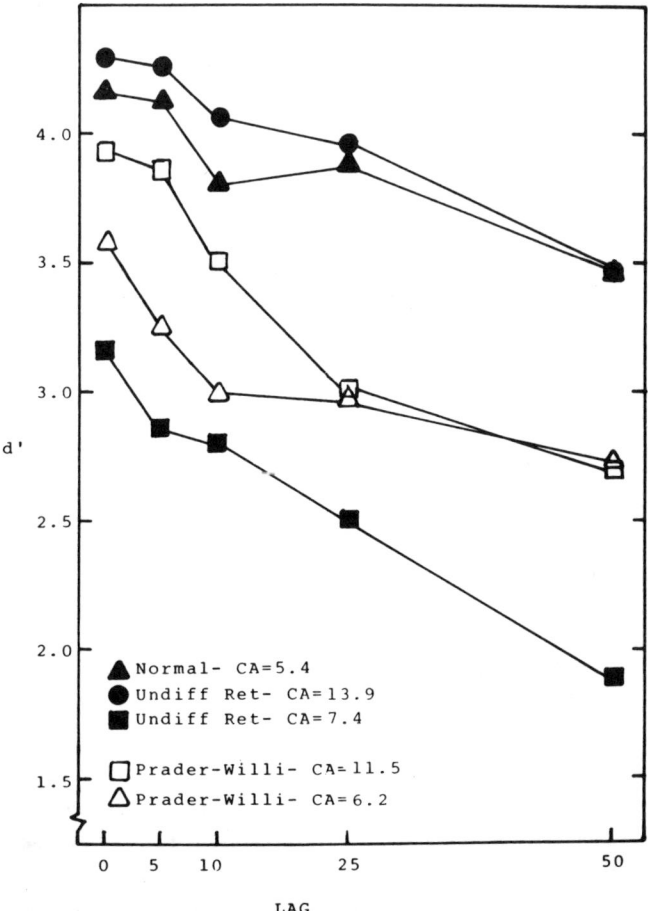

Figure 12.1. Mean group d' rates at each lag for experiment 1

effect was not significant. There was a significant day × lag interaction ($p = 0.04$) with the lag effect appearing more pronounced on the second day of testing. None of the other interactions was significant.

Post hoc testing on the group mean scores combined over day and lag indicated that the younger and older P-W groups performed equivalently. By contrast the performance of the younger undifferentiated retarded, while comparable to that of the P-W children, was significantly different from the older undifferentiated retarded children and the normal preschoolers.

Performance of the preschool children was correlated with CA ($p = 0.02$) and more strongly with MA ($p = 0.004$). The undifferentiated retarded group also showed significant correlations of d' with CA ($p = 0.008$) and with MA ($p = 0.01$). Thus, in the normal and undifferentiated retarded samples, picture recognition performance improved with increasing age and overall ability. However, memory strength in P-W children was not significantly correlated with either CA or MA ($p = 0.37$ and 0.19, respectively).

Discussion

These data suggest that the development of picture recognition memory is substantially different in P-W children than in undifferentiated retarded subjects. The performance of P-W youngsters did not improve with CA or MA as it did in the control groups. In addition, P-W subjects were unable to achieve the accuracy levels displayed by the lower MA normal group, as could the older undifferentiated retarded children.

The lack of a group × lag interaction is striking. It suggests that, in simple tasks, whatever differences exist in picture recognition memory are immediately detectable, even with no interfering pictures. The poor performance of P-W children thus appears not to be caused by differential rates of forgetting but by some other failure of the recognition system.

It is notable that performance by all subjects in the first experiment was quite good, at times close to ceiling levels for some individuals. Thus, while it was apparent that group differences existed, it was not possible from the first study alone to estimate how impaired the P-W subjects actually were.

EXPERIMENT 2

The second study, which used less easily discriminated pictures as stimuli, was designed to test the replicability of the effects seen in experiment 1, to clarify the developmental trends involved in picture recognition performance, and to estimate the magnitude of the group differences. The picture recognition task was made more difficult by using distractor items that were similar to the target pictures. For instance, a swing set might appear several times during the session, once unoccupied and later being used by different individuals. The goal was to create a relatively short task that would be moderately difficult for all subjects.

Method

Subjects Children with P-W syndrome were matched as closely as possible for MA and IQ with a group of undifferentiated retarded subjects. An additional adolescent with P-W syndrome who was of normal intelligence (IQ > 105) was also tested. Her scores are considered separately. Five different age groups of normal subjects were also tested. Subject characteristics for all age groups are shown in Table 12.2

Stimulus Materials A total of 250 color slides made up the stimulus set. There were 100 duplicate pairs and 50 distractor items. As in experiment 1, the slides were ordered so that the duplicate picture recurred after a certain number of intervening items had been viewed. To make the task

Table 12.2. Subject characteristics for experiment 2

Group	MA (years)	CA (years)	IQ
Retarded Subjects			
Prader-Willi	7.8	13.1	63.0
(n = 11)	SD = 2.8	SD = 3.2	SD = 24.4
Undifferentiated	7.4	11.7	64.8
(n = 11)	SD = 2.7	SD = 1.9	SD = 21.7
Normal Subjects			
5-year-olds	6.7	5.0	126.4
(n = 12)	SD = 0.76	SD = 0.64	SD = 14.9
7-year-olds	9.6	7.6	121.6
(n = 10)	SD = 1.3	SD = 0.49	SD = 12.5
10-year-olds	12.5	10.1	115.5
(n = 10)	SD = 2.1	SD = 0.61	SD = 12.2
13-year-olds	15.0	13.3	112.8
(n = 10)	SD = 0.67	SD = 0.67	SD = 9.2
			WPC Verbal	WPC Quantitative
		CA		
College[a]		19.6	56.4	56.5

[a] IQ test scores were not available for these subjects. They had, however, taken the Washington Pre-College (WPC) Entrance Exam in their junior year of high school. This test, similar to other college entrance examinations, has a mean of 50 and a standard of 10 (Technical Manual, Washington Pre-College Testing Program, 1977).

more difficult, the number of distractor pictures, or lag, was increased and set at either 0, 10, 30, 50, or 100 intervening slides. There were 20 tests at each lag that were distributed as evenly as possible.

Procedure After a brief pretraining session, each subject was tested individually in a single session. Again, children were asked to determine whether or not they had already seen each slide.

Results

The performance of each group at each lag is shown in Figure 12.2. The lag factor is highly significant ($p < 0.001$) with longer lags being more

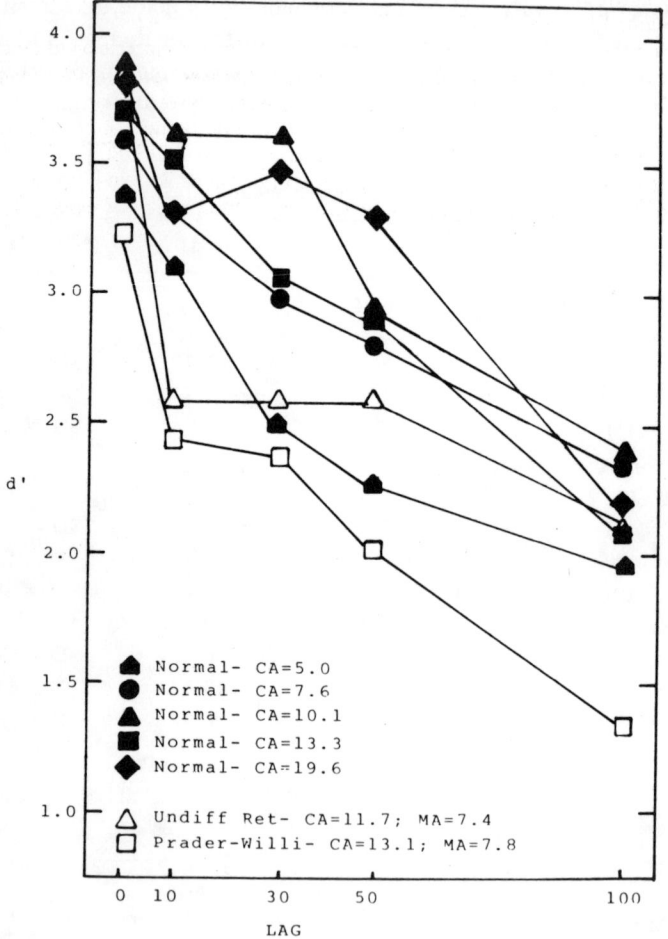

Figure 12.2. Mean group d' rates for experiment 2.

difficult for all subjects. There was also a significant group effect ($p < 0.01$). Post hoc analysis showed that all the normal groups performed comparably, with the exception of the 5-year-olds whose scores were significantly below those of the 10-year-olds and college students. The scores of the undifferentiated retarded children were significantly better than the P-W group and were comparable to normal children of equal CA. P-W subjects did not perform as well as equal CA controls. They scored comparably to the lower MA preschoolers but not as well as the higher MA 7-year-olds.

The group $\times$ lag interaction was significant ($p < 0.01$). Post hoc testing indicated that the performance of P-W youngsters became increasingly discrepant from the other groups as the lag interval increased, until at a lag of 100 items the performance of P-W youngsters was clearly less than that of any other subjects. Thus, P-W subjects appear to have particular difficulty with memory at the longest lag.

Within the normal control groups, picture recognition performance was only related to age when the preschool group was included in the analysis (d' with CA $p = 0.006$ and d' with MA $p = 0.004$. When the younger children were excluded from the analysis, the correlations failed to reach significance.

In order to assess better the developmental trends, another 22 undifferentiated mildly retarded children were tested. The total group of 33 children then had a mean IQ of 68.8 with a mean CA of 10.5 years and a mean MA of 7.2 years. Performance of the undifferentiated group was significantly correlated with both CA and MA ($p < 0.001$ in both cases). This pattern was not apparent in the P-W group, whose accuracy levels correlated with neither CA nor MA.

Figure 12.3 shows the accuracy levels of each group at each age. Performance of each P-W child is shown individually. Normal children appear to achieve adult levels of picture recognition memory by age 7. The recognition memories of undifferentiated retarded children seem to mature later than do those of normals, although by age 11 the two groups have comparable performance levels. P-W and undifferentiated retarded children have similar recognition levels until about age 9 or 10 when the undifferentiated group begins to surpass the non-improving P-W children. The performance of the sole P-W subject with normal intelligence is of particular interest. Although her most recent IQ score (117) is easily comparable to the college sample, her recognition memory proved to be well below not only that of college students but also that of older undifferentiated retarded and normal children. Thus, the failure of the recognition memory system demonstrated here seems to be a syndrome-specific problem that affects all persons with the disease regardless of their general level of functioning.

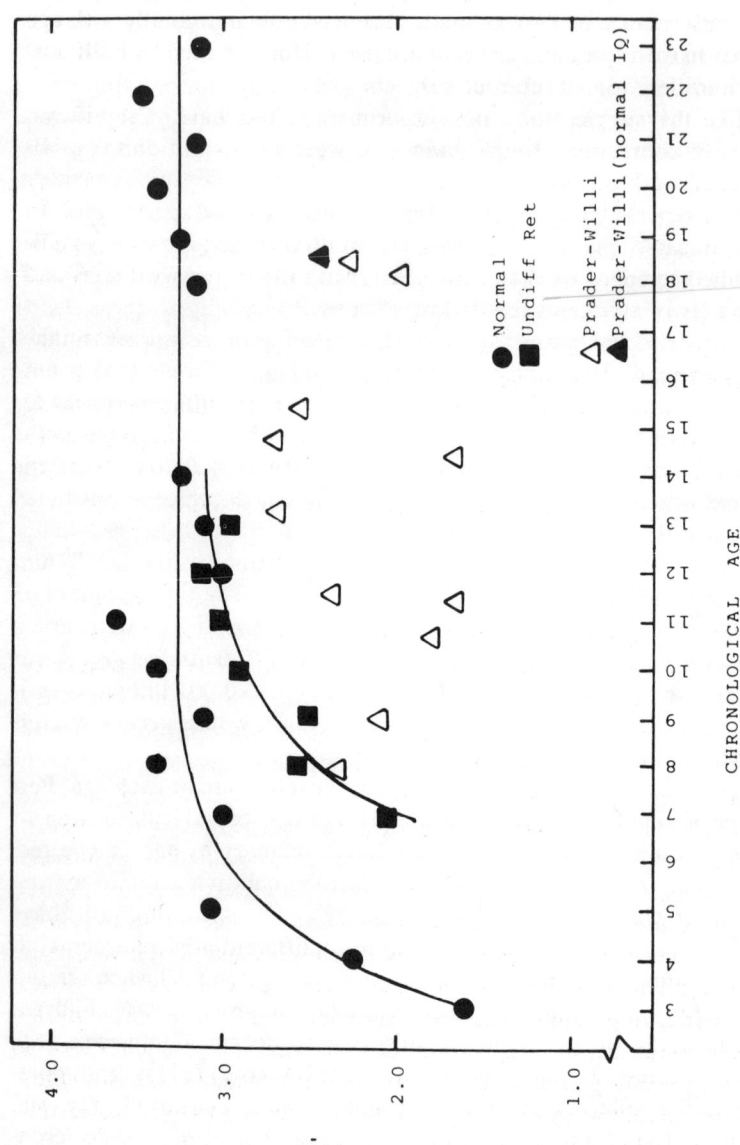

Figure 12.3. Plot of individual d' scores by age.

Discussion

The results of the second study replicate and extend the findings of experiment 1. Performance of P-W subjects improved only marginally with age in contrast to the increasing levels of accuracy demonstrated by both normal and undifferentiated retarded subjects.

Unlike the simple first task, experiment 2 did have a significant group × lag interaction. The difference between the two studies is probably the result of the greater demands of the second test. The initial memory impairment reported in experiment 1 is also suggested in experiment 2. In addition, the P-W group had a steeper retention function, with significantly more memory loss than any other group when many pictures and much time had elapsed between the repetitions.

The results of the two picture recognition studies suggest some impairment in memory functioning in children with P-W syndrome that is not apparent in an undifferentiated retarded group. P-W subjects appear to show both a greater loss of information over time and difficulties with immediate memory. Although these problems are unlikely to be related to possible differences in strategy usage, it is not possible to be more specific about what processes might be impaired without further research.

EXPERIMENT 3

The picture recognition experiments suggested that P-W children have some difficulty with short term memory processes. These subjects showed evidence of memory impairment even when items were repeated at very short intervals, in addition to demonstrating greater loss over time than their undifferentiated retarded peers.

One critical component of short term memory is the speed at which individuals are able to review the contents of their immediate memories. An experimental paradigm to study this rate of short term memory (STM) scanning was developed by Sternberg (1966) and has been used with both normal and retarded subjects. A series of digits is presented, followed after a brief pause by a probe digit (e.g., 3 9 7 2 ... 7?) The task is to determine as rapidly as possible whether or not the probe item appeared in the series. The dependent variable is typically the reaction time (RT) for the response, accuracy being virtually perfect. RT is usually found to be a linear function of the number of digits being scanned. The slope of this function is considered the scanning rate for individual digits.

The intent of the third experiment was to determine whether P-W children differed from undifferentiated retarded subjects in their STM scanning rate.

Method

Subjects A group of children with P-W syndrome was studied along with two groups of undifferentiated retarded subjects. Four age groups of normal children were also tested. Subject characteristics are shown in Table 12.3.

Apparatus and Stimulus Materials Stimulus slides were composed of the digits 1 through 9 printed in black on brightly colored backgrounds. The slides were presented sequentially at the rate of one every 1.5 seconds, using a carousel slide projector.

Procedure Subjects were tested individually in three sessions about 1 week apart. A series of one to four slides was presented followed by two blank slides after which the probe digit was shown. Subjects indicated by pressing a button whether or not the probe digit had been in the stimulus set. RT was measured from the onset of the probe to the subject's response, and accuracy information was also recorded. A total of 112 trials was presented on each of the 3 test days.

Results

Typically, RT is the dependent variable in memory scanning experiments since accuracy is usually perfect. However, an analysis of the group error rates revealed significant group differences ($p < 0.010$), with P-W subjects having significantly more errors than any other group. Error rates for the normal and undifferentiated retarded subjects were comparable and low. This is shown in Figure 12.4. Although there was no effect of day of

Table 12.3. Subject characteristics for experiment 3

Group	MA (years)	CA (years)	IQ
Normal			
7-year-old ($n = 10$)	7.6	9.1	116
10-year-old ($n = 10$)	10.0	12.0	114
13-year-old ($n = 10$)	13.5	15.2	113
19-year-old ($n = 10$)	19.5[a]		
Retarded			
Prader-Willi ($n = 7$)	12.7	8.4	68
Young undifferentiated ($n = 10$)	11.7	8.1	68
Old undifferentiated ($n = 10$)	14.5	10.7	75

[a] Results of the Washington Pre-College (WPC) Entrance Exam: verbal = 57; quantitative = 56.

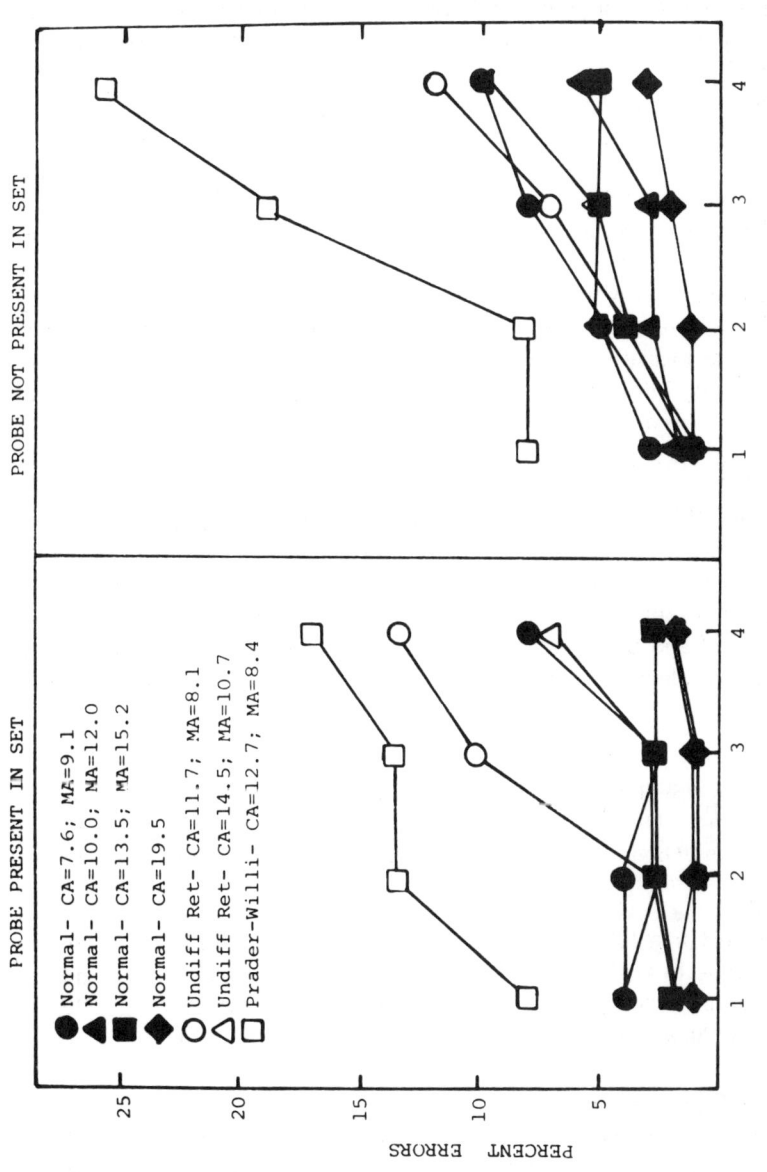

Figure 12.4. Mean percent errors at each set size.

testing on error rate, set size was highly significant ($p < 0.001$) with larger stimulus sets producing more errors. The group × set size interaction was also significant ($p < 0.01$). P-W subjects had significantly more errors at all set sizes than any other group. When three digits appeared in the stimulus set, the younger undifferentiated retarded children and the normal 7-year-olds displayed more errors than all other groups except the P-W group. At set size 4, both retarded groups and the normal 7-year-olds had more errors than the other normal group.

There was a slight trend for trials to be more difficult ($p = 0.09$) where the probe had not been present in the set, although probe condition did not interact with group. Condition did interact with set size ($p < 0.01$), and errors increased more across set sizes when the probe had not been in the stimulus set.

The group × condition × set size interaction was also significant ($p < 0.01$). Errors for P-W subjects rose much more sharply with increasing set size on trials where the probe had not been seen in the stimulus set. This would be expected since on one-half of the set size 4 trials, where the set included the probe, the probe was present in the last two positions. To respond accurately the subject had only to recall the last two digits, whereas when the probe was not within the set he had to recall all four stimuli.

Because of the poor performance of P-W children, an analysis of their RT data was not pursued. As a result of the extreme number of errors they accumulated, its interpretation would not have been clear.

Discussion

The difficulty experienced by P-W children in responding accurately when more than two stimuli were presented was extreme. When asked to recall three or four items their error rates were 9% and 26%, respectively, far above that seen in the undifferentiated retarded sample.

One-item sets constitute a special case and the performance of P-W children on these was also notable. In many ways, positive trials are comparable to the 0 lag items in the picture recognition studies. A stimulus is presented, a few seconds pass, and then the same item appears again. P-W children manifest the same difficulties with one-item sets as they do with picture recognition at short lags: Their error rate is almost 8%.

It might be argued that the differences between P-W and retarded subjects were not related to STM deficits but to group differences in attention. P-W children might have been more distracted or bored and might not have attended to the stimuli as well as the undifferentiated group. Two informal observations are relevant. First, many subjects in all the groups named the stimuli as they were presented. This was equally true of the P-W group. Frequently, P-W subjects were heard to name a stimulus that subsequently appeared as a probe. Often they still mistakenly indicated that the item had not been in the set. Inattention is unlikely to cause such errors. Second, one of the P-W children with a high error rate (13%) on day 1 was offered pennies rather than poker chips on days 2 and 3. It was understood that he could keep the pennies after the study was over. Errors on later days of testing, however, continued to be high, 12.5% and 22%.

Within this experiment it is probably not possible to distinguish whether the deficits of P-W children are in scanning speed or some other component of STM processing. It could be that P-W children scan items so slowly that items are lost through decay or interference before they are reviewed. Alternatively, there may be major differences between P-W and undifferentiated retarded subjects in the capacity of STM, in the rate of decay of items in short term storage, or in their susceptibility to interference.

What does seem clear is that some component(s) of STM in P-W children is impaired compared to undifferentiated retarded children.

EXPERIMENT 4

It is possible that the high error rates of P-W subjects on the STM scanning task do not reflect differences in STM processing, but in some other component of STM. If subjects fail to identify the stimulus accurately during the brief display period, error rates would increase. Thus, the high error rate of P-W subjects may reflect differences in access times to long term memory (LTM) information (the names of the digits or colors) rather than problems with STM processing.

Posner, Boies, Eichelman, and Taylor (1969) developed a letter comparison task which measures how quickly subjects can access well known information in their long term memories. Subjects are asked to decide whether two letters have the same name. The stimuli are physically identical (AA), identical in name but not physical characteristics (Aa), or different (AB). A large amount of data is available about adult performance on this task (Hunt, Frost, & Lenneborg, 1973; Posner, 1973). Typically it has been found that college subjects require an extra 80 milliseconds to make the "same" judgment when the letters have only name identity (NI) in common as opposed to both name and physical identity (PI). The additional time is presumed to be an index of the time necessary to access a highly overlearned piece of information—the name of a letter—from LTM.

If P-W subjects were able to perform as well as their undifferentiated retarded peers, it would strengthen the argument that their high error rates on the scanning task reflect differences in STM processing. The goal of the fourth experiment, therefore, was to determine whether P-W and undifferentiated retarded children had comparable LTM access speeds.

Method

Subjects Three types of subjects were tested: P-W, undifferentiated retarded, and normal children. Subject characteristics are shown in Table 12.4

Apparatus and Stimulus Materials Stimulus slides contained two letters printed on a white background. The slides were presented with a carousel projector and reaction time was recorded from the onset of the slide to the response.

Procedure Subjects were tested individually in three sessions approximately 1 week apart. On one-half the trials the two letters had different names (AB). In the remaining trials, one-half the items were physically identical (AA). The other items shared the same name but were physically different (Aa). Subjects pressed buttons to indicate whether or not the two letters had the same name. A total of 96 trials was presented on each test day.

Results

Error Analysis Errors for all groups were rare, and there were no group differences in error rates. All subjects made more errors in the name identical (Aa) condition.

RT Analysis PI (AA) condition means were subtracted from the NI (Aa) condition means in order to yield a measure of the extra time required for access of the LTM code. Figure 12.5 shows the RTs for each

Table 12.4. Subject characteristics for experiment 4

Group	CA (years)	MA (years)	IQ
Retarded			
Prader-Willi	12.5	7.8	68
($n = 6$)	SD = 2.9	SD = 1.6	SD = 12.3
Older undifferentiated	14.3	10.4	65
($n = 10$)	SD = 9.0	SD = 1.7	SD = 9.6
Younger undifferentiated	11.5	7.3	74
($n = 10$)	SD = 1.2	SD = 1.2	SD = 9.1
Normal			
7-year-olds	7.4	8.7	114
($n = 10$)	SD = 0.35	SD = 1.3	SD = 14.6
10-year-olds	10.4	13.6	118
($n = 10$)	SD = 0.64	SD = 2.3	SD = 14.4
13-year-olds	13.4	15.1	112
($n = 10$)	SD = 0.62	SD = 0.77	SD = 9.0

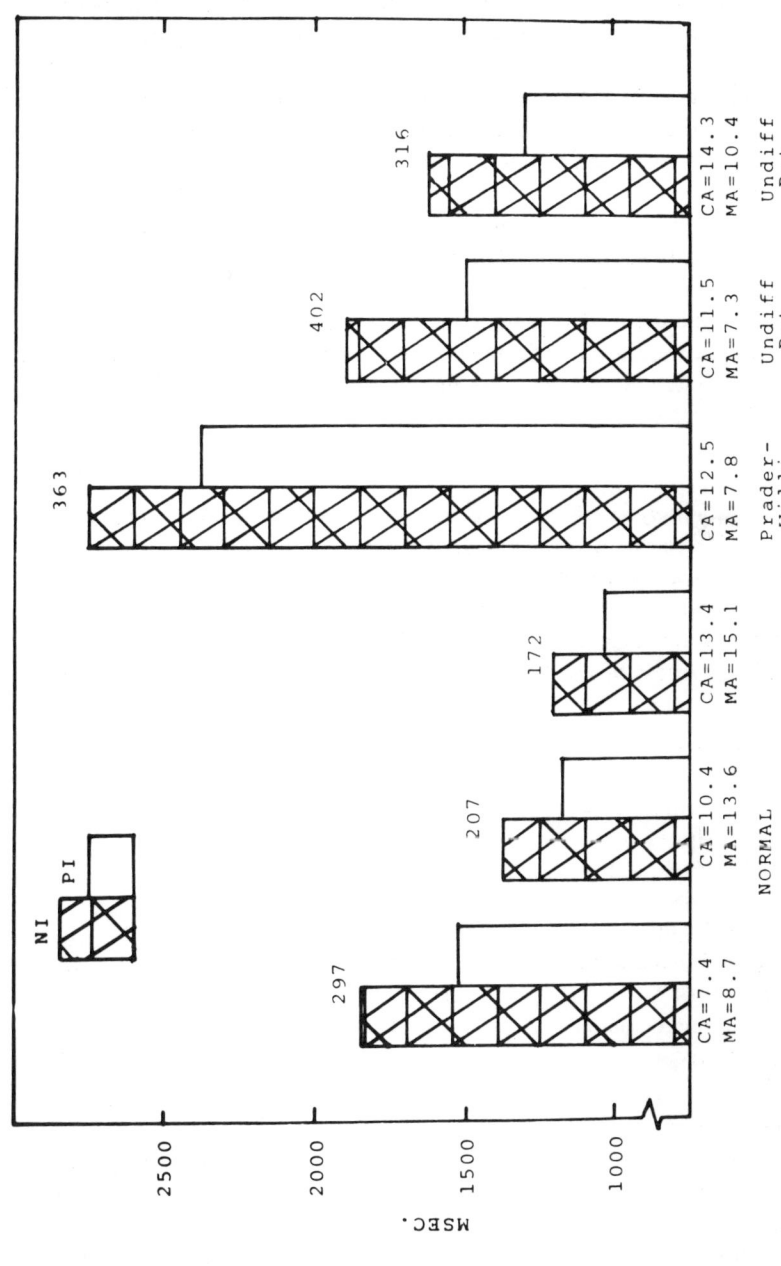

Figure 12.5. NI-PI comparisons for each group.

condition with the difference score printed at the top of each group's bar graph. It is these difference scores that are relevant to the question of LTM access speeds since the RT in both NI and PI conditions alone is obviously colored by each subject's gross RT. The group difference was significant ($p < 0.01$), but the retarded groups did not differ from one another and performed comparably to the 7-year-old normal children. Neither the day effect nor the group × day interaction was significant.

Discussion

No significant differences in LTM access speeds were detected between P-W and undifferentiated retarded subjects. Although reaction time for both PI and NI conditions varied widely across groups, with P-W children having the largest RTs, the difference between PI and NI scores appeared similar for all retarded groups. It is of course possible that the small size of the P-W group precluded the detection of significant group differences. The possibility of faster or slower LTM access by the P-W syndrome children cannot be discarded at this time. Further tests with more subjects are necessary.

It does seem likely that the difficulty P-W children experience with STM processing is related to particular deficits in encoding. Error rates for P-W subjects were generally low, as they were for all groups. The severe syndrome-specific problems seen in the previous experiments were not apparent when LTM access speeds were studied.

GENERAL DISCUSSION

The goal of these experiments has been to determine whether there are systematic differences in the cognitive capabilities of retarded individuals that vary with the etiology of their retardation.

Individuals with P-W syndrome appeared to have a pattern of cognitive processing different from what their global IQ score alone might predict. These mildly retarded children seemed to have particular difficulty with short term memory processing. They made mistakes identifying pictures that had just been presented. When required to hold three or four stimuli in STM, their error rate became substantial. Further tests are necessary in order to distinguish those aspects of STM that are impaired. Additionally, P-W subjects lost more information from memory over time. Previously seen items were not as familiar to them as to an undifferentiated retarded group. Their recognition memories did not manifest the characteristic developmental improvement seen in most children. On the other hand, the speed of their long term memory access to well known information seemed comparable to that of the undifferentiated retarded children of equivalent age.

It should be noted that the observed differences between the cognitive processing abilities of P-W and undifferentiated retarded children were not found after an arduous search through many experimental paradigms. Given the relative ease in identifying such striking deficits in so small a sample, it can only be hypothesized that many more differences between P-W and other retarded children exist.

REFERENCES

Brown, A. Context and recency cues in the recognition memory of retarded children and adolescents. *American Journal of Mental Deficiency,* 1972, *77,* 54-58.

Hunt, E., Frost, N., & Lenneborg, C. Individual differences in cognition: A new approach to intelligence. In G. Bower (Ed.), *The psychology of learning and motivation* (Vol. 7). New York: Academic Press, 1973.

Posner, M. Coordination of internal codes. In W. Chase (Ed.), *Visual information processing.* New York: Academic Press, 1973.

Posner, M.I., Boies, S.J., Eichelman, W.H., & Taylor, R.L. Retention of visual and name codes in single letters. *Journal of Experimental Psychology Monographs,* 1969, *79,* 1-16.

Sternberg, S. High-speed scanning in human memory. *Science,* 1966, *153,* 652-654.

chapter 13
SPEECH AND LANGUAGE CHARACTERISTICS OF CHILDREN WITH PRADER-WILLI SYNDROME

Cynthia Branson

> In this chapter Ms. Branson reports that she did not find enough common elements in the speech and language problems of 21 Prader-Willi syndrome patients to make possible the design of treatment strategies that could be generalized for the whole group. Individualized assessment and therapy, singly or in compatible small groups, is necessary.—*Eds.*

One objective of a speech and language evaluation is to determine whether an individual differs linguistically from age-mates. If linguistic differences are found, the speech and language pathologist is called upon to detail the nature of those differences in order to permit development of intervention plans. In examining a special population like the Prader-Willi (P-W) syndrome group, the evaluation process goes beyond analysis of individual data and attempts to identify common features typical of the group. If common speech and language behaviors can be found, treatment strategies that have proved effective can be generalized across subjects and therapy progress can be better predicted.

The following sections detail the speech and language findings for 21 youngsters diagnosed as having P-W syndrome. These children appeared heterogeneous in language comprehension and production abilities but showed some common features in speech-sound production skills.

Assessment strategies used in the evaluation of P-W youngsters varied as a function of age and developmental differences. The special linguistic characteristics of children at different functional levels demanded individually tailored evaluation procedures in order to test acquisition of linguistic milestones predicted for age or general level of functioning. Despite differences in methodology, the speech and language evaluations of the P-W population were consistent in terms of linguistic characteristics assessed. Comprehension and production of grammatical forms, word knowledge and ability to process major semantic notions carried in verbal input, and speech-sound production skills were evaluated in each case.

LANGUAGE SKILLS

Collective findings show the P-W group to be heterogeneous in terms of linguistic abilities. Slightly more than one-half of the youngsters seen (52%; $N = 11$) demonstrated comprehension and production abilities generally compatible with their overall cognitive level. Three of these subjects had language skills within the normal range; other members of this group showed language delays ranging from 1 to 4 years below their chronological ages. Older subjects differed most from age-mates in terms of the level of abstraction of information understood and produced.

The remaining P-W subjects ($N = 10$) presented uneven profiles characterized by comprehension skills (receptive language) significantly in advance of production skills (expressive language). With three noteworthy exceptions, analysis of production data from this group yielded no general patterns that might explain the discrepant receptive and expressive abilities.

The verbal performances of three youngsters from this high comprehension–low production group were exceptional. Two were diagnosed as apraxic, that is, production of speech was compromised by motor planning problems. In addition to manifesting many of the speech-sound production characteristics of developmental apraxia, these youngsters demonstrated the seriously delayed expressive language skills described as a feature of the disorder (Yoss & Darley, 1974). A third youngster showed marked word recall problems and disordered syntax. This child demonstrated delays as long as 18 seconds in length in picture-naming tasks where the stimuli had been practiced. Inability to recall needed verbal labels had impact on verbal fluency as seen in repetitions, additions, and circumlocutions in spontaneous speech. The youngster's disorganized syntax suggested the possibility of difficulty in recalling syntactic rules as well as specific verbal labels, although the fragmented nature of the utterances emitted made it difficult to separate the syntactical problems from the word-recall difficulties.

SPEECH-SOUND PRODUCTION SKILLS

The articulation skills of the P-W group are notable for the high frequency of problems. Seventeen of 21 subjects demonstrated atypical speech-sound production skills. Severity of articulation problems varied considerably, with some showing problems serious enough to render speech unintelligible most of the time and others presenting problems so subtle that listener understanding was unimpeded. The nature of the articulation deficits represented by the P-W group varied as well. Analysis of the data yielded two distinctive patterns of errors.

Pattern 1: Distortions Characterized by Nasal Air Emission

This pattern is interesting because of its unusual nature. Seven subjects showed nasal air emission in association with articulation of selected phonemes, namely sounds from the fricative (e.g. "f," "s"), affricate (e.g., "ch"), and ocassionally the plosive (e.g., "p," "b," "t") sound categories. This type of distortion error was noted inconsistently in most subjects, with no obvious cause. In the majority of cases presenting this type of articulation problem (four of seven), articulation of other consonants and vowels was not problematic.

In considering possible causes of this type of distortion error, two avenues were explored: structural deviations and faulty articulator placement. Part of the difficulty in determining which factor(s) might be contributing to inappropriate nasal air emissions is the invisibility of the sounds involved. For example, one is unable to directly examine articulatory contacts in the mouth during production of "ch" without sophisticated instruments. As a result, it was necessary to make some inferences about adequacy of velopharyngeal closure in connected speech based on performance of discrete speech-related tasks, such as sustained phonation of |a|, and listener judgments of resonance characteristics in connected speech. Six of the seven subjects were judged as having appropriate oral-nasal resonance balance. The single subject who was judged hypernasal in connected speech showed posterior movement of the velum on phonation of |a|, but the examiner was unable to observe whether there was adequate participation of the lateral and posterior pharyngeal walls in effecting closure, thus raising a question of velopharyngeal incompetency. Examination of bony structures in subjects showing this articulation pattern showed these structures to be adequate for speech-sound production.

Two additional subjects not evaluated by this examiner were reported as having hypernasal voice qualities particularly noticeable in connected speech. An oral peripheral exam was not completed on one of these subjects; therefore, no conclusions can be drawn regarding adequacy of velopharyngeal closure. The other subject's oral structures were examined and were found adequate for speech and language purposes.

There remains the question of faulty placement of the articulators for production of the fricative, affricate, and plosive sounds in question. While direct evidence is not available for the P-W population, a study by Peterson (1975) suggests a strong possibility that nasal air emission such as that noted in the P-W group is an artifact of articulator placement.

Lateral cephalometric films completed on Peterson's subjects with inappropriate nasal emission showed faulty tongue positioning with the dorsum elevated and the tongue tip malpositioned.

Pattern 2: Oral-Motor Difficulties

In eight of the subjects a significant oral-motor component was evident that had an impact on articulation proficiency. In six out of eight of these subjects there appeared to be a significant relationship between oral-motor coordination and speech-sound production skills. Intelligibility in connected speech was limited because of poor ability to perform rapid alternating tongue movements. Subjects had particular difficulty coordinating the finely graded articulatory gestures required in syllable-sequencing tasks where place and manner of articulation features varied. Regarding this oral-motor incoordination problem, the P-W group's history of hypotonia and fine motor problems is of interest.

Two children demonstrated motor-speech disorders of a different type. These subjects were diagnosed as apraxic, showing speech-sound production characteristics compatible with diagnostic criteria in the literature, namely, limited phonological repertoires for age, difficulty in sequencing novel phoneme combinations, inconsistent speech-sound errors, high frequency of omission errors, high frequency of multiple feature errors, and poor imitative skills. As previously noted, effectiveness in communciation of the apraxic children was very seriously compromised by their articulatory difficulties.

Other Articulation Deficits

Two children presented articulation problems without inappropriate nasal air escapage or oral-motor difficulties. Misarticulations evidenced by this group appeared to represent a mixture of delayed phonological development and faulty learning. These subjects had misarticulations that represented phonological processes seen in the speech of children approximately 2 to 3½ years of age. These types of errors, well described by Ingram (1976), illustrate systematic attempts by young children to simplify speech. Other misarticulations seen in this group are not so easily classified and do not so simply reflect delayed phonological development. These misarticulations, many of which differed drastically from target phonemes, exemplify faulty learning, the etiological basis for which remains unexplained.

MANAGEMENT IMPLICATIONS

Diagnostic experience with a large number of P-W youngsters shows that there are no generalizable treatment strategies for the language problems of this group because the language profiles of most of the youngsters lack common features. If one can assume that the academic programs of P-W children have language development as an emphasis, classroom intervention is probably appropriate for those who show language abilities commensurate with their general cognitive level. For those youngsters who show discrepant comprehension and production skills, individual or compatible small group speech and language therapy is warranted to develop expressive skills. Specific program goals should be individually tailored, and decisions regarding articulation therapy should be individually considered, based on the severity of the problem. In many youngsters distortion errors characterized by nasal emission, if present, may be clinically insignificant since speech intelligibility is not compromised. For those youngsters presenting oral-motor difficulties, speech therapy can be effective in improving precision of speech-related oral movements.

REFERENCES

Ingram, D. Current issues in child phonology. In D.M. Morehead & A.E. Morehead (Eds.), *Normal and deficient child language*. Baltimore: University Park Press, 1976.

Peterson, S.J. Nasal emission as a component of the misarticulation of sibilants and affricates. *Journal of Speech and Hearing Disorders,* 1975, *40*, 106-114.

Yoss, K.A., & Darley F.L. Developmental apraxia of speech in children with defective articulation. *Journal of Speech and Hearing Research,* 1974, *17*, 399-416.

chapter 14
A BEHAVIORAL APPROACH TO TREATMENT OF PRADER-WILLI SYNDROME

Barringer D. Marshall, Jr., Charles J. Wallace, John Elder, Karen Burke, Tim Oliver, and Richard Blackmon

> This chapter describes a successful weight reduction program for Prader-Willi syndrome clients in an institutional setting. The program is especially noteworthy because it does not involve a special diet or extensive staff time.—*Eds.*

Obesity and its associated complications pose the greatest threat to the health of individuals with Prader-Willi (P-W) syndrome. It is generally believed that P-W persons require fewer calories than the average non-affected person to lose weight or maintain an appropriate weight. Weight reduction, while often extremely difficult, has been accomplished by means of caloric restriction. Maintenance of weight loss has generally been less than satisfactory, although it is possible with continued careful control of the diet (Holm & Pipes, 1976; Pipes & Holm, 1973). Counseling of P-W children and responsible adults in areas of dietary restriction and limited access to food between meals has been stressed (Holm & Pipes, 1976). A "protein-sparing modified fast" has been recommended for weight reduction and maintenance (Bistrian, Blackburn, & Stanbury, 1977). Dextroamphetamine has been prescribed to control hyperphagia in certain clients and phenmetrazine has been said to be superior to amphetamines in this regard (Dunn, 1968; Zellweger, 1969). Simple behavior therapy procedures, such as social reinforcement, have been employed, but their overall contribution to the treatment is unclear in the absence of supportive data (Bistrian et al., 1977; Holm & Pipes, 1976). One report of the systematic application of behavioral techniques was extremely costly and

---

The opinions stated in this article are those of the authors and do not reflect the official policy of the California Department of Developmental Disabilities or of the Regents of the University of California.

ultimately had limited success (Thompson, Kodluboy, & Heston, 1980).

The primary goal of the authors in the development of a behavioral weight reduction program for hospitalized P-W adults was the modification of food-related behaviors both during and between meals. This was accomplished by contingent application of available reinforcers, in particular, food. P-W residents were given maximum responsibility for limiting their own food intake, and staff supervision was limited. Calorie counting and weighing devices were not employed because of the limited intelligence of some P-W individuals. Ingestion of unauthorized foods was anticipated and taken into consideration in the development of the program. After satisfactory weight loss was obtained, the program was modified in an attempt to provide generalization of treatment effects to other settings where supervision could be further reduced and where expertise in behavior therapy was not available.

METHOD

Setting

The treatment was developed and conducted at the Clinical Research Unit (CRU) of the Camarillo State Hospital-UCLA Neuropsychiatric Institute. The CRU is a 12-bed coed unit designed for the intensive treatment of persons with a variety of behavioral disorders. Additionally, research in the areas of psychopharmacology and behavior therapy has characterized the unit since its inception. Nursing personnel are responsible for the delivery of all treatment procedures. Fourteen nursing staff members provide average daily coverage of three personnel for day and evening shifts and two for the night shift. Additional staff include a full-time psychiatrist, a social worker, and a recreation therapist. Consultation is available from numerous other behavioral experts, including psychiatrists, psychologists, and research associates. The CRU now forms part of the Mental Health Clinical Research Center for the Study of Schizophrenia, recently established through a grant from the National Institute of Mental Health.

Standardized treatment programs apply to all CRU admissions. These programs were utilized in the treatment of P-W residents and included:

1. *Assault and property destruction.* Any observed incident of assault and/or property destruction resulted in from 15 minutes to 1 hour of timeout from reinforcement in a locked quiet room.
2. *Daily living skills.* A credit-incentive system (token economy) provided residents with increasing responsibility, autonomy, and privileges as they rose through the five levels of the system. Credits were given for

satisfactory task performance. A special meal program provided brief plate removals and fines for certain program violations. Credits earned were exchanged for privileges and tangible reinforcers.

3. *Personal hygiene.* Bathing was rated on three levels with credit given only for top performance. Grooming included washing the face and hands, oral hygiene, combing the hair, shaving (males), dressing neatly, and wearing matching socks with shoes tied. Credits were given for satisfactory performance without repeated prompting.

4. *Interpersonal behavior.* A rap group for residents and staff met twice each week. The first session provided an opportunity for participation in the development of programs and for dealing with problems among peers and staff. The second weekly session was a data review with feedback given on program performance and promotions and demotions made in the credit-incentive system. In assessing social interaction, the staff observed the residents and engaged them in conversation four times each day. Social behaviors and verbal and nonverbal conversational skills were rated.

In addition to the standard unit programs, the CRU has always maintained the capability to develop and apply highly individualized behavior programs for all residents. Thus, at times, the staff may be required to master nearly a dozen different treatment programs. Reliable data collection systems are fundamental to all CRU programs. All data are graphed nightly.

Subjects

Descriptive data concerning the four P-W residents are presented in Table 14.1. All four had histories of neonatal hypotonia, feeding problems, delayed developmental milestones, and onset in early childhood of hyperphagia and obesity. Each exhibited short stature, mental deficiency, self-abuse, ingestion of abnormal foods, small hands and feet, cryptorchidism and hypogonadism (males), obesity, and personality problems.

The first subject (S1) was discharged against medical advice before many of the program's components could be implemented. Therefore, much of the data pertain to three subjects only. Informed consent of each resident, or, if appropriate, guardian or conservator, was obtained prior to entry into the program. Individual approval for each subject was given by the hospital's Human Rights Committee.

Treatment Elements

Meal Program The program used the standard hospital meal minus gravies and high calorie salad dressings. Fresh or dietetic fruits were substituted for the usual high calorie desserts. The treatment consisted of

Table 14.1. Descriptive characteristics of subjects

Subject	Age	Sex	IQ	Height	Weight	
					Pretreatment	Posttreatment
S1	21	M	80	56 in. (142.24 cm)	180 lb. (81.8 kg)	102 lb. (46.36 kg)
S2	21	F	70	56 in. (142.24 cm)	170 lb. (77.27 kg)	88 lb. (46 kg)
S3	20	F	60	60 in. (152.4 cm)	219 lb. (90.09 kg)	125 lb. (56.82 kg)
S4	26	M	50	58 in. (147.32 cm)	235 lb. (107.72 kg)	100 lb. (45.45 kg)

four phases. In the initial phase the staff member divided the meal and chose the half-portion that the resident was to consume. In subsequent phases the resident assumed the responsibility for dividing food and choosing and consuming no more than one-half of any portion. In all phases the resident's meal was under the control of a surpervising staff member, the monitor. Division of food portions began only at a signal from the monitor, and the resident was not allowed to eat any half-portion until told to do so by the monitor. Decisions made by the monitor concerning violations of this program were final and discussion was not permitted.

The meal program was determined by the hospital dietitian to provide approximately 1,000 cal per day including 100 g of carbohydrate, 55 g of protein, and 40 g of fat. The dietitian calculated a potential calcium deficit and 60 mg of calcium supplement was provided each day in the form of one 325-mg calcium lactate tablet. Supplemental vitamins were also prescribed on a daily basis. Ground privileges were permitted on a weekly basis and were contingent upon a weekly weight loss of at least 1 pound and no more than two violations of the meal program in the preceding week. When residents had ground privileges they were also eligible for bedtime snacks and could purchase, through credits, one dietetic treat per day from the unit canteen. Division of snacks was also required. Caloric content of approved snacks was not calculated. At times, P-W residents regurgitated and rechewed their food; meals were then limited to tea and toast for 24 hours, as is the case in the CRU for all residents with gastrointestinal upset.

Phase 1 The monitor divided one separate portion of food at a time from the resident's meal onto each of two separate empty dinner plates. One of these plates was placed directly before the resident in normal meal position and the other was placed immediately adjacent. The monitor chose the half-portion to be consumed and this was placed on the plate immediately before the resident. The resident consumed each half-portion, one at a time, as it was divided. The extra half-portions were allowed to accumulate on the adjacent dinner plate and were later discarded. Before the start of the meal, beverages were divided and selected or, where appropriate, a mark was made no more than halfway down the side of the beverage container. Beverages were then consumed at the resident's own pace during the meal. The resident was permitted to indicate the order in which portions were to be divided and consumed.

Phase 2 This phase proceeded exactly as did phase 1 with the major exception that the resident was responsible for the division of food and for choosing the appropriate half-portions. Thirty seconds were allowed for division of each portion.

Phase 3 Only one empty dinner plate was employed and this was placed directly before the resident. The resident divided one portion at a time onto this plate leaving at least one-half of each portion on the plate originally containing the meal. Division of each portion was checked before the next was divided, but no food was consumed until the entire meal had been divided. The plate containing the excess food was placed adjacent to the plate in normal meal position during the consumption of food.

Phase 4 This phase proceeded exactly as did phase 3 except that all portions were divided and chosen before inspection by the monitor. A total of 30 sec per portion (e.g., five portions equals 2½ minutes) was permitted.

Contingencies Violations of the meal program resulted in the application of one of several contingencies as described in Table 14.2. The principal reinforcer applied in the P-W meal program was food. Con-

Table 14.2. Meal program—violations and contingencies

Phase	Violation	Contingency
1	a. Began to eat before being told to do so	Lost portion
	b. Ate food from adjacent plate	Meal terminated
	c. Ate food from monitor's plate	Meal terminated and next meal lost
	d. Drank from second beverage container or below mark on container	Meal terminated
	e. Ate food from any other source during meal (table, other resident, etc.)	Lost remainder of meal and next meal
	f. Ate unauthorized food between meals	Lost next meal
2	a. through f.	Same as phase 1
	g. Began to divide before being told to do so	Lost portion
	h. Took more than 30 seconds	Lost portion
	i. Mixed portions	Lost portions mixed
3	a.	Lost entire meal
	e., f.	Same as phase 1
	g., i.	Same as phase 2
4	a.	Same as phase 3
	c., f.	Same as phase 1
	i.	Same as phase 2
	j. Took more than total of 30 seconds per portion to divide	Lost meal

tingencies included loss of part or all of a meal depending upon the violation. The loss of more than two meals consecutively was specifically prohibited.

Generalization Program The goal of the generalization program was to maintain appropriate eating behaviors and to stabilize the weight of each subject within an appropriate range. The program attempted the gradual reduction of monitoring and the ultimate termination of monitoring and all meal contingencies.

Phase 5 The resident took a plate containing the full meal and an empty plate to a table in a separate area of the dining room away from the staff. Division proceeded unmonitored as in phase 4 of treatment. The resident indicated the completion of division to a staff member and, unless otherwise instructed, carried both plates and rejoined the other residents at the regular dining table. At seven randomly scheduled meals per week an individual staff member unobtrusively observed the time required for division and then monitored results of division before the resident left the dividing table. Meal contingencies applied only to the seven randomly scheduled meals.

Phase 6 This phase proceeded exactly as did phase 5 except that while data were collected on the seven monitored meals no meal contingencies applied.

Phase 7 No monitoring of eating was done. No food-related data were collected except weekly weight.

Food Selection In addition to the meal program, residents were given instructions in discrimination among high, medium, and low calorie foods. This was accomplished in a single session by discussion and demonstration of the relative caloric values of various types of food (e.g., beef, pork, vegetables, fruits, desserts, dairy products, and cereals) and of foods with different characteristics (e.g., fried versus broiled, oily versus dry). Pictures of foods were used.

Exercise Program A program of gradually increasing exercises was designed to improve the general physical condition of each subject and to aid weight loss. Exercises consisted primarily of daily walking and/or jogging. During baseline the physical activity of the residents consisted primarily of daily cleanup tasks. During the exercise phase residents gradually increased their daily walking distance from several hundred meters to 3 kilometers. Distances were increased weekly and limited by the tolerance of the residents, who were instructed that exercise is good for the heart, lungs, muscles, weight, and emotional state. After each exercise period they recited these reasons, were praised, and were given credits. Thrice weekly stretching exercises and calisthenics were recently added.

Requests for Positive Social Reinforcement Once each week (the day before weigh-in) for 6 weeks, residents were engaged in a 30-minute role-play session designed to instruct them in appropriate means of requesting social reinforcement for weight loss. For example, "I lost___ pounds! Don't I look thinner?"

Assessment and Data Collection

Weight Residents were weighed once each week on rising, in their pajamas and after voiding.

Meal Violations A separate letter of the alphabet was assigned to each distinct violation of the meal program. At each meal, the monitor recorded, in the appropriate space on the data sheet, the letter for each violation that occurred.

Food Selection Prior to instruction in the discrimination of foods, residents were given pictures of various foods and asked to sort them into groups of high, medium, and low calories. After instruction the same test was administered.

Exercise Program Once each week a step test was administered to each resident. A single 8-inch step was placed against a wall and a mark was made on the floor 3 feet from the step. Residents stood at the floor mark, walked to the step, mounted it, then stepped backward off the step and returned to the floor mark without turning around. They repeated this activity for exactly 5 minutes and were encouraged to move as rapidly as could be tolerated. Residents rested for 30 seconds after completion of the test and the posttest 30-second pulse rate was determined.

Requests for Positive Social Reinforcement Residents were unobtrusively observed one morning each week for 5½ hours after weigh-in. The number of requests for positive social reinforcement for weight loss was noted. Baseline and posttraining data were recorded.

Aggression Incidents of observed acts of assault and/or property destruction were recorded on a daily data sheet for each resident.

Metabolic Effects Once weekly, on the morning that the residents were weighed, a urine sample was obtained from each subject and semiquantitative determinations of urinary glucose and ketones were made.

RESULTS

Weight Loss

Weight loss data are presented in Figure 14.1. The mean weight loss per resident was 97.5 pounds (44.32 kg). There was an average rate of weight loss of 7.1 pounds (3.23 kg) monthly for each resident for the first 12 months of treatment.

Meal Violations

S1 averaged 19.5 violations of the Prader-Willi meal program per month,

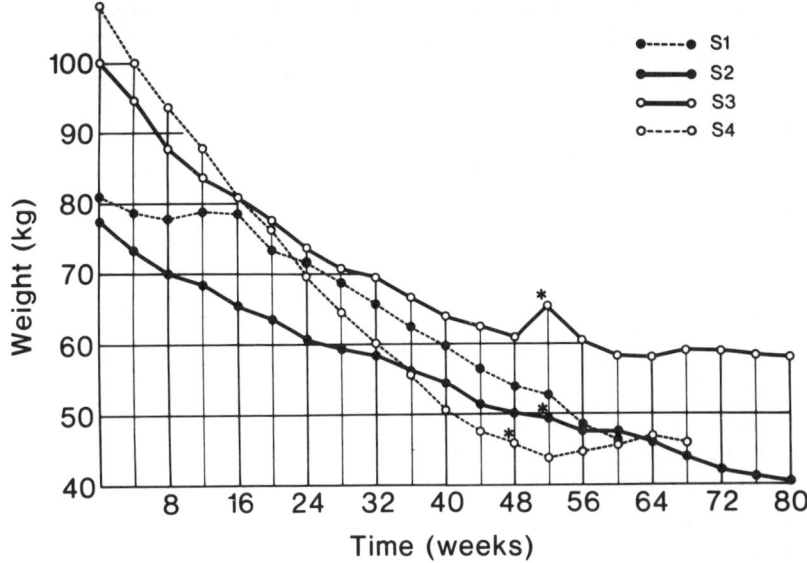

Figure 14.1. Weight loss of subjects during 80 weeks of therapy *(began generalization phase.)

while S2, S3, and S4 averaged 9.0, 3.9, and 14.5 monthly violations respectively.

Food Selection
Table 14.3 presents the pre-post results on the calorie-sorting test. All residents improved from pre- to posttest, even though pretest scores were unexpectedly high.

Exercise Program
Individual results of the weekly step test are presented in Table 14.4. The overall mean 30-second pulse rate for these three patients was 46.09 during the baseline phase and 40.3 for the treatment phase.

Requests for Positive Social Reinforcement
Table 14.5 shows that the number of requests for reinforcement made after each Thursday morning weigh-in increased, after role-played training sessions, for each resident.

Aggression
The mean number of monthly incidents of assault and/or property destruction for all residents was 4.3. Individual monthly averages were 3.5

Table 14.3. Food selection—percent correct responses on calorie-level sorting test

Subjects	Pretest	Posttest	Increment
S2	62.5	87.5	+25.0
S3	67.5	90.0	+22.5
S4	62.5	70.0	+7.5

Table 14.4. Mean 30-second pulse rate

Subject	Baseline	Exercise Phase	Change
S2	46.2 ($n = 5$)[a]	42.8 ($n = 13$)	−3.4
S3	43.6 ($n = 6$)	39.4 ($n = 19$)	−4.2
S4	48.3 ($n = 15$)	38.7 ($n = 11$)	−9.6

[a] n, number of sessions per phase.

Table 14.5 Mean number of requests for social reinforcement

Subjects	Baseline	Posttraining	Change
S2	3.5 ($n = 2$)[a]	9.1 ($n = 7$)	+5.6
S3	1.0 ($n = 5$)	6.8 ($n = 10$)	+5.8
S4	12.0 ($n = 8$)	16.5 ($n = 8$)	+4.5

[a] n, number of sessions per phase.

for S1, 3.5 for S2, 0.90 for S3, and 12 for S4. The incidence of these behaviors intensified slightly over time for S4, remained essentially unchanged for S1, and showed a gradual but definite reduction for S2 and S3.

Metabolic Effects

A trace of ketonuria was detected in the urine of S4 on a few occasions. Ketones were not observed in the urine of any other resident. Glycosuria was not evident.

Self-help Skills

On admission to the unit, task performance was usually limited by shortness of breath, but weight reduction and gradual increase of exercise tolerance ultimately led to outstanding execution of chores ranging from room cleanup to folding laundry to mopping halls. Table manners, grooming, and bathing, often deficient on admission, were promptly remediated and maintained at a high level as a result of the credit economy. Personal hygiene was a problem in two areas—incontinence and toothbrushing. Residents were often incontinent of urine or feces or both, but weight loss was usually sufficient to resolve this problem. On the other hand, severely inadequate oral hygiene was extremely resistant to improvement. Promotion within the credit economy was at times limited as a result of fines levied in response to aggression, self-abuse, or other inappropriate behaviors. Mendacity and artifice characterized attempts to avoid the application of contingencies for unseemly behaviors.

DISCUSSION

Experience with this program indicated that food-related behaviors of adult P-W residents can be modified through the contingent application of food as the reinforcer. Weight reduction was satisfactorily accomplished with a prescribed diet of some 1,000 calories daily without continuous monitoring for unauthorized food intake. In spite of the fact that excess food was left on the table during meals as a form of temptation, the staff monitor did not need to maintain continuous contact with the residents but was able to move about the dining room observing other patients while continuing to monitor P-W residents. Residents clearly tolerated the dietary restriction with little psychological or metabolic difficulty.

Occasional disruptive temper tantrums occurred following the application of meal contingencies, but these usually took place when the resident had been previously agitated by some non-meal-related incident. It is also clear that P-W residents were capable of assuming at least limited responsibility for choosing appropriate quantities of food in the presence of supervision and effective contingencies. The program is low in cost, and the staff required limited training for its delivery. One staff member can easily monitor three or four P-W residents during meals, and continuous observation of between-meal behavior is not required. Extensive laboratory studies are not necessary as long as urinary ketone determinations and simple hematologic and urine studies reveal no significant abnormalities. Residents should have periodic physical examinations and a physician should establish the appropriate targeted weight range for each P-W person.

Significant behavioral excesses, not entirely resolved by treatment interventions, included temper tantrums, aggression, theft, and self-abuse. Real or imagined slights, injustices, or frustrations, even when apparently insignificant, often led to extreme bellicosity. The behavior of the residents escalated within minutes or hours from loud verbal hostility to self-abuse and acts of aggression and/or property destruction. These temper tantrums, more often than not unrelated to food, persisted up to several hours and were ignored except when it was necessary to consequate belligerent acts. In addition to food, stolen objects usually consisted of money or clothing. Residents were rarely caught in the act of theft of nonfood items. The behavior was infrequent and not significantly affected by any contingencies. Head banging, self-inflicted bites, face slapping, and highly abortive "suicidal" gestures often accompanied tantrums, but the most common form of self-abuse was gouging and picking at skin. This behavior, often surreptitious, occurred as often as several times a day and frequently was not associated with flare-ups of temper. Partial suppression was effected with credit fines.

A number of other highly interesting sidelights and problems have developed during this study with P-W residents, particularly with regard to parental involvement. Following publication of a previous article briefly outlining this program (Marshall, 1978), the parent of one young P-W adult called the CRU for further information and employed the meal program in her home. Preliminary reports indicated at least partial success. In spite of family counseling and training of parents in the meal program, P-W residents often gain weight during home visits. A mother, mildly obese herself, took advantage of her daughter's half-portion program during home visits by consuming no food except the remaining one-half of her daughter's meal. Regrettably, this same parent stated quite frankly, "I just cannot deny her any food." A P-W resident on a home visit forfeited a meal when she ate garbage but was then given a piece of birthday cake. The parent of one resident sends bags of candy to her son, ostensibly for him to give to his girl friend. The boyfriend of another resident, also a Camarillo State Hospital resident, prefers that she remain obese and often finds means of providing her with large quantities of candy even when she is restricted to the unit. A parent, after stating repeatedly his determination to have his son lose weight and complete the program, removed his son from treatment before this was fully accomplished.

A difficulty with this meal program is its inflexibility. The program was especially designed to avoid calorie counting and individualization of diets. It is not appropriate for children and young adolescents because specificity of diet under careful supervision is necessary to meet their growth requirements (Holm & Pipes, 1976; Pipes & Holm, 1973). This is an important limitation because it can be expected that the most effective long term treatment would require early intervention in childhood. While it appears that the majority of adult P-W residents will achieve weight reduction with the dietary program described in this chapter, it is clear that there were wide variations in rate and stabilization of weight loss. Some of this diversity may be accounted for by individual variations in the amounts of unauthorized foods consumed, but it is doubtful that this fully accounts for the differences. For example, a dietary supplement of 700 cal per day was required to prevent excessive weight reduction for S4, whose weight loss was extreme. Food supplements were employed because effective generalization was considered more likely if the specific meal program was not modified. On the other hand, it was found necessary to accept a weight of approximately 125 pounds (56.82 kg) for S3 whose appropriate weight would be 100 to 105 pounds (45.5 to 47.7 kg). She had fewer violations of the meal program and therefore had fewer dietary restrictions. Also, of all residents treated, she showed the least interest in weight loss.

The generalization program employed in the CRU has met with mixed success. S2 completed this program without difficulty and maintained her appropriate weight for several weeks without supervision, restriction, or contingencies. S3 and S4, both with somewhat lower IQs, had difficulty. S3 never completed generalization and it was necessary to maintain all contingencies to prevent weight gain. On the other hand, S4 had early difficulties with generalization but ultimately maintained his appropriate weight for 4 months without restriction or contingencies.

Once it was demonstrated that weight loss could be accomplished in the CRU, the major area of concern was off-unit generalization of treatment effects. All residents have now been discharged. S1, who experienced no generalization procedures in the unit and was placed in a totally unsupervised residential care facility, regained 64 pounds (29.9 kg) in 1 year. S2, placed in a work/training center with no mealtime supervision, was, most unfortunately, given a job working in a kitchen. She regained 54 pounds (24.54 kg) in 10 months. She has, however, requested readmission to the CRU for another opportunity to lose weight. S3 was transferred to an open unit for the mentally retarded at Camarillo State Hospital. The P-W meal program was not implemented and no contingencies were placed on her food-related behaviors or weight. A 17-pound (7.72 kg) weight gain occurred during 2½ months. S4 was transferred to a locked mental retardation unit with strong staff leadership. He continues to divide his food scrupulously without specific contingencies or consistent supervision; however, his ground privileges have been made contingent upon maintenance of appropriate weight. A 3-month follow-up revealed no net gain or loss of weight.

Persons affected by P-W syndrome suffer the cardiopulmonary problems and disorder of carbohydrate metabolism typically associated with morbid obesity. One P-W person, 63 inches (160.02 cm) tall and weighing 360 pounds (163.63 kg), died suddenly while awaiting admission to the CRU. Another CRU referral, height 58 inches (147.32 cm), weighed 270 pounds (122.32 kg), developed severe heart failure before she could be admitted. All subjects evinced marked restriction of exercise tolerance and shortness of breath even at rest. Certainly, the long term prevention or relief of complications can best be accomplished by effective, lasting weight control. While the problems associated with weight loss and maintenance have not been fully resolved, some tentative conclusions are suggested by the experiences in this study:

1. Adult P-W residents can be assisted to lose weight even without their full cooperation.
2. The interest of P-W residents in, and personal reinforcement from, weight loss and maintenance may be significant, particularly if this enthusiasm is maintained after completion of treatment.
3. The success of the early phases of generalization is probably important but prolonged maintenance of appropriate weight in the treatment setting, without formal and overt reinforcement contingencies, may be essential for an ultimately successful outcome.
4. Once the residents leave the CRU it is doubtful that treatment effects can be maintained without at least minimal supervision and contingencies. This would appear to be fundamental to the ultimate success of the program, but it is not known whether any community-based residential care facility in California exists where this can be accomplished.
5. With minimal training the program can probably be applied in any setting capable of providing the limited supervision and control necessary.
6. The best long term results should be accomplished by avoiding hospitalization and implementing the program at the P-W person's place of residence.
7. Sufficient experience or data have not yet been accumulated to determine the characteristics of P-W individuals that may be associated with variations in outcome.

ACKNOWLEDGMENTS

The authors gratefully acknowledge the contribution of the Clinical Research Unit nursing personnel to the development of this program, and to its effective consistent delivery. Their unflagging efforts, frequently under very trying circumstances, have made this chapter possible. The support and encouragment of Clinton Rust, M.P.A., and Doug Van Meter, B.S. (Executive Director and Clinical Director, respectively, of Camarillo State Hospital), have been vital to the authors.

REFERENCES

Bistrian, B.R., Blackburn, G.L., & Stanbury, J.B. Metabolic aspects of a protein-sparing modified fast in the dietary management of Prader-Willi obesity. *The New England Journal of Medicine,* 1977, *296,* 774-779.

Dunn, H.G. The Prader-Labhardt-Willi syndrome: Review of the literature and report of nine cases. *Acta Paediatrica Scandinavica,* 1968, Suppl. 186, 2-38.

Holm, V.A., & Pipes, P.L. Food and children with Prader-Willi syndrome. *American Journal of Disease of Children,* 1976, *130,* 1063-1067.

Marshall, B.D. Behavioral treatment of Prader-Willi syndrome. *The Gathered View,* 1978, *4,*(6), 4-5.

Pipes, P.L., & Holm, V.A. Weight control of children with Prader-Willi syndrome. *Journal of the American Dietetic Association,* 1973, *62,* 520-524.

Thompson, T., Kodluboy, S., & Heston, L. Behavioral treatment of obesity in Prader-Willi syndrome. *Behavior Therapy,* 1980, *11,* 588-593.

Zellweger, H. The HHHO or Prader-Willi syndrome. *Birth Defects: Original Article Series,* 1969, *5*(2), 15-17.

chapter 15
MAINTENANCE OF PROGRAMMED WEIGHT LOSS IN PATIENTS WITH PRADER-WILLI SYNDROME

Glenn Hirsch and Karl Altman

In this chapter the authors describe a weight loss and weight maintenance program involving caloric restriction, self-monitoring, and contingency-contracting that was used for two Prader-Willi syndrome adolescents. Contingency contracting was found to be necessary for long term maintenance of the weight losses.—*Eds*.

Attempts to control the obesity of individuals with Prader-Willi (P-W) syndrome have involved either dietary management alone or dietary management with the use of behavior modification techniques. Most programs using dietary restrictions alone have successfully produced short term weight loss but have been less successful in altering the atypical eating behaviors associated with the syndrome (Coplin, Hine, & Gormican, 1976; Evans, 1964; Jancar, 1971; Juul & Dupont, 1967; Laurance, 1967). Programs using dietary restriction and behavior modification have produced both short term weight losses (Heiman, 1978) and an increase in the frequency of behaviors incompatible with inappropriate eating, e.g., exercise and daily self-monitoring of weight and caloric intake (Altman, Bondy, & Hirsch, 1978). While it is possible to produce short term weight loss in P-W individuals, it is difficult to maintain the loss over time. Both Evans (1964) and Laurance (1967) reported failure of their subjects to maintain weight losses. Following termination of dietary restriction many of their subjects gained back all of the weight lost and, in some cases, became even more obese. However, Holm and Pipes (1976) and Pipes and Holm (1973) reported on 14 P-W individuals, 12 of whom maintained weight losses of 3 to 40 kg (6.6 to 88 pounds) for periods

---

Salary support for this project was provided by DHEW Grants MCT-000407-20-0 and MCT-5PO1HD00870-14. Space in which to conduct the project was made possible by NIH Grant HD-0258/10.

ranging from 10 months to 6 years, 7 months. In addition, Altman et al. (1978) produced long term weight losses totalling 29 kg (65 pounds) and 14 kg (30 pounds) in two P-W subjects over a 2-year, 9-month period.

In summary, programs using dietary restriction alone or dietary restriction plus behavior modification have produced short term weight losses in P-W individuals. However, only two studies have reported long term maintenance of these losses.

Because obesity and inappropriate eating behaviors are lifelong complications of P-W syndrome (Holm & Pipes, 1976; Pipes & Holm, 1973) it is important that any weight loss and improved eating behavior in these individuals be maintained over time. While such maintenance has been demonstrated in two weight loss programs, the variables responsible for maintenance were not isolated.

Stokes and Baer (1977) suggested that maintenance will most likely occur if specific maintenance strategies are built into behavior-change programs. Adult weight loss programs have demonstrated the effectiveness of several such maintenance strategies, including self-monitoring of daily weight and caloric intake and contingency contracting (Abramson, 1977). These techniques have proved effective in producing weight loss in P-W individuals (Altman et al., 1978), but the value of these techniques for maintaining weight loss was not fully demonstrated.

The purpose of this report is to review the weight loss strategies used in the Altman et al. (1978) weight loss program, to describe the incorporation of these techniques into a 3-year maintenance program, and to assess the effectiveness of these techniques for producing maintenance of weight loss.

METHOD

Subjects

At the time of initial referral the first subject (S1) was 18 years old, had a height of 145 cm, weighed 111 kg (244 pounds) and produced test scores in the mildly retarded to dull-normal range of intelligence. She had spent 6 months prior to referral in transactional analysis therapy during which she maintained a weight of 91 kg (200 pounds). When referred, S1 exhibited symptoms of anoxia, and it was the "opinion" of the referring physician that continued weight gain could result in her premature death.

The second subject (S2) was 13 years old at the time of referral, had a height of 130 cm, and weighed 55 kg (121 pounds). Testing showed her to be functioning in the moderately retarded range of intelligence.

Based on clinical findings (e.g., infant hypotonia, early onset of obesity, autogenic skin lesions, food stealing, and mental retardation), a diagnosis of P-W syndrome was made for both subjects.

Procedure

S1 and S2 were involved in both weight loss and maintenance programs.

Weight Loss Program

The weight loss program, described in detail by Altman et al. (1978) is only summarized here. Table 15.1 lists subject behaviors monitored and consequated during the weight loss and maintenance programs. Program components were gradually introduced across four program phases as described below.

Phase 1: Baseline Both subjects were weighed weekly by a parent or caregiver but were not encouraged to weigh independently or take an interest in their own weight.

Phase 2: Self-Monitoring Subjects monitored their own morning weight, daily caloric intake, and exercise, while parents or caregivers recorded food-stealing frequency. For self-monitoring of caloric intake a system was used that converted calories to food-point equivalents (*Kilocalorie controlled diets*, Note 1). This system enabled the subjects to record each food item consumed and its calorie-point value. Also, behavioral contracts (DeRisi & Butz, 1975) specifying consequences for appropriate and inappropriate *self-monitoring* behavior were introduced. Subjects could earn reinforcers of their own choosing by meeting contract-specified criteria.

Phase 3: Reinforced Decreased Caloric Intake and Weight Loss Reinforcement for decreased caloric intake and weight loss was introduced gradually. Contracts were first revised so that decreased caloric intake for one meal was reinforced. After 1 week, reinforcement was introduced for staying within total daily caloric intake limits (1,000 cal for S1; 1,275 cal for S2) and for weekly weight loss (0.45 kg for both subjects). The contract of S1 also included reinforcement for 15 minutes of daily exercise.

Punishment for food stealing was introduced. Punishment involved aversive consequences (e.g., public apologies, monetary fines, and loss of privileges) which were delivered immediately following each food-stealing incident.

Phase 4: Reinforced Weight Loss Subjects continued daily monitoring of exercise, caloric intake, and weight, but only weekly weight loss and exercise (S1 only) were reinforced. Because S2 had failed to lose weight in the last 5 weeks of phase 3, her daily caloric intake was reduced to 1,125 cal. Food stealing continued to be punished.

Table 15.1. Behaviors monitored and consequated during weight loss program

Program	Phase	Monitored behavior	By whom	Frequency	Consequences
Weight loss	1	Weight	Parent/caregiver	Daily	None
	2	Weight	Subject	Daily	Reinforcement for accurate monitoring
		Caloric intake	Subject	Daily	Reinforcement for accurate monitoring
		Exercise (S1 only)	Subject	Daily	Reinforcement for accurate monitoring
	3	Weight	Subject	Daily	Reinforcement for weight loss
		Caloric intake	Subject	Daily	Reinforcement for decreased caloric intake
		Exercise (S1 only)	Subject	Daily	Reinforcement for increased exercise
	4	Food stealing	Parent/caregiver	Daily	Punishment
		Weight	Subject	Daily	Reinforcement for weight loss
		Caloric intake	Subject	Daily	None
		Exercise (S1 only)	Subject	Daily	Reinforcement for sustained exercise
Maintenance	Pre-goal weight attainment	Food stealing	Parent/caregiver	Daily	Punishment
	Post-goal weight attainment (S2 only)	Same as in phase 4 above			
		Weight	Subject	Daily	Periodic verbal reinforcement
		Caloric intake	Subject	Daily	None
		Food stealing	Parent/caregiver	Daily	Punishment

Maintenance Program

The maintenance program was introduced after reinforced weight loss had been in effect for 8 weeks. Maintenance was initiated by fading contact between subjects and therapists. Weekly phone contact was faded to twice, then once a month, and home visits were reduced from once a month to every 3 to 4 months. This fading substantially reduced the amount of professional time required to carry out the program.

At the beginning of the maintenance program, long term goal weights of 40.9 kg (90 pounds) and 38.6 kg (85 pounds) were selected for S1 and S2, respectively. Goal weights were based on the upper age limit of the height-weight percentile chart developed at the Children's Medical Center, Boston (Vickers & Stuart, 1943) and were determined by choosing the weight corresponding to the height percentile of each subject. Acceptable goal weight ranges (goal weight ± 1 kg) were also specified at this time.

Before goal weight attainment, procedures used in the reinforced weight loss phase were continued in the maintenance phase (self-monitoring of daily weight and caloric intake, reinforcement for weekly weight loss, and punishment for food stealing). When goal weight was attained (S2 only), reinforcement was gradually faded. For 4 weeks following goal weight attainment, S2 was reinforced for weekly maintenance of goal weight while her daily caloric limit was gradually increased to and maintained at 1,275 cal. After 4 weeks, contingency contracting was discontinued and reinforcement was faded to periodic verbal praise for weight maintenance. Self-monitoring of daily weight and caloric intake and punishment for food stealing continued. Weight checks were made once every 3 months by the family physician of S2 or the therapist involved in the maintenance program.

One year after contingency contracting was discontinued, S2's weight returned to a level above the goal weight range. Consequently, the daily limit of 1,125 cal and contingency contracting were reintroduced.

Setting

S1's weight loss and maintenance programs were carried out in three settings: an inpatient hospital ward (phases 1, 2, and 3), a residential home for retarded adults (phase 4 and the first 16 months of the maintenance program), and the home of the parents (2-month baseline phase 3 and 4 and maintenance program months 17 to 41). S2's weight loss and maintenance programs were carried out in the home of her parents.

Design

A multiple baseline design and a reversal (S1 only) were used to evaluate weight loss program effectiveness. The occurrence of both unprogrammed reversals (S1) and programmed fading of techniques (S2) allowed for evaluation of procedures used during the maintenance program.

RESULTS

Reliability checks for daily weight and caloric intake were made periodically throughout the maintenance phase. Subject data were compared with data recorded independently by parents or caregivers, and reliability was calculated for each sample by dividing the number of agreements by the total number of comparisons and multiplying the quotient by 100. For eight reliability samples with S2, the mean reliability was 100% for weight (all samples had 100% agreement) and 90% (range 80% to 100%) for caloric intake. Mean reliability for S1's nine reliability checks was 83% for weight (range 0 to 100%) and 100% for caloric intake (all samples had 100% agreement).

Results of the weight loss program were presented previously (Altman et al., 1978) and are summarized here.

For S1 the weight loss program resulted in a loss of 19 kg (41.8 pounds), 17% of her baseline weight of 111 kg (244 pounds). Figure 15.1 illustrates S1's body weight over 39 months of the maintenance program. Over the first 32 months of the maintenance program, S1 lost 14 kg

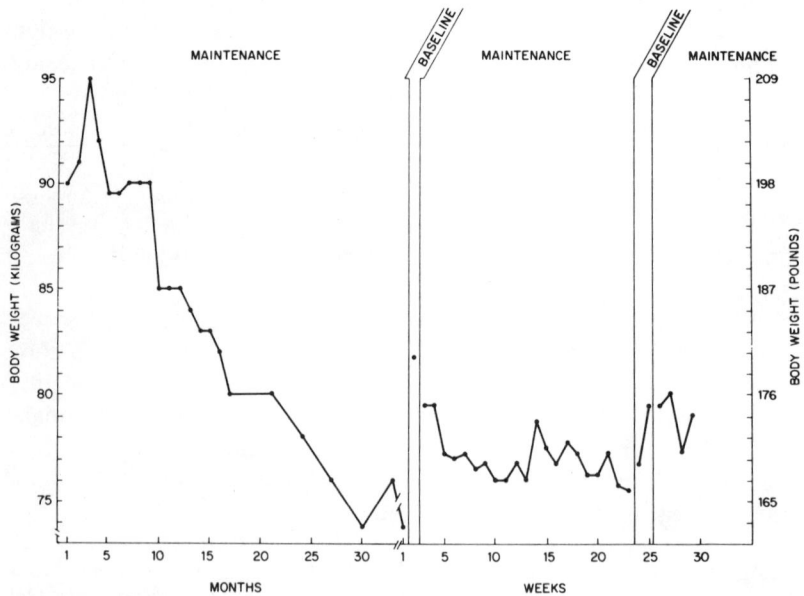

Figure 15.1. Body weight for S1 across consecutive program months and weeks for alternating maintenance and baseline conditions.

(30.8 pounds). During a 1-week return to baseline (no program was in effect), S1 gained 8 kg (17.6 pounds) from the low weight of the previous week. Following reinstatement of the maintenance program, S1 lost 6.25 kg (13.75 pounds). A second 2-week return to baseline resulted in her gaining 4 kg (8.8 pounds). Reintroduction of maintenance procedures produced a loss of 0.5 kg (1.1 pounds) over a 4-week period.

During the weight loss program S2 lost 9 kg (19.8 pounds) or 16% of her baseline body weight of 55 kg (121 pounds). Figure 15.2 shows S2's body weight over 35 months of the maintenance program. Self-monitoring plus contingency contracting produced a loss of 5.5 kg (12.1 pounds). S2 achieved her goal weight of 38.6 kg (85 pounds) over a 7-month period.

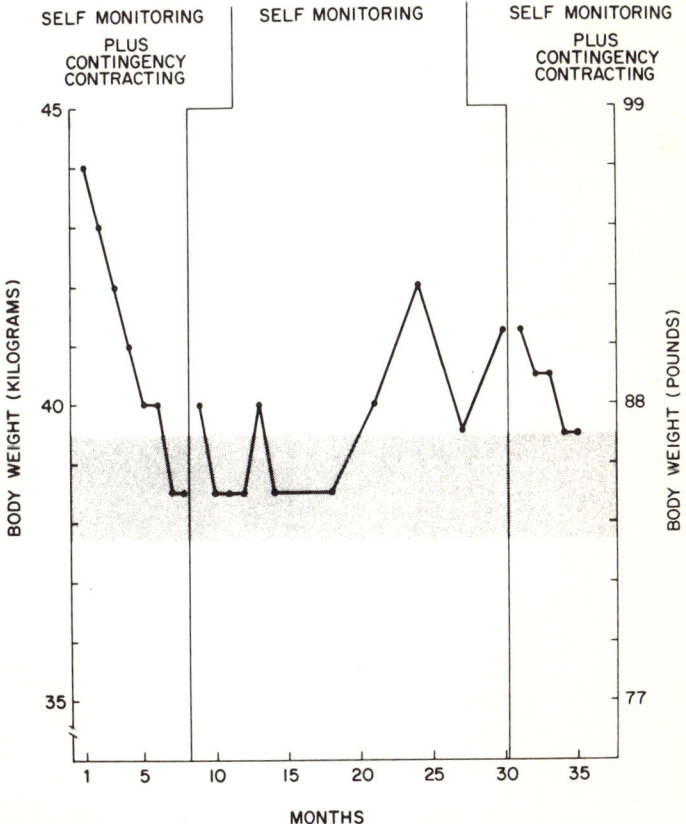

Figure 15.2. Body weight in kilograms for S2 during consecutive maintenance program months of self-monitoring and contingency contracting, self-monitoring alone, and a return to self-monitoring with reintroduction of contingency contracting conditions. Shaded area represents the goal weight range.

For 10 months following discontinuation of contingency contracting, S2's weight was maintained between 38.6 kg (85 pounds) and 40 kg (88 pounds). However, following this 10-month period, her weight increased and was maintained above the goal weight range, fluctuating between 39.5 kg (86.9 pounds) and 42 kg (92.4 pounds). Reintroduction of contingency contracting produced a loss of 1.75 kg (3.85 pounds) over a 4-month period.

DISCUSSION

Reduced caloric intake combined with self-monitoring and contingency contracting produced long term weight loss as well as maintenance of that weight loss for two adolescents with P-W syndrome. Both subjects lost weight during a 9-month weight loss program. During the 3-year maintenance program, S1 continued to lose weight while maintenance procedures were in effect. Two reversals to baseline, with no maintenance procedures, resulted in S1 showing marked weight gain. Thus, the weight maintenance procedures, reduced caloric intake combined with self-monitoring and contingency contracting, were essential for maintenance of S1's weight loss.

S2 reached her goal weight after 7 months on the maintenance program. Following discontinuation of contingency contracting, calorie restriction and self-monitoring alone resulted in S2 maintaining her weight within, or just above, her goal weight range for 10 months. For the next 9 months, however, she maintained her weight above the goal weight range. Reintroduction of contingency contracting resulted in gradual weight loss to the upper limit of her goal weight range. Thus, for S2 a more precise statement can be made about the procedures necessary for weight maintenance. Self-monitoring and caloric restriction maintain weight loss for some time; however, in the long run and/or under special circumstances, short term contingency contracting seems necessary for weight maintenance.

It is not clear why S2's weight increased above her goal weight range after 9 months of self-monitoring. However, her weight gain did coincide with her father's hospitalization for a back injury. The family reported having less time following the hospitalization to monitor S2's maintenance program, particularly when she was being cared for by friends or relatives. It is likely that S2 frequently exceeded her allowable daily caloric intake during this period.

Previous studies found self-monitoring to be an important but not sufficient condition for producing weight loss in children (Brownell & Stunkard, 1978), in adolescents with P-W syndrome (Altman et al., 1978), in normal adults (Abramson, 1977), and in retarded adults (Joachim &

Korboot, 1975). Results of the current study suggest that self-monitoring can be a valuable *maintenance* strategy but may need to be supplemented with contingency contracting to produce weight maintenance during high risk periods (e.g., substitute caregivers and vacations).

Self-monitoring may facilitate weight maintenance in several ways. First, self-monitoring can serve to provide common stimuli and responses in both weight loss and maintenance programs. Wooley, Wooley, and Dyrenforth (1979) and Stokes and Baer (1977) have suggested that maintenance is enhanced when both treatment and maintenance programs contain similar behavioral components. Self-monitoring can serve as a common component continuing to control overeating while foods denied during weight loss programs are slowly reintroduced during maintenance. Second, self-monitoring places maintenance responsibility on the subject and provides him/her with feedback about program success. Feedback to subjects and subject/caregiver responsibility for maintenance have been shown to be potent strategies for enhancing maintenance (Abramson, 1977; Brownell & Stunkard, 1978). Third, self-monitoring may improve eating habits by increasing the time needed to acquire and consume food and by requiring subjects to assess what they eat. Such habit change may be the most effective way of producing and maintaining weight loss in adolescents (Weiss, 1977).

Of particular importance to the P-W population is the incompatibility of self-monitoring with food stealing. Recorded food consumption makes the subject accountable for what is eaten, and provides the opportunity to choose appropriate foods and consumption amounts. For example, S2 periodically ate unauthorized food when she got home from school. This was controlled by providing her with a variety of appropriate snack foods (e.g., frozen yogurt and diet pop), teaching her to use measuring cups to determine appropriate serving size, and periodically having her mother monitor the foods and amounts consumed. (She was already self-monitoring her food intake.) When S2 learned to select appropriate snack foods and measure her servings accurately, unauthorized after-school eating ceased. Data from attempts to decelerate other behaviors also confirm the value of providing acceptable, alternative responses (Azrin & Holz, 1966; Baumeister & Rollings, 1977).

When self-monitoring alone is not sufficient to produce weight maintenance, contingency contracting can be implemented. Contingency contracting replaces eating with other reinforcing events, increases the probability that diet-compatible behaviors will be performed, and ensures that these behaviors will be followed by reinforcing consequences. Common contracting errors made by both families involved reinforcing subjects only for large weight losses (2 to 3 kg), and replacing short term, easily delivered contingencies with long term contingencies (e.g., a trip to the Caribbean for losing 15 kg). These strategies usually failed to produce weight loss, probably because they decreased the frequency of reinforcement for appropriate dieting. Weight loss was produced by reintroducing small weight loss goals and short term contingencies. Readily achievable goals and short term contingencies give subjects more immediate feedback as well as frequent reinforcement for engaging in diet-compatible behaviors daily. Contract negotiation sessions help ensure that the parents understand the program and will provide subjects with positive feedback for program compliance (Tharp & Wetzel, 1969).

While self-monitoring and contingency contracting were important components of the maintenance program, punishment for food stealing was also used. Punishment was effective in reducing stealing frequency and, consequently, eliminated the need to make all food unavailable to subjects (e.g., locking food storage).

Several additional strategies may be useful during periods where subjects are at high risk for inappropriate eating (e.g., having guests for a meal and eating out). Family guests should be instructed not to give any food to the subject without first getting permission from parents or caregivers. If food served to guests cannot be made compatible with the subject's diet, a special meal should be prepared for the subject. Substitute caregivers (babysitters, grandparents, etc.) should demonstrate that they can carry out the weight management program correctly before being allowed to supervise the subject independently. This is particularly important because of the rapidity with which P-W individuals seem to gain weight when program procedures are not implemented.

The most effective strategy developed by the families for eating out involved choosing restaurants offering a choice of diet-compatible foods (e.g., salads, lean meats, and fish). When eatng out, S2 and her family weighed and measured food just as was done at home.

Inappropriate eating proved most difficult to control during vacations, presumably because of the difficulty in controlling the nutritional environments of the subjects. On a 1-week trip to Hawaii, for example, S1 gained 8 kg (17.6 pounds). Nevertheless, both families developed strategies for minimizing inappropriate eating behavior while on vacation. On one trip, the family of S2 weighed her daily, stocked a portable cooler with diet soft drinks and fruit for easy access while traveling, and had at least one sit-down meal daily during which appropriate diet foods were ordered.

The parents of S1 and S2 were asked to fill out a weight program questionnaire to assess their satisfaction with the weight management programs. Both sets of parents expressed satisfaction with the techniques used and the program outcome. As one parent stated:

> The program got the results we were after. Our daughter was a very sad picture when we started. We couldn't fit her properly in clothing, and it broke

our hearts to see her eating constantly. Her medical health was in jeopardy. We had tried numerous diet programs with no success. Only this one program ... could achieve our goal ... The program was at (our daughter's) own level. She understands it and knows what to do with it.

Both families, however, felt that their life-styles had been moderately altered and made more difficult by the program. For example, the families considered it difficult to continuously provide appropriate foods for their children and dislike having to forego certain family activities (e.g., trips to the ice cream parlor). The families also experienced difficulty in finding potent reinforcers for their children. Both subjects satiated quickly on reinforcers, which necessitated frequent contract negotiations. One strategy that proved effective with S1 involved developing a list of 10 reinforcers and allowing her to choose one or two weekly to be received contingent upon weight loss.

Both families expressed frustration at the relatively slow weight loss rates of the subjects during the maintenance program (0.66 kg/1.45 pounds per month for S2 and 0.39 kg/0.85 pounds per month for S1). However, this slow loss rate may be appropriate given the recent finding associating slower weight loss with better maintenance (Wooley et al., 1979). Summarizing research on both humans and animals, Wooley and his colleagues suggested that if the rate of weight loss is slow, organisms are less likely to initiate compensatory metabolic changes that slow weight loss and weaken maintenance (e.g., decreased metabolic rate). These compensatory metabolic changes may also be avoided by alternating periods of weight loss and weight maintenance. Such strategies may be particularly useful with P-W individuals, given the documented metabolic differences between P-W individuals and normal individuals (Holm & Pipes, 1976).

Prior to initiated weight loss programs with P-W individuals, subjects and their parents or caregivers should be informed that the rate of weight loss will be slow. During initial program phases subjects should be reinforced for appropriate dieting behavior, even if weight loss has not yet begun. Several adjustments in daily caloric intake, such as exercise rates, may be needed before weight loss is produced.

Alternating weight loss and maintenance periods may be attempted if weight loss has ceased or if environmental conditions are periodically unfavorable to continuing the weight loss program. However, this technique should be monitored closely because its effectiveness in promoting weight loss and maintenance has not been demonstrated.

In summary, calorie restriction plus self-monitoring and contingency contracting are effective techniques for producing weight loss and long term maintenance in P-W individuals. While some combination of these techniques is necessary for long term maintenance, it is not clear whether self-monitoring and contingency contracting should be used concurrently during all program phases for all subjects. Whenever program elements are eliminated, caregivers must be especially watchful for the reappearance of behaviors that are incompatible with weight maintenance. Should such behaviors reappear, immediate program reinstatement may be necessary to preclude rapid weight gain. Finally, the expected rate of weight loss and difficulties of a long term in-home behavior modification program should be carefully considered by the clinician, subject, and subject's family before a behavioral weight control program is begun.

ACKNOWLEDGMENTS

The authors wish to thank Andrew Bondy for assisting in designing and implementing the weight loss program for S1 and Royce Wilcox for her invaluable assistance in preparation of this manuscript.

REFERENCE NOTE

1. *Kilocalorie controlled diets*. Topeka, Kan.: Kansas Dietetic Association, and Kansas City, Kan.: University of Kansas Medical Center, 1969, 1972, 1977.

REFERENCES

Abramson, E. Behavioral approaches to weight control: An updated review. *Behavior Research and Therapy*, 1977, *15*, 355-363.

Altman, K., Bondy, A., & Hirsch, G. Behavioral treatment of obesity in patients with Prader-Willi syndrome. *Journal of Behavioral Medicine*, 1978, *1*, 403-412.

Azrin, N.H., & Holz, W.C. Punishment. In W.K. Honig (Ed.), *Operant behavior: Areas of research and application*. New York: Appleton-Century-Crofts, 1966.

Baumeister, A., & Rollings, J.P. Self-injurious behavior. In N.R. Ellis (Ed.), *International review of research in mental retardation*. New York: Academic Press, 1977.

Brownell, K., & Stunkard, A. Behavioral treatment of obesity in children. *American Journal of Diseases in Childhood*, 1978, *132*, 403-412.

Coplin, S.S., Hine, J., & Gormican, A. Outpatient dietary management in the Prader-Willi syndrome. *Journal of the American Dietetic Association*, 1976, *68*, 330-334.

DeRisi, W.J., & Butz, G. *Writing behavioral contracts*. Champaign, Ill.: Research Press Co., 1975.

Evans, P.R. Hypogenital dystrophy with diabetic tendency. *Guy's Hospital Reports*, 1964, *113*, 207-222.

Heiman, M.F. The management of obesity in the post-adolescent developmentally disabled client with Prader-Willi syndrome. *Adolescence*, 1978, *13*, 291-296.

Holm, V.A., & Pipes, P.L. Food and children with Prader-Willi syndrome. *American Journal of Diseases of Children*, 1976, *130*, 1063-1067.

Jancar, J. Prader-Willi syndrome. *Journal of Mental Deficiency Research*, 1971, *15*, 20-29.

Joachim, R., & Korboot, P. Experimenter contact and self-monitoring of weight with the mentally retarded. *Australian Journal of Mental Retardation*, 1975, *3*, 222-225.

Juul, J., & Dupont, A. Prader-Willi syndrome. *Journal of Mental Deficiency Research*, 1967, *11*, 12-22.

Laurance, B.M. Hypotonia, mental retardation, obesity, and cryptorchidism associated with dwarfism and diabetes in children. *Archives of Diseases in Childhood*, 1967, *42*, 126-139.

Pipes, P.L., & Holm, V.A. Weight control of children with Prader-Willi syndrome. *Journal of the American Dietetic Association*, 1973, *62*, 520-524.

Stokes, T., & Baer, D. An implicit technology of generalization. *Journal of Applied Behavior Analysis*, 1977, *10*, 349-367.

Tharp, R. & Wetzel, R. *Behavior modification in the natural environment*. New York: Academic Press, 1969.

Vickers, V.S., & Stuart, H.C. Anthropometry in the pediatrician's office. *Journal of Pediatrics*, 1943, *22*, 155-170.

Weiss, A. A behavioral approach to the treatment of adolescent obesity. *Behavioral Therapy*, 1977, *8*, 720-726.

Wooley, S., Wooley, D., & Dyrenforth, S. Theoretical, practical and social issues in behavioral treatments of obesity. *Journal of Applied Behavior Analysis*, 1979, *12*, 3-25.

chapter 16
A RETROSPECTIVE STUDY OF THE BEHAVIOR OF PRADER-WILLI SYNDROME VERSUS OTHER INSTITUTIONALIZED RETARDED PERSONS

Ruth Turner and Rogelio H. A. Ruvalcaba

> Drs. Turner and Ruvalcaba compared the behavior of Prader-Willi syndrome and non–Prader-Willi syndrome patients in an institution. They found that the Prader-Willi syndrome group was more verbally aggressive, self-assaultive, and regressive, while the control group exhibited more inappropriate sexual behavior.—Eds.

Persons with Prader-Willi syndrome have been described as pleasant and placid, but there have been references in the literature to severe temper tantrums or rage reactions (Hall & Smith, 1972; Zellweger & Schneider, 1968). The purpose of this study was to analyze and compare the recorded behavior of Prader-Willi with non–Prader-Willi residents institutionalized at Rainier School for the physically and mentally handicapped at Buckley, Washington.

METHOD

Groups of 10 Prader-Willi (P-W) and 10 control subjects were compared. The control group was matched for age, sex, and degree of mental deficiency (Table 16.1). Excluded from the control group were known psychotics, patients with seizure disorders, those with known, specific syndromes, and those with chromosomal anomalies. The mean age of P-W patients was 21.2 years, with a range of 12.2 years to 29.9 years, while that of the control group was 22.7 years, with a range of 12.1 years to 30.5 years. P-W patients had a mean IQ of 46.5, which is compatible with

Table 16.1. Characteristics of patients studied

Prader-Willi (case no.)	Sex	Age (years)	IQ	Control (case no.)	Sex	Age	IQ
1	F	12.2	35	1	F	12.1	35
2	F	27.8	62	2	F	27.8	55
3	M	29.9	46	3	M	30.5	54
4	F	17.9	22	4	F	20.2	19
5	M	24.5	51	5	M	24.9	49
6	F	27.9	30	6	F	27.9	38
7	F	18.1	40	7	F	19.2	33
8	F	23.9	39	8	F	23.0	30
9	F	24.6	58	9	F	24.5	51
10	F	15.5	62	10	F	16.9	63
Mean		21.2	46.5			22.7	47.7

previous reports in the literature of IQs in the range of 40 to 60. The mean IQ of the control group was 47.7.

As a matter of institutional policy, attendant personnel are required to document all undesirable behaviors on a prescribed behavioral incident report form that is then reviewed and initialed by the Hall Supervisor before filing in the resident's main file. These reports are frequently scrutinized by administrators and state officials; therefore, Hall Supervisors are conscientious and consistent in filing them accurately. Two hundred forty-two behavioral incident reports of P-W patients and 121 reports of the control subjects were analyzed.

Because of the policy of deinstitutionalization, it was difficult to match the two groups on length of institutionalization. The control group did, in fact, have more opportunity to display the behaviors investigated during a period of 1,157 months as opposed to 923 months for P-W patients. Mean age at time of institutionalization was 12.7 years for the P-W group and 12.3 years for the control group. Investigation suggests that the behaviors studied did not result from institutionalization, but were documented during the intake interviews as having occurred prior to institutionalization. In the P-W group the behaviors had often been what led to institutionalization, along with the difficulty parents found in curbing food intake.

The classification of the behaviors studied was developed following a study of the literature concerning P-W syndrome, a study of the intake interviews and behavioral reports of both groups, discussion with medical and attendant staff, development and monitoring of a behavior modification program for a female P-W patient, and observation of both P-W and other retarded residents at Rainier School in a variety of settings. Behavioral incidents were tabulated into nine categories: physical aggressiveness (toward persons or property), verbal aggressiveness (including prolonged screaming), self-assaultiveness (including head banging, hair pulling, inflicting wounds on limbs, face, and scalp, slapping own face, and cutting self with sharp objects), negativism, stealing, hoarding, sexual inappropriateness (including public display of sexual impulses, such as masturbation and attempted rape), regressiveness (a decline in performance of mental age–appropriate behavior, such as a decline in toileting skills, resulting in public urinating, defecating in clothing, smearing feces on self, walls, furniture, or others), and passiveness (a lack of motor responses or intellectual initiative or assertiveness).

RESULTS

The results of chi-square analyses of the behavioral categories are summarized in Table 16.2. P-W patients presented significantly more verbal aggressiveness directed toward staff and peers than controls ($p < 0.001$). Equally significant was the difference in self-assaultive episodes ($p < 0.001$). Another highly significant difference was observed in regressive behaviors ($p < 0.001$). P-W patients displayed significantly less sexually inappropriate behavior than did the control subjects ($0.05 > p > 0.02$). No behavioral reports were maintained that documented passive or hoarding behaviors, although both types of behaviors have been described by parents in the intake interviews and have been observed. Behaviors specifically related to food seeking were not studied.

Table 16.2. Chi-square values and significance levels of the behaviors studied

	χ^2 values	Areas of significance
Physical aggressiveness	2.252	$0.20 > p > 0.10$
Verbal aggressiveness	15.677	$p < 0.001$
Sexual inappropriateness	4.742	$0.05 > p > 0.02$
Self-assaultiveness	26.615	$p < 0.001$
Negativism	0.008	$p < 0.90$
Stealing	0.121	$0.70 > p > 0.50$
Regressiveness (immature)	12.603	$p < 0.001$
Hoarding	(No behavioral reports)	
Passiveness	(No behavioral reports)	

SUMMARY AND DISCUSSION

The behavior of a group of 10 institutionalized patients with P-W syndrome was analyzed and compared to that of a control group. P-W patients were found to be significantly more verbally aggressive, self-assaultive, and regressive than the control group, while the latter displayed more inappropriate sexual behaviors.

The use of behavioral reports in a study such as this imposes limitations, but long term data were not otherwise available. In addition, because of community placement of many residents from Rainier School, the length of institutionalization could not be controlled in the study, even though an attempt was made to do so whenever possible.

Although there is probably no systematic bias in the hall records of behavioral incidents, it must be noted that the data in this study had no reliability checks and were filed by many different Hall Supervisors, who were unaware that the information would subsequently be part of a study. However, the high degree of statistical significance of the results and their consistency with the behaviors reported by others in this book support the contention that these data do provide a reasonably accurate picture of the behavior of P-W persons in an institutional setting.

ACKNOWLEDGMENT

The authors are grateful to Helen Gross, Ph.D., for assistance with statistical analysis.

REFERENCES

Hall, B.D., & Smith, D.W. Prader-Willi syndrome: A resumé of 32 cases including an instance of affected first cousins, one of whom is of normal stature and intelligence. *The Journal of Pediatrics*, 1972, *81*, 286-293.

Zellweger, H., & Schneider, H.J. Syndrome of hypotonia-hypomentia-hypogonadism-obesity (HHHO) or Prader-Willi syndrome. *American Journal of Diseases of Children*, 1968, *115*, 588-598.

chapter 17
RELAXATION TRAINING WITH YOUNGSTERS WITH PRADER-WILLI SYNDROME

Stevan L. Nielsen and Stephen Sulzbacher

In this chapter Mr. Nielsen and Dr. Sulzbacher report their success in using relaxation training to provide Prader-Willi syndrome patients with a tool for preventing anxiety-related temper tantrums.—*Eds.*

Although obesity and mental retardation are the most noticeable features of Prader-Willi (P-W) syndrome, the characteristic non-compliant and acting-out behaviors that are also often present represent a very disturbing and difficult feature of the disorder. The poor self-control and judgment apparent in their eating behavior, which often includes scavenging from waste containers or gorging, can be as disturbing as the obesity that follows. Even when obesity is prevented or controlled with careful supervision of the diet, and when mental retardation does not reach severe levels, acting-out and non-compliance problems often persist. Many parents of P-W children report that their children's frequent, unpredictable temper tantrums are a major concern.

In an attempt to investigate strategies for dealing with these behaviors, a training program in relaxation training for self-control was undertaken with two P-W children. The self-control desensitization and coping skills training program described by Goldfried (1971) and later by Goldfried and Davison (1976) was modified slightly and presented to these children. This program consists of training the children in systematic muscle relaxation (Jacobsen, 1929) and then training them to apply the relaxation response to stressful situations. Parents of P-W children have reported an increase in signs of anxiety and tension in their children prior to difficult periods. This anxiety may serve as a proprioceptive cue for aggressive behavior. The relaxation response has been useful in controlling anger and aggressive responses in non-retarded populations (Navaco, 1975). The training undertaken here was therefore seen as a possible alternative response to the anxiety that seems to precede tantrums in P-W children. To document the effectiveness of the relaxation training, biofeedback measurements were taken for frontalis muscle tension.

METHOD

Relaxation Exercises

A simplified set of 10 relaxation instructions followed by training in meditation was given to each child. Five training sessions were undertaken with one child and six with the other. The relaxation procedures consisted of systematic flexing and relaxing of specified muscle groups. Muscles were flexed for 5 to 10 seconds, and the tension was released for 5 to 10 seconds, while the patient received instruction to concentrate on the feelings of relaxation. Again, the muscle group was tensed and relaxed and the patient concentrated on the feelings of relaxation a final time. The instructions given were as follows:

1. Point your toes like a dancer. Hold (slow count to five). Now relax your muscles. Think about what your toes feel like. (Pause and repeat entire procedure.)
2. Pull your toes back as if you are trying to touch them to your knees (slow count to five). Let go and think about what your legs feel like. (Pause and repeat entire procedure.)
3. Make your legs as straight as you can and make your thighs hard. (The thigh muscles were pointed out, and this tension was held for the slow count to five.) Let go and feel the relaxation. (Pause and repeat.)
4. Make your stomach as hard as you can; as hard as steel like Superman's (slow count to five). Let go and feel the relaxation. (Pause and repeat.)
5. Push your palms together in front of you. Let's see which arm is strongest (slow count to five). Let your arms drop and feel the relaxation. (Pause and repeat.)
6. Imagine that you have a lemon in each hand. Squeeze that lemon until there is no juice left. Squeeze! (slow count to five). Let the lemon drop and feel the relaxation. (Pause and repeat.)
7. Make a muscle like this (demonstration of biceps flex). See if you can make it big and hard like Superman's (slow count to five). Let your arm drop and rest on the chair. (Pause and repeat.)
8. Can you look at your Adam's apple? Try! As hard as you can! (slow count to five). Now relax. (Pause and repeat.)
9. Imagine you have a bullet between your teeth and, like Superman, you're going to bite it in half. Squeeze the bullet (slow count to five). Now let go of the bullet and feel what it's like to relax. (Pause and repeat.)
10. Imagine the sun is shining brightly in your eyes. Close your eyes as tightly as you can so that no light can get through (slow count to five). Open your eyes and think about how it feels to relax. (Pause and repeat.) I'm going to talk about what we did and I want you to think about how relaxed the part of your body feels that I talk about. Close

your eyes and when I talk about part of your body think about it and about how relaxed it feels. First, you pointed your toes (brief pause). Then you pulled your toes back as far as you could and released them (brief pause). You made your legs as straight as you could (brief pause). You made your stomach as hard as you could, like Superman, and then you relaxed (brief pause). You pushed your hands together to see which one was strongest, then you let go and felt your chest relax (brief pause). You squeezed all the juice out of two imaginary lemons (brief pause). You flexed the muscles in your arms (brief pause). You tried to look at your Adam's apple (brief pause). You bit a bullet in half (brief pause). Finally, you closed your eyes as tightly as you could so that no light could get through (brief pause). This is what it feels like to relax.

Meditation

The patient was then instructed in the meditation format described by Benson (1975). This consisted of repeated deep, regular breathing accompanied by covert repetition of the word "calm." These instructions were given:

> I want you to sit quietly and take deep slow breaths. When you breathe out I want you to say the word *calm* inside your head. Say it to yourself so that nobody else can hear you, not even me. Don't let any other words or pictures come into your head. If you start to think about something else, just tell yourself to say the word *calm* and relax.

The period of meditation lasted for about 5 minutes. The total time for the relaxation and meditation training period was 15 to 20 minutes.

The relaxation and meditation instructions were recorded during the first training session. The patients were asked to listen to the relaxation tape at home each weeknight immediately before or following dinner. The patients' parents were asked to be responsible for monitoring compliance with this instruction.

Measurement

A J&J Enterprises model M-55 electromyograph biofeedback unit was used to monitor frontalis muscle activity. Electrode placements were made on the forehead in the manner described by Budzynski, Stoyva, Adler, and Mulleney (1972). Earphones were used with one of the patients to provide auditory feedback on the level of relaxation achieved as an additional measure of response to training.

RESULTS

Case 1

The first patient was an 11-year-old male P-W child. The patient and his mother agreed that he might benefit from learning to control his temper better. At the time therapy began he was having one or two tantrums each day. This boy's IQ is in the mildly retarded range and he was at the 7th percentile for height and 85th percentile for weight at the time of the study.

The patient was seen six times for training. During the first four training sessions, he was prepared for electrode placement, the electrodes were placed, and he was asked to relax and sit quietly for 10 minutes. The relaxation and meditation training was carried out as described above, and the patient was asked to relax and sit quietly for 10 minutes longer. During the pre- and post-relaxation training periods, measurements of frontalis muscle activity were made every 30 seconds. Following the post-relaxation measurement period, the patient was given earphones that provided feedback on the level of muscle activity. This relationship was demonstrated for the patient and he was challenged to slow the feedback signal as much as he could (reducing the level of frontalis activity) for 4 minutes. Five microvolts root mean square (μV RMS) was defined as the criterion level under which the needle was to be deflected.

The patient's average electromyogram (EMG) reading for pre- and post-relaxation training periods and the patient's lowest EMG deflection achieved during the 4-minute biofeedback period are presented in Figure 17.1. As can be seen in the figure the patient's frontalis muscle activity decreased from the pre- to post-relaxation measurement periods during sessions 1 and 2. This effect is reliable, $t(64) = 2.29$, $p < 0.03$. During sessions 3 and 4 the pre- and post-relaxation measurements did not differ. However, it was found that the post-relaxation measurements of frontalis activity in sessions 3 and 4 were reliably lower than those in sessions 1 and 2, $t(56) = 2.83$, $p < 0.02$. It can also be seen in Figure 17.1 that the patient's lowest EMG deflection decreased during each successive session. The duration of EMG deflections beneath 5 μV RMS is presented in Figure 17.2. The number of seconds below this criterion level increased for each successive session.

During session 5 the patient was trained in an imagination-controlled relaxation technique taken from Tai Chi (Huang, 1973). He was instructed to imagine that his weight was being supported by a string and, since the string was holding him up, to relax completely, using his breathing and relaxation skills. This instruction was repeated in both sitting and standing positions. Following the instruction the patient was asked to sit in a relaxed position with his head held erect and later to stand up in a relaxed position. EMG measurements were taken during these two 5-minute periods. The patient was then told to sit in the same position while imagining the string supporting his weight and later to stand while imagining the string supporting his weight. EMG measure-

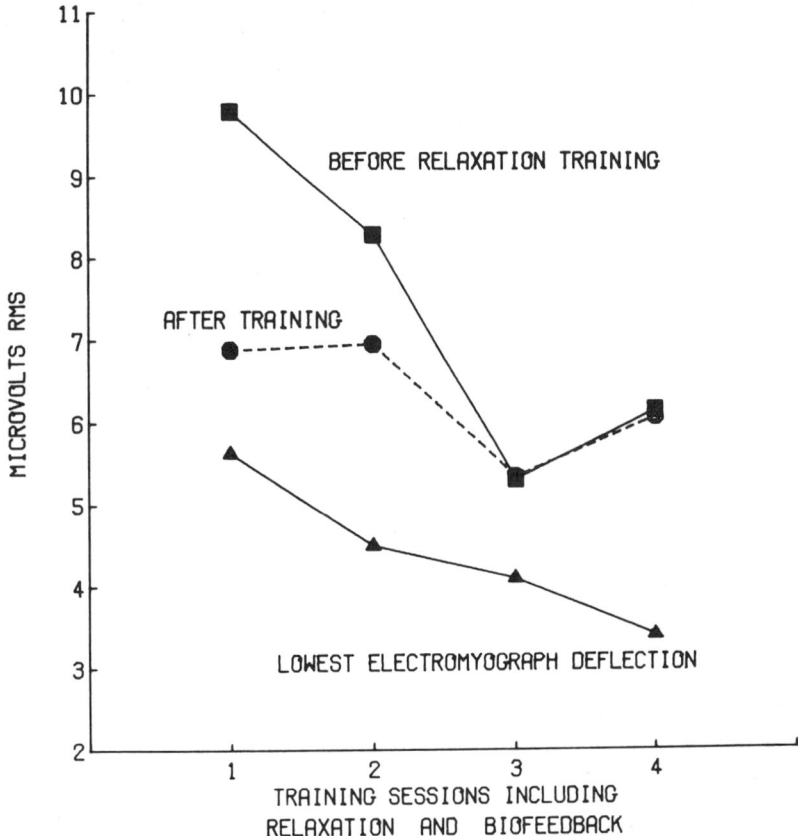

Figure 17.1. Comparison of EMG reading before and after progressive muscle relaxation, with lowest EMG deflection occurring during 4 minutes of auditory biofeedback training, during sessions 1, 2, 3, and 4.

ments were also taken during these Tai Chi periods. Frontalis muscle activity during these periods is presented in Figure 17.3. Average muscle activity was found to decrease reliably in the Tai Chi versions of standing and sitting, $t(42) = 2.90$, $p < 0.01$.

The patient was trained in the use of his newly attained relaxation skills during sessions 4, 5, and 6. He was asked to demonstrate the use of various skills (e.g., relaxation, breathing, and Tai Chi standing) in role-play problem situations. The patient's mother participated in the role playing during session 6. Following session 1 she had begun to count the number of tantrums occurring at home. The number of tantrums occurring over an 8-week period are presented in Figure 17.4. Following session 4, instructions for dealing with anger and role-play situations

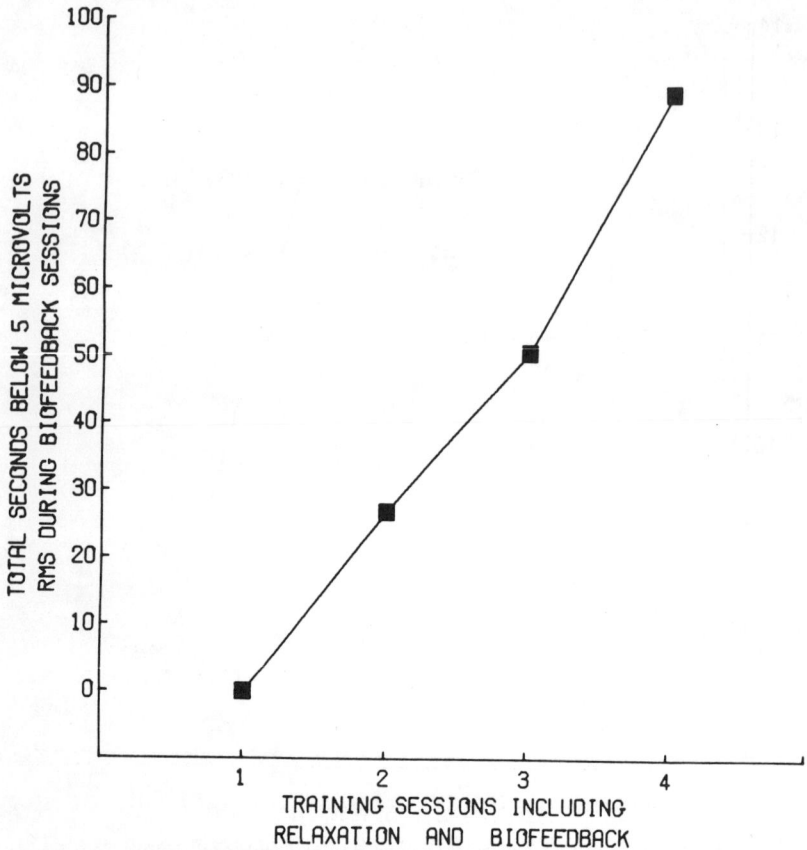

Figure 17.2. Total seconds when EMG deflection was below a criterion level of 5 μV RMS during 4 minutes of auditory biofeedback.

approximating potential tantrum-causing situations at home were begun. A significant decrease in the frequency of tantrums occurred, that is, the number of tantrums from the fifth week of training on was less than the number during weeks 2, 3, and 4, $\chi^2(2) = 25.65$, $p < 0.001$. The patient's mother also reported that the weeks following week 4 were uncharacteristically pleasant. During the subsequent months, the mother neglected to record the data, but she reports that tantrums have decreased further, to approximately less than one per week, while the patient has been in school.

Case 2

The second patient was a 16-year-old P-W male who had been experiencing episodes of violent acting out in response to ordinary educa-

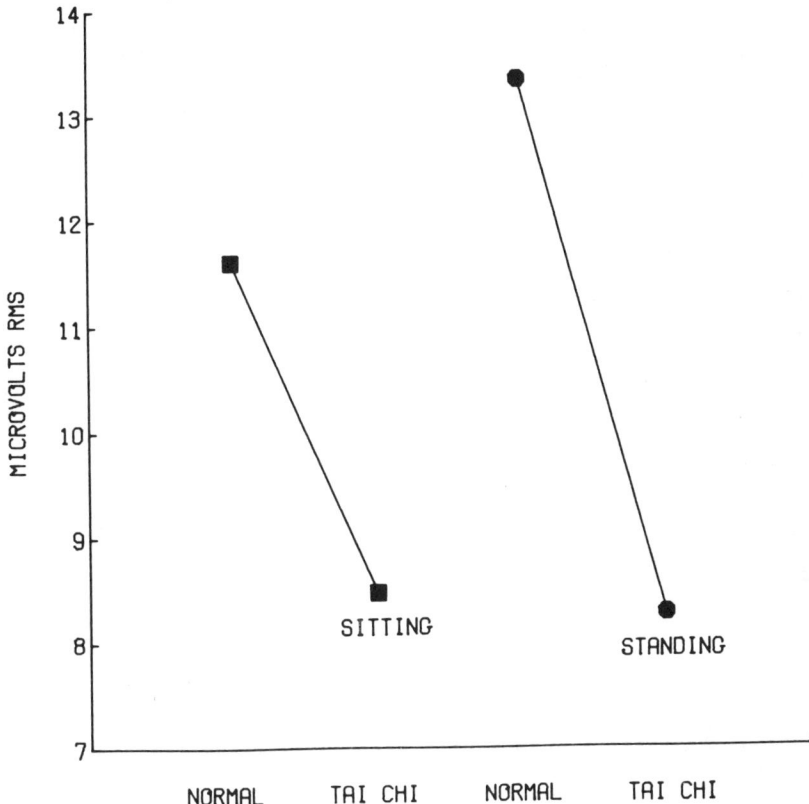

Figure 17.3. Response to Tai Chi posture training in standing and sitting positions. Tai Chi training was carried out in session 5.

tional and family experiences. His weight and height were both below the 5th percentile for his age. His intellectual functioning is in the mild to moderate range of mental retardation. The relaxation procedures described above for the first patient were employed with the exception of the Tai Chi image-controlled relaxation and the biofeedback measurements. A baseline EMG measure was taken, followed by five relaxation training sessions. During the training it was discovered that a resistance defect in an electrode resulted in unreliable EMG readings. It can be reported, however, that during the third session of relaxation training, the patient responded by falling asleep. The first three relaxation training sessions were administered with the patient in a reclining position; the final two sessions were administered with him sitting. During the last of the sitting training sessions the patient also fell asleep. A surprising aspect of the patient's response to the training is that he fell asleep

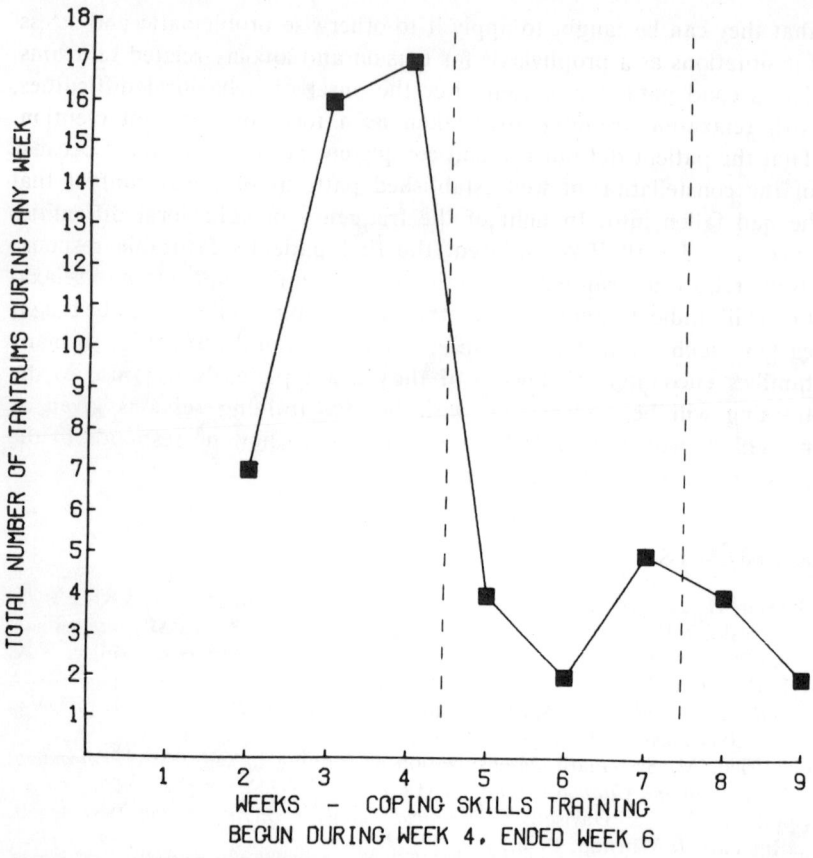

Figure 17.4. Number of tantrums recorded by the patient's mother. Tantrums recorded occurred during the week *preceding* the indicated point of measurement.

despite repeated protests that he did not like the training and that it was painful for him to flex his muscles. The patient's parents also reported that he fell asleep repeatedly at home while listening to his practice tape.

Before training in the application of the relaxation response could begin, the patient had run away from home several times. Relaxation training and practice had become a compliance issue at home. The patient's parents decided that they were unable to control his behavior sufficiently to continue with the training. At the writing of this chapter, the second patient is awaiting placement in a group home.

DISCUSSION

The results of these case studies seem to indicate that P-W children can be taught the relaxation response and, in the case of the first patient, that they can be taught to apply it to otherwise problematic and stressful situations as a prophylaxis for tension and anxiety-related tantrums. The second patient was seen after the onset of behavioral difficulties, with relaxation training undertaken as a form of crisis intervention. That the patient did not respond completely can be understood because of the constellation of well established patterns of social conflict that he had fallen into. In light of the frequency of behavioral difficulties encountered with P-W children, the first patient's favorable response to the relaxation training and to the training in the application of relaxation skills indicates that this and other stress-coping skills should be taught early to such youngsters to help ease the behavioral difficulties so many families encounter. Follow-up of the second patient's response to the training will be undertaken, with booster training sessions given as needed. It will be especially interesting to see how he responds to the pressures of the adolescent years.

REFERENCES

Benson, H. *The relaxation response.* New York: William Morrow & Co., 1975.
Budzynski, T.H., Stoyva, J.M., Adler, C.S., & Mulleney, D.J. EMG biofeedback and tension headache: A controlled outcome study. In N.E. Miller, T.X. Barber, L.V. Di Cara, J. Kamiya, D. Shapiro, & J. Stoyva (Eds.), *Biofeedback and self-control, 1973:* An Aldine annual on the regulation of bodily processes and consciousness. Chicago: Aldine, 1972.
Goldfried, M. Systematic desensitization as training in self-control. *Journal of Consulting and Clinical Psychology,* 1971, *37,* 228-234.
Goldfried, M., & Davison. G. *Clinical behavior therapy.* New York: Holt, Rinehart, & Winston, 1976.
Huang, W.S. *Fundamentals of Tai Chi Ch'uan.* Hong Kong: South Sky Book Co., 1973.
Jacobsen, E. *Progressive relaxation.* Chicago: University of Chicago Press, 1929.
Navaco, R. *Anger control: The development and evaluation of an experimental treatment.* Lexington, Mass.: D.C. Heath & Co., 1975.

chapter 18

IMPLICATIONS OF PRADER-WILLI SYNDROME FOR THE INDIVIDUAL AND THE FAMILY

Jurgen Herrmann

> Dr. Herrmann discusses the preliminary results from his survey of Prader-Willi syndrome families. These results indicate that the primary impact of the syndrome is caused by behavioral problems and social attitudes rather than medical problems.—*Eds.*

Our health care system is set up primarily to take care of normally healthy individuals with temporary ailments. Genetic disorders and birth defects conflict with this medical model in two major ways: They are lifelong and they involve other family members as well as the patient. This involvement of other family members occurs because they also may be genetically at risk and, further, because they share in the long term care of the patient.

It is important that patients, family members, and health professionals recognize the limitations of the prevailing medical system so that they can anticipate problems and deal with conflicts constructively. Frequently this is not the case and unrealistic expectations of health professionals are harbored by the families. The health profession has done little to discourage this or to define the limits of its activities.

Medical and non-medical characteristics and needs vary in different disorders. Non-medical professionals may be of help to the patient and the family under different circumstances to establish for individual disorders the type and magnitude of non-medical needs.

For most birth defects and genetic disorders, little or no specific information is available that describes the burden for the family, the magnitude of non-medical issues, and the needs for and availability of non-medical resources. As such information becomes available, the role of the medical professionals can be defined better, patients and families can be assisted in using appropriate non-medical resources, and the disorder can be treated more comprehensively and effectively. These aspects for Prader-Willi (P-W) syndrome are discussed in this chapter.

PRADER-WILLI SYNDROME QUESTIONNAIRE

To collect information, questionnaires were sent to over 250 families who have a child with P-W syndrome. The questionnaire is printed as Appendix A. Following is a partial evaluation of the first 50 responses received.

The recipients of the questionnaire were primarily families of P-W syndrome patients from the Clinical Genetics Center in Madison, Wisconsin, from the Genetics and Birth Defects Center at Milwaukee Children's Hospital, and members of the Prader-Willi Syndrome Association.

Two questionnaires that raised the problem of diagnosis of P-W syndrome are not included in this study. In all other instances the description of the problems by the family does not raise any doubt about the diagnosis.

In the first 50 families that responded, the patient was a male in 23 cases, a female in 24, and of unstated sex in three. The questionnaire was filled out by the mother in 40 instances, by the mother with other family members in six instances, and by other family members in four instances. Therefore, the following comments reflect primarily the opinions of the mothers of persons with P-W syndrome. The mean age of P-W persons involved was 13.2 years (SD = 7.88). Eight patients (17%) were under 5 years, 15 (31%) were between 5 and 10 years, 8 (17%) were between 10 and 15 years, and 17 (35%) were older than 15 years.

RESULTS

Diagnosis

In 46 instances the age at the time of diagnosis was given. (The mean age at the time of diagnosis was 7.25 years (SD = 5.88).) Only one-half the children were diagnosed before school age, and one-third were diagnosed at the age of 13 or later.

There was not only the problem of delayed diagnosis, but also of the manner in which the diagnosis was made and how the implications were explained to the parents. In 15% of the cases the diagnosis was not made by professionals but by the parents themselves after reading an article in a popular non-medical magazine. Only 40% of the parents felt that the diagnosis was appropriately explained to them. In 33% of the cases the implications of the syndrome were inadequately explained, either because they were not discussed at all or, at the other extreme, because an overly pessimistic picture was painted. Another 13% of the parents felt that the doctor handled the diagnosis especially poorly by being defensive, accusatory, ignorant, or egotistical. On learning the diagnosis parents felt relieved (27%), worried (17%), helpless (16%), sad (13%), upset (9%), angry (8%), and puzzled (8%).

Burden to the P-W Syndrome Person

The significance of P-W syndrome is different for various family members. As expected, the impact from medical problems is more severe for P-W persons themselves than for their parents or siblings. Approximately 20% to 30% of the problems for P-W persons are medically related, while this figure for parents and siblings is about 12% and 5%, respectively. This indicates that the problems in these families, although originally due to a medical disorder, are in fact mostly non-medical.

In a more specific listing (Table 18.1) of the types of problems for groups of persons inside and outside the family, it is indicated that for P-W persons 31% of the problems are related to obesity, 20% to other medical problems, and 28% to behavior, and that the percentage of other types of problems (lack of knowledge about P-W syndrome, lack of understanding, impatience, financial problems, etc.) is individually not higher than 7% and combined less than 25%.

The two principal problems, obesity and behavior, show distinct patterns of impact, however. Weight problems are mostly confined to P-W persons, affecting the mother and father to some extent, but peers, school personnel, and the public relatively little. Behavioral problems, on the

Table 18.1. Types of Prader-Willi syndrome-related problems for persons within and outside Prader-Willi families

	a	b	c	d	e	f	g	h	Total[a]
P-W Person	37	34	5	9	7	24	2	4	122
Mother	18	28	18	14	18	17	5	8	126
Father	12	26	16	10	15	11	7	3	100
Siblings/relatives	5	26	13	20	18	5	—	—	87
Peers	7	15	17	26	14	2	—	1	82
School	7	18	23	19	9	1	1	4	82
Public	4	7	28	24	10	1	—	1	75
Total[a]	90	154	120	122	91	61	15	21	674

[a]The numbers are the frequency of responses; usually there were multiple responses by one family or person.
Interpretation of code entries above:
a. Obesity; b. behavior; c. lack of knowledge; d. lack of understanding; e. impatience; f. medical problems; g. lack of financial resources; h. other.

other hand, very markedly affect the mother, father, siblings, other relatives, peers, school personnel, and the public.

Problems stemming from obesity and behavior combined with the problem of delayed development often lead to impaired peer relationships. In fact, 58% of P-W children are said to have moderate or severe difficulties with peer relationships, while 22% are reported to have few such difficulties and only 20% none. Specifically, the parents indicated lack of friends, absent or decreased play activities with other children, and teasing or being taken advantage of by others. In addition, P-W persons may have diminished self-image: It is reported that for 32% the ability to like themselves is moderately or severely affected, for 30% there is little impairment, and for 37% there is none.

Burden to Parents in Terms of Time and Effort

This aspect changes with the age of the P-W person. Many families spend considerable time and effort in the management of feeding and medical problems during infancy. When the children gain noticeable strength, usually during the second year of life, the feeding problems lessen or disappear. But other problems develop or become apparent at this time, causing the parents to take their children to the doctor for delayed development, increased weight, strabismus, undescended testes, unusual behavior, temper tantrums, or skin infections. Thus, while medical visits become less intense, they usually continue for a variety of reasons. At the same time, non-medical aspects of the syndrome, in particular dietary management, special education, and behavioral problems, become more and more important.

At least 10% of the families that responded felt that medical contacts represent a major threat to normal family life. Initially, the medical involvement is very extensive and largely related to physical problems, while later it becomes somewhat less extensive, and dietary, behavioral, and educational matters, as well as problems with interpersonal relationships, predominate. Many parents stated that it would be helpful for them to have facilities available to share temporarily in the care of their P-W children.

Financial Burden

The impact of P-W syndrome on family finances was reported as follows: 31% of the families reported none, 20% little, 29% moderate, and 20% severe impact. This is in part because of medical bills, but also because of expenses for special education, transportation, physical and speech therapy, summer camps, and, eventually, group home placement.

Family Living

Many families described how profoundly their P-W syndrome child influenced their family living, causing many changes too numerous to mention individually. When asked to place the major problems in four categories (medical, financial, family living, and personal-social), the response was: medical 33%, financial 4%, family living 8%, personal-social 56% for P-W persons; and medical 14%, financial 30%, family living 21%, and personal-social 34% for parents. Only 6% of the families indicated no unusual disruption of normal family living, while 28% reported severe, 40% moderate, and 26% little disruption.

The types of adaptive changes made reflect to some degree how the P-W child is being accepted as having special problems. Acceptance may proceed at a different rate for each parent. One key factor is diagnosis. In all families adaptive changes had occurred before the diagnosis was made, but after the diagnosis concrete expectations were set and adaptive changes became more specific. A situation of generally increased stress, which prevailed in 34% of the families before the diagnosis was made, often decreased afterward. In two families, a separation or divorce was probably, in part, the result of difficulties stemming from the P-W child. In many other families, however, the P-W child brought the parents closer together.

In at least 16% of the cases the family had instituted adaptive changes before diagnosis that related to food, eating habits, and the P-W child's or sibling's behavior. After diagnosis was made and the specific nature of P-W syndrome was described, 18% of the parents reported greater acceptance of the child, and 44% described improved diet management and eating habits. Many families reported that while diagnosis of the condition does not change the P-W child, it does lead to better adaptation of the family to his or her problems. Diagnosis allows the parents to recognize their P-W child as one who has very specific problems that can be dealt with rather than as an individual who is helplessly handicapped.

It is particularly important that parents receive adequate information on the syndrome. When asked about "your biggest need from health professionals" at the time the diagnosis was made, 84% wanted more medical information on P-W syndrome, 82% asked for information on living skills, 68% asked for information on non-medical resources available, and 36% pointed out the need for more compassionate understanding. When parents were asked what information they required earlier, 56% said they needed knowledge of the prognosis and management of the eating problem, 22% wanted information on behavioral problems, 12%

on the general aspects and prognosis of P-W syndrome, 8% on the medical problems, 6% on resources, 4% on exercises, and 2% wanted to be made aware that most physicians are not very knowledgeable about the syndrome. All implied, and 62% stated spontaneously, that they wanted to know everything about P-W syndrome. Two families acknowledged that it was initially painful to learn about the mental retardation and decreased life expectancy.

Parents were asked to rate severity of the impact of P-W syndrome on the diet, eating habits, activities, and recreation of family members. A moderate-to-severe impact was indicated by 50% to 70% of the families for each of the four categories, and very few families reported no disturbance. The figures for these categories are not significantly different, but the impact of P-W syndrome was slightly higher on family eating habits and somewhat lower on family recreation.

Siblings, Peers, School, and the Public

Table 18.1 shows the frequency of problems for the P-W person, family members, and outsiders occurring in conjunction with specific features of the syndrome. The numbers are the absolute frequency of the responses for each category; usually there were multiple responses. Chi-square analyses performed on the data in Table 18.1 show significant differences (at the 0.001 level) between P-W persons and other persons. Perceptions of mother and father (but not of siblings) differed from those of peers, school, and public. The responses of peers, school, and public were not significantly different from each other.

DISCUSSION

The responses of P-W persons differ primarily because of increased obesity and medical problems. In fact, it is remarkable that obesity does not play a bigger role with siblings, peers, school personnel, and the public. It seems to involve mainly the P-W person and his or her parents. It might be helpful for the P-W person to know that it is not the obesity that creates problems with outside persons, but the behavior problems. The mother, father, and siblings feel that most problems are related to the behavior of the P-W person. This is also the opinion of peers in school, although to a lesser extent. Parents characterize the problematic behavior as involving repetitive or incessant activities (talking, playing with puzzles, hair pulling, and picking sores), overconfidence and boasting, a manipulative personality, tiring easily and not having enough strength to keep up with peers, snitching food and other items, frequent temper tantrums, and communication difficulties because of speech delay.

The reactions of the siblings to the P-W child have been mixed (see also Leconte, Chapter 19, this volume). In some families tension arises because of temper tantrums and other behavior problems, and in other families siblings become especially protective and supportive. Frequently, parents have found it helpful to apply different standards to their P-W child and their other children for those behaviors (food snitching, temper tantrums, and repetitive activities) that are related to the syndrome.

Many P-W children suffer from lack of friends during the school years, contributing to the cycle of decreasing stimulation-decreasing activity-less peer contact, a cycle which perpetuates their isolation. Several families have been successful in breaking this pattern by getting their P-W child involved in church activities, YMCA programs, and special neighborhood or school programs.

A common theme in the responses to this questionnaire is the lack of knowledge about P-W syndrome and the lack of understanding by relatives and persons outside the family. In fact, Table 18.1 shows that lack of knowledge and understanding is the major cause of problems with peers, in school, and in public. Those families that have been successful in this regard generally have educated peers, school teachers, therapists, neighbors, and other relevant persons concerning P-W syndrome, thereby creating an environment of knowledgeable and understanding persons for their child. This relieves the pressure on the P-W person and other family members as well, who are sometimes blamed by outsiders for "not trying hard enough," for "letting the child get away with everything," for "being inconsistent," etc. Table 18.1 indicates that the school and the public particularly lack knowledge and that peers, siblings, and more distant relatives specifically lack understanding. In general, there seems to be a definite progression from knowledge to understanding to acceptance of the patients.

Like parents of all handicapped children, parents of P-W children hope that their child will be able to live independently. Acquisition of skills for independent living is a long process during which both the family and the P-W child have to be educated. It is usually difficult because of lack of knowledge and understanding on the part of outsiders (including medical professionals), lack of facilities, and apathy. The important role of the Prader-Willi Syndrome Association in providing support, publicity, information, and referral was pointed out by many parents. Of immeasureable help are local parent groups, particularly if they have been successful in establishing summer camps or group homes. Where facilities specifically for P-W persons are not available, parents have had to search carefully to find a suitable home or institution. Several of the parents who had placed their older P-W child or young adult in a group home commented that a structured setting had a good influence and was very appropriate.

This survey shows that the main burdens of P-W syndrome are not caused by medical factors but by the personal-social aspects of the disorder. Let us then consider P-W syndrome as a social rather than a medical disorder. Body functions, which from a biological standpoint are neutral, nevertheless may have distinctly different social values. For instance, a sneeze and a burp can be considered equal from a biological standpoint, while obviously each has different social implications.

Social values differ from country to country and change with time. Among parents of P-W children and among readers, some argument might be expected as to the specific values of those social features that relate to the syndrome, namely obesity, delayed development, and certain behavioral patterns.

In the estimation of the author, P-W syndrome does not fare well as a social disorder. Were it associated with lower-than-normal weight and thin appearance, it is suspected that persons with P-W syndrome would be more highly regarded in our society. As it is, being overweight puts P-W persons at a disadvantage socially because their appearance does not conform to our social ideal. On the other hand, it is probable that if P-W persons lived in a culture which looked more kindly on obesity, they would be more highly recognized.

The delayed development of the P-W syndrome child has a similar effect. Children in our society are generally educated and adults are often encouraged to reach the highest level of achievement. There are few psychological mechanisms and educational facilities for those who must be content with less. Like all handicapped persons, children with P-W syndrome and their families find out eventually that the social structure and the institutions of society may be of only limited value or not appropriate for their needs. On a personal level, even well meaning people are often not sure of what to say and how to act in the presence of a person with an obvious handicap. This usually leads to awkward situations, uncomfortable feelings, decreased interaction, and therefore contributes to the handicap.

Certain behavior patterns that are a part of the syndrome should be considered in their proper context, especially food snitching. In any other person this would be called "stealing" and would be considered unethical. I would not encourage such behavior on the part of P-W persons; nevertheless such behavior is not the same in a P-W syndrome person as in others and it should be dealt with differently. Therefore, in P-W persons this behavior should be referred to as "snitching" rather than "stealing." (Eds. note: We refer to this behavior as "foraging.")

The purpose of looking at P-W syndrome as a social rather than a medical disorder is to allow P-W persons, their families, and outsiders caring for them to make appropriate and constructive changes.

RECOMMENDATIONS

1. Create a more positive image for P-W syndrome. Often P-W persons are portrayed as human garbage pails rather than individuals who have an eating disorder and other problems. The prognosis is often described as very pessimistic while it is, in fact, clear that much can be done, that much help is available, and that extraordinary progress has been made in many instances.
2. Early diagnosis. Diagnosis is late in most instances. Physicians and health professionals must realize that diagnosis of P-W syndrome should be seriously considered in all infant patients with severe feeding difficulties and that it is possible to make the diagnosis before the onset of obesity. Early diet restriction appears to be effective in preventing obesity.
3. Education of the public and professionals. It may not be realistic to expect everybody to know about this syndrome, but general publicity has led to diagnosis, appropriate referral, and helpful information for parents in numerous instances. Pediatricians, neurologists, geneticists, neonatologists, nutritionists, physical and occupational therapists, speech pathologists, and special education teachers must receive specific education regarding P-W syndrome.
4. Parent training. Parents who defer to professionals are frequently not as effective in securing help or establishing successful programs for their children as parents who are more assertive. Parents must provide information to medical and non-medical professionals about P-W syndrome, and then work with them to develop programs and materials.
5. Support of the Prader-Willi Syndrome Association. This association has a vital role in publicizing the syndrome, pulling information together, supporting individual families, developing printed materials, and communicating with professional groups. (Eds. note: The address of the Prader-Willi Syndrome Association is 5515 Malibu Drive, Edina, Minn. 55436.)
6. Emphasize non-medical needs of P-W persons and families. Most of the negative impact of the syndrome on affected persons and family members is the result of non-medical problems. To a large extent this is attributable to the social values of our society. Recognition of this fact, and increased knowledge of P-W syndrome by family members,

peers, and other persons outside the family will lead to better understanding and acceptance of P-W persons and to improvement of their lives.

ACKNOWLEDGMENTS

I thank the families for their willing response, John M. Opitz, M.D., and Sean Phipps, M.S., for discussion and information, and Julie Harmon for secretarial assistance.

APPENDIX A

Prader-Willi Syndrome Questionnaire

Name _____ Age _____ Sex _____

Address _____

Phone _____

Please feel free to answer this questionnaire any way you see fit by adding separate pages or by indicating questions or by providing comments. If it is so indicated by you, I will be glad to call you for an explanation or for a discussion. The term Prader-Willi Syndrome is abbreviated PWS in this questionnaire.

Number of older sibs _____ Number of younger sibs _____

1. One or several family members may each answer the questions on this single questionnaire by using pens of different color. Then please indicate who is using what color. Please indicate whether questionnaire is being filled out by:
   a. Person with PWS _____
   b. Mother of person with PWS _____
   c. Father of person with PWS _____
   d. Other _____

2. How old was the person with PWS when the diagnosis was made? _____

3. Did parents know earlier that something was wrong? _____ Please explain.

4. Had parents previously been reassured that nothing was wrong? _____ Please explain.

5. Had parents been told that the person with PWS would eventually outgrow his or her problems? _____ Please explain.

6. How did the person with PWS/mother/father feel when the diagnosis was made: a) sad, b) angry, c) relieved, d) upset, e) puzzled, f) worried, g) helpless, h) other.
(Circle as appropriate.) Please explain.

7. Did the fact that the diagnosis of PWS was made in any way change the person with PWS? ____ Please explain.

8. a. Was the fact that you have/your child has been diagnosed as having PWS changed your family life? ____ Please explain.

   b. Had family life been changed before the diagnosis was made? ____ Please explain.

9. What about PWS would you like to have been told earlier than you learned it? ____ Please explain.

10. What information about PWS would you like to have been told later or not at all? Please explain.

11. When the diagnosis was made, what do you feel were your biggest needs from the health professionals involved?
    a. More medical information about the condition ____
    b. Information on daily living skills—such as handling diet ____
    c. Information about services available—schools, programs, etc. ____
    d. More compassion and understanding, to have somebody to listen to your problems ____
    e. Need to be left alone for awhile ____
    f. Others ____

12. How in general was the explanation of the diagnosis handled? How could it be improved? Please explain.

13. Have the following medical problems been of concern?

		No Concern	Slight Concern	Moderate/ Severe Concern
a.	Breathing difficulties	——	——	——
b.	Feeding difficulties as a baby	——	——	——
c.	Constipation	——	——	——
d.	High blood pressure	——	——	——
e.	Overweight	——	——	——
f.	Heart problems	——	——	——
g.	Undescended testicles	——	——	——
h.	Kidney problems	——	——	——
i.	Eye problems	——	——	——
j.	Other (name)	——	——	——

Comment:

14. Does the condition have an impact on the following aspects of the life of the person with PWS and his family?

		None	Little	Moderate	Severe
a.	Self-image/ability to like oneself	——	——	——	——
b.	Peer relations	——	——	——	——
c.	Grandparents relations	——	——	——	——
d.	School placement	——	——	——	——
e.	Daily school habits	——	——	——	——
f.	Family finances	——	——	——	——
g.	Daily family activities	——	——	——	——
h.	Family eating habits	——	——	——	——
i.	Family members diet	——	——	——	——
j.	Family recreation activity	——	——	——	——
k.	Others	——	——	——	——

Comment:

15. Do you think the major problems associated with PWS in your family have been:

	Medical	Financial	Family	Personal/ Social
a. For persons with PWS	___	___	___	___
b. For father/mother	___	___	___	___
c. For other relatives	___	___	___	___

Comment:

16. Problems have mostly been due to: a) overweight, b) behavior, c) lack of knowledge about PWS, d) lack of understanding, e) impatience, f) medical problems, g) lack of finances, h) other. Please use letters a-h to describe the most important problems for the following:

    For person with PWS _____
    For mother _____
    For father _____
    For sib/other relative _____
    For peers _____
    For school personnel _____
    For public _____
    For other _____

    Comment:

17. Do you think that in the future the present problems for the person with PWS in your family will be related to:
    a. Overweight _____
    b. Medical problems _____
    c. Behavior _____
    d. Lack of finances _____
    e. Lack of peer relationship _____
    f. Lack of independence _____
    g. Lack of support in or from public _____
    h. Lack of schooling _____
    i. Other _____

       Comment:

18. As the person with PWS has gotten older, which areas have become more problematic? Which less so?

   a. For person with PWS _____

   b. For mother _____

   c. For father _____

   d. For sib/other relatives _____

   e. For peers _____

   f. For school personnel _____

   g. For others (name) _____

   Comment:

19. Do you think more research on PWS needs to be done? ____ What areas?

20. Do you know other persons with PWS? Yes ____ No ____

   a. Was or is it helpful to know them? Please explain.

   b. Was it *in any way* not helpful or associated with difficulties to have gotten to know them? Please explain.

21. What advice would you give another person or parent of a person with PWS? Please explain.

22. Lack of understanding of PWS by certain persons can cause problems for the PWS family. How have you found the level of

understanding of PWS by the following persons? What type of problem has their lack of understanding caused? In what areas do they most need to be educated?

a. Health professionals _____

b. School professionals _____

c. More distant relatives _____

d. General public _____

e. Other specific groups _____

Comment:

chapter 19
SOCIAL WORK INTERVENTION STRATEGIES FOR FAMILIES WITH CHILDREN WITH PRADER-WILLI SYNDROME

Judith M. Leconte

> In this chapter Ms. Leconte discusses the role of the social worker in meeting the needs of families with Prader-Willi syndrome children. She stresses that the needs of the entire family must be considered if the needs of the Prader-Willi syndrome child are to be adequately met, and that the interventions required by the syndrome often create additional problems.—*Eds.*

Prader-Willi (P-W) syndrome presents a unique constellation of needs that demand equally unique responses from families and professionals. To date, the literature on this syndrome has been either descriptive in nature or oriented to researching specific medical or nutritional characteristics. Management of this total collection of needs in a social context has been only peripherally addressed (Dunn, 1968; Hall & Smith, 1972; Holm & Pipes 1976; Pipes & Holm, 1973). Effective medical services for an individual affected by P-W syndrome requires full cooperation from the primary caregivers (parents, foster parents, and group home staff). Professionals rely heavily on families to carry out dietary, nutritional, medical, and social changes in the individual's environment. Therefore, assessment and management of the needs of the total system of interaction surrounding the P-W person are critical. Professionals must develop methods that will enhance and strengthen the role of the caregivers. What follows is a scheme for assessing the needs of the total system surrounding the P-W person and examples of interventions used by families who have children with P-W syndrome.

This chapter is based on clinical experience over a number of years with parents and siblings of children in the Prader-Willi Syndrome Clinic at the University of Washington. Within the clinic setting, work has been carried on with parents and siblings to mediate between the often conflicting demands of normal family life and those of a P-W child.

PARENTAL NEEDS

Since parental cooperation is essential in carrying out various methods of intervention to assist in the growth and development of the P-W child, assessment and management of the needs of parents is a critical factor in being able to serve the P-W child. Too frequently parents are labeled as the problem when the reality is that only the needs of the child have been considered.

Frameworks developed for management of parental needs in other handicapping conditions (such as cerebral palsy and mental retardation) do not address the unique aspects of this syndrome. The model proposed by Menolascino (1977; also see Wolfensberger, 1967) for helping parents of mentally retarded children assists in many areas faced by the P-W family. Rosen's (1955) study of maternal understanding of mental retardation provides a management model based on stages in accepting the diagnosis of mental retardation. But this model has limited clinical use for families facing a P-W syndrome diagnosis because the children involved in Rosen's study were more severely retarded and had no physical handicap. A further limitation is that the model is based on the experience of mothers only, rather than on that of whole families. Farber's (1960;1968) sociological studies of families with mentally retarded children have proved helpful in understanding the parents of P-W syndrome children but they do not provide practical management strategies for the P-W child in a family.

Clinical experience with P-W children has taught that parents must share their experiences. Many of them have developed techniques of management that may or may not be related to theory but that are often effective. The professional should be open to individual solutions to problems and should continuously search the literature for techniques that might be feasible for a particular P-W child or parent.

Parental Response to Diagnosis

A major task for professionals is helping parents deal with their initial response to a P-W syndrome child. Frequently, parents report complete shock when their P-W child is born. The extreme hypotonia and failure to thrive in early infancy were inconsistent with the expectations of the parents; they often mention that they were frightened by the child's floppiness and almost total lack of responsiveness during this period. They report feeling inadequate to care for the child. In most cases the need for diagnostic information and appropriate treatment to help the child was not adequately met, leading to a sense of confusion, guilt, anger, and helplessness. There were continuing searches for information from doctors, medical centers, and libraries. Comments such as "he'll never walk," "therapy won't help," "maybe he should be institutionalized," or "I don't see that anything will help at all," were often made by professionals during the first year of the child's life. Parents find that the time period between knowing something is wrong (at birth) and a final diagnosis is one of great anxiety and emotional turmoil.

The diagnosis of P-W syndrome was not made until rather late for many children. Symptoms were sometimes confused with those of other conditions. Many parents report feeling somewhat bewildered when a diagnosis of P-W syndrome was finally presented because the behaviors described as typical for this syndrome seemed so bizarre. They often report a sense of disbelief and, at the same time, some sense of relief when discovering that their child's condition is known but can't be cured. Menolascino (1977) describes the initial reaction of parents to the diagnosis of mental retardation in their child as "novelty shock." This can be brief or relatively long depending on the situation and circumstances surrounding diagnosis and the support that is given at the time of diagnosis. Parents of P-W children do, indeed, experience this shock and need support from professionals, relatives, and friends.

A unique feature of P-W syndrome is that as the severe hypotonia and failure to thrive disappear, developmental milestones finally appear and overeating begins. The latter symptom is frequently attributed to parental mismanagement if the syndrome has not been correctly diagnosed. The guilt produced by this assumption is overwhelming. The major intervention suggested by Menolascino (1977) for professionals is to tell the facts regarding the diagnosis in a very direct but supportive way. He cautions against pushing parents at this stage and suggests continuing to look for concrete symptoms that confirm the diagnosis. In the case of P-W syndrome, it has been the experience of the author that if the children are quite young when the diagnosis is made, parents find it difficult to accept not only that their expectations for a normal child are not met, but that their young, passive, underweight child will later develop tantrums and obesity. In cases where the diagnosis is made later, the appearance of behaviors such as extreme overeating and temper tantrums has usually begun and the parents feel relieved that a specific diagnosis does exist. Parents of older children often find it helpful to observe other children with the same disorder so they can make comparisons. In summary, the older the child when diagnosed, the more flexibility one has in approaching a discussion of diagnosis with the parents.

An example of the problems in explaining the P-W diagnosis to the parents of a young child is the experience with Jimmy. He was sent to the

University of Washington's Prader-Willi Syndrome Clinic at the age of two by his pediatrician for further exploration of the diagnosis of P-W syndrome. From birth he displayed feeding problems and slow weight gain coupled with severe hypotonia that resulted in delayed motor milestones. Previous diagnoses had included severe mental retardation, severe neurological impairment, and central nervous system disease. During the last assessment a little known neurological disease had been suggested as a possibility for the child's deficit in feeding and motor skills. The parents were dubious about coming to the P-W Clinic because they felt that the last diagnosis was correct. Evaluation at the clinic led to the diagnosis of P-W syndrome, which the parents found difficult to accept. Facts about P-W syndrome were explained to them, and similarities between Jimmy and other P-W children were pointed out. They were given further information about diet control and behavior management. Their response was to terminate contact with the clinic.

The professionals involved gave the parents written material on P-W syndrome and informed them that they had been managing the diet well and had been doing everything possible to stimulate motor development. The clinic staff accepted the fact that the family was not ready to participate in the clinic. Contacts have been made with the family periodically to assist them in pinpointing changes in the child's motor development, behavior, or eating patterns. There is no need for further intervention, because only Jimmy's further growth and development will confirm the diagnosis. The staff handled the family in a supportive way, acknowledging the fact that the parents chose to accept another diagnosis, although they followed all of the interventions appropriate for the child at that time. In situations like this it is critical not only to give honest information but also to provide support appropriate for the child's symptoms.

An example of parental acceptance of diagnosis is Harriet, who was 8 years old when she came to the Prader-Willi Syndrome Clinic. Her mother had read an article in a newspaper about P-W syndrome. Harriet's developmental milestones were severely delayed; she did not crawl until she was almost 14 months old, and she did not begin walking until 2½ years. She had displayed failure to thrive in the first year of life, with increased eating in the second year. During her fourth year she began to show a less passive style of relating to other people and began having tantrums, often involving food. Her mother reported being "beside herself" at the thought of Harriet getting older because of her obesity and behavior problems. She said that her daughter had begun taking food from neighbor's houses and was almost impossible to manage. Harriet was examined by the clinic staff and found to be a mildly retarded child with severe obesity and other physical and behavioral problems that confirmed the diagnosis of P-W syndrome. When the mother was told of the diagnosis and the interventions that would be required, she expressed relief that she had finally found individuals who did not blame her for her child's behavioral problems and unusual eating patterns. She welcomed returning to the P-W Clinic where she could get acquainted with other parents and their P-W children. In this case the mother was very open to the diagnosis of P-W syndrome as opposed to "having nothing at all to blame Harriet's behaviors on." Her husband and mother-in-law were not as easily convinced. Both thought that the mother was grasping at straws to explain bad parenting behavior. They were invited to the clinic to discuss the diagnosis. Physical similarities between Harriet and other P-W children were pointed out. Both father and grandmother were dubious at first, but on exposure to other P-W children they saw the similarities and were convinced.

Value Conflicts

Most parents of P-W children come to accept that their child is different from others, and that slow mental development, the tendency to overeat, and other behavioral problems are permanent. At this point, value conflict, as described by Menolascino (1977), often develops. Cultural or subcultural values and beliefs mold an individual's perception of the world and set standards for acceptable behavior and thoughts to which a handicapped child often does not conform. Each parent has unique experiences and values. Raising a handicapped child may make it necessary to forsake old values and assume new, more functional ones. This is a long term process, never easy, and always uniquely personal.

Spouses are often in conflict about their values because of the behavior presented by their P-W child. Parents sometimes wonder if the task of keeping the child thin is worth the effort required. These values can sometimes be traced back to their own family value systems of "productivity is good" or "if you are not intelligent, you are not worth anything." At times, parents feel that the efforts they have made toward keeping their child thin or managing school programs or attempting to resolve behavioral problems is "a waste of time." Parents are shocked and horrified at these feelings. Such value conflicts are often brought up when the parents are exposed to situations in which their child looks normal but behaves abnormally. On the other hand, they also occur when comments are made by the general public or relatives on the appearance or behavior of the child. Many situations in daily living can generate internal value conflicts in the parents.

Another problem sometimes encountered is that values of spouses differ. One parent may think that their P-W child should eat anything wanted in order to be "happy," while the other may believe that longevity and good health are important, and therefore restrict the diet. It is important to distinguish between the internal value conflict of one parent that may cause ambivalent or non-functional behavior toward the child and the conflict that arises from the different values of both parents. The aim in internal value conflict is to clarify for the individual what values are held and how they affect behavior towards the child, while in conflicts between spouses communication and resolution of the conflict are important.

In parents of P-W children value conflicts sometimes result in rejection of treatment or rejection of the child. Parents often express guilt over negative feelings that are a normal response. Intervention consists of discussing their feelings, tracing their roots to values held by relatives, the community, or close friends, and talking about ways in which the values might be modified. Beyond this, discussion of value systems might best be managed in a group of parents holding similar values. In the University of Washington's Prader-Willi Syndrome Clinic, the P-W parent group is open to free discussion and allows parents the chance to explore value systems with others who are also affected by the syndrome. Parents have revealed that they have found these groups most helpful when they have not focused exclusively on managing diet behavior and on medical concerns. It is important to allow the parents time to share feelings toward their P-W children and the disruption the children cause in their lives.

For example, one discussion within the parent group revolved around whether P-W children should be grouped together in schools and other programs or placed with other developmentally disabled individuals. Some were afraid that the children's developmental levels would be worsened if they were placed with children with more severely handicapping conditions. One mother thought that her child should have as much exposure to "normal people" as possible because his developmental level was in the high mildly retarded range. She disliked the thought of having him placed with individuals from whom she felt he "could not learn." A discussion followed about values concerning mental retardation and intelligence. It soon moved toward valuing happiness above learning. Then some parents began discussing their feelings that the child needed to be productive and strong; others discussed feelings about the importance of independence and ability to survive.

Therapeutic intervention directs families to focus on their own values and how strongly rooted they are in the past. One parent said that in the previous week her own mother had indicated that she hoped her grandson would not be one of those people who cannot contribute to society by working and "carrying his own weight." Others agreed that they had often heard this kind of statement. They discussed ways in which these values can be changed or modified to fit the futures that their children may have. Parents are usually willing to participate in this kind of discussion, although they are not always aware that in this way they are changing their values.

Several parents in the P-W Clinic have turned to their churches or religious counselors for support of new and different values regarding mental retardation and obesity. One parent is an active church member and is involved in its social activities. Her P-W child accompanies her to church functions where food is often available. The members of the church have been told of this child's problems and assist her in supervising his eating behaviors at church gatherings. They have accepted this child and allow him to function within the church. This exemplifies the idea that each individual can participate in the whole community regardless of handicap.

Reality Stress

The concept of reality stress as presented by Menolascino (1977) has great relevance to parents of P-W children. Symptoms of stress may result from the demands placed on the parent for the child's daily care. The pressure created by the need for specialized programs, a rigorously controlled diet, behavioral control, and therapy appointments is far greater than that related to the raising of a normal child, or even a child who is mentally retarded. Once parents are established in the P-W Clinic, the intervention strategies used by the clinic staff will probably increase reality stress.

Major areas of stress for parents are management of food intake and food-related behavior problems. Food management places restrictions on all family members, and therefore creates stress for the parents who are responsible for it. The P-W Clinic diet, which requires low calorie recipes that must appeal to the whole family, locking up all foods, and making alterations in habits of eating out, presents considerable problems for the parents. As the child gets older the problems around food become more difficult because the developmental level allows more alternatives in obtaining food. The 8- or 9-year-old child can take food from neighbors, eat out of garbage cans, or shoplift in stores. In adolescence the problem becomes worse as the P-W syndrome individual seeks food from peers, strangers, or through delinquent acts. Children in the P-W Clinic have run away to police stations in order to get meals and have stolen from large grocery stores. Parents have also reported behavioral problems regarding food that caused considerable embarrassment in public. This is difficult for parents because they are looked upon as the ones who should be in control. Parents report being sanctioned by others for not controlling their child and, at other times, for attempting to control him. This is a heavy burden to bear.

Another major area of stress for parents results from the needs of their normal offspring. Frequently, parents express frustration and guilt over meeting the P-W child's needs at the expense of their normal children. The constant monitoring of the P-W child preoccupies parents and this seems to pass on to other family members as well. A lack of recreational facilities for younger children often causes parents to require that siblings play with the P-W child.

For the teenage P-W child, this lack of social experiences and recreational opportunities continues and worsens because of motor deficits, temper outbursts, and eating behaviors. Recreational programs rarely demonstrate the willingness to manage the behaviors displayed by these individuals when they want food. Therefore, more and more demand is placed on the family to give the child social experiences. These stresses can be greater than those associated with most handicapping conditions in children. Often, P-W children have been excluded from programs or resources because they are not just mentally retarded. This increases the burden for parents.

The level of stress maintained over a period of time in dealing with the P-W child has considerable impact on all family members. Parents frequently find themselves exhausted and have reported giving up the diet in order to place their child in recreational programs. Fears about what the future will hold add to the stress caused by current realities.

Intervention for reality stress varies considerably depending on the parent and child in question. Concrete services are the usual response. The process used in the P-W Clinic assists the parents in identifying areas of stress. Frequently, stress is generalized and not related to specific events. The major focus for intervention is to find the specific areas of concern that are most stressful to the parent. It was found that diet management and medical problems are most important when the child is between 1 year and 5 years of age. Stresses from 6 years to 9 years tend to relate to school and social behavior. Between the ages of 10 years and 18 years the most critical behaviors are overeating, temper tantrums, poor social skills, and some delinquent behaviors surrounding food, such as running away, foraging for food, and stealing money to buy food.

In addition to identifying specific areas of stress, it is important to acknowledge that professional intervention cannot solve every existing problem. The services provided at the P-W Clinic can only address a limited amount of the stress parents face in raising a child with P-W syndrome. Since so little is known about the behaviors and their causes, interventions that are suggested may not completely resolve the issue. When other interventions have not been helpful in providing relief for parents in their daily contacts with their child, one can use respite or recreational care services. The use of these methods is illustrated by the following example.

Tommy, age 13, has been known to the P-W Clinic since 6 years of age, when the diagnosis of P-W syndrome was made. In the past, Tommy kept his weight down through the assistance of his mother and the nutritionist. His behavior was manageable except for brief episodes of temper tantrums, usually the result of being denied food. Then Tommy began running away from home whenever he had been sneaking food or had gone off the diet. All family members increased monitoring of behaviors when food was accessible to him. His mother came to the clinic more frequently. She was haggard in appearance and reported losing weight. Her husband began staying away from home more frequently in the evenings. Her two younger daughters, ages 9 and 12, were constantly fighting with Tommy and with each other. The nutritionist became concerned because Tommy had begun gaining weight. In an interview Tommy's mother began to talk about the future and her concern that there will be no one to care for Tommy as he gets older. She expressed fears that Tommy's intolerable behavior might become worse. She began to cry and said that she felt she could not go on.

At this point, there were several areas in which help could be offered. Tommy's behavior problems were not going to disappear, but it was possible to control how they occurred. The initial intervention was respite care for Tommy on weekends. In addition, a recreation program was found for Tommy in the afternoons. This lessened the time his mother spent with him, and allowed her to spend more time with the girls. The third service was to provide a behavior management program for Tommy that included both parents. It was made quite explicit in explaining the realities that it was not possible to stop the cravings Tommy had for food, nor his foraging for food, but that some competing behaviors could be introduced to reduce the time he had to think about food. These three services allowed the family to gain control over their situation and lessened the impact of Tommy's behavior on them.

SIBLINGS

The author's clinical experience with brothers and sisters of P-W children indicates that the syndrome also has considerable impact on siblings. Although their role is not as vital as that of the parents in the care of the P-W child, they are an important part of the total picture. Parents often think that the primary problem is that the other children do not understand their P-W sibling. Brothers and sisters need to understand the reasons for limiting food intake and that the P-W child is mentally as well as physically handicapped. Parents feel that their children are missing a normal childhood and that their lives are greatly disrupted by the needs of the P-W child. They feel guilty because the other children in the family must assume responsibility for caring for the P-W child in the parents' absence.

Grossman (1972) interviewed college-age siblings of the mentally handicapped. She found that mentally handicapped children who were of the same sex as their siblings, very deformed in appearance, and older than their siblings tended to be resented more and were difficult to cope with. The clinical experience of the author indicates that siblings of the P-W child are far more intruded upon by their P-W sibling than by the child who is only mentally handicapped. Locking up food and restrictive diets are intrusive upon all family members. Reports from siblings often indicate their embarrassment at being in the same school with their P-W sibling and having to be identified with that child in the school environment. Siblings also report that they feel a heavy sense of responsibility for the eating behaviors and temper tantrums of their P-W sibling because these behaviors make their parents very angry; they have associated the P-W child's eating behaviors and tantrums with parent upset and disruption of family plans. The older siblings appear to be able to cope better with the P-W child than younger siblings, which is similar to Grossman's findings with siblings of the mentally retarded.

A series of group sessions involving siblings 11 years to 14 years of age whose P-W syndrome brothers are older proved to be a valuable experience. All of the children who participated indicated that meeting other children with similar life experiences was most helpful to them. The aim of these sessions was to increase the knowledge of the children regarding P-W syndrome, to increase their ability to express positive and negative feelings about having a sibling with the syndrome, and to help them to become aware of other siblings and their problems. Information given about P-W syndrome covered mental retardation and normal intellectual functioning, physical characteristics such as motor development and growth patterns, and nutritional needs and the hunger drive.

A checklist of true/false questions about P-W syndrome was furnished before the series of groups sessions. These questionnaires indicated that most siblings in the group were fairly well informed about the general characteristics of the syndrome. Yet, during discussions of each of the areas covered, the siblings demonstrated less specific knowledge of how these characteristics related to daily functioning. The siblings were most interested in relating syndrome characteristics to everyday life situations in their families. For example, in discussing low muscle tone, Susan, 14 years of age, reported that her brother tended to walk downstairs very slowly and would yell at others if they came up behind him or passed him. She did not notice the same kind of nervousness or yelling when he was walking upstairs, which he tended to do much faster. The review of motor development helped Susan to recognize her brother's slowness as part of his delayed motor development rather than simply as irritating behavior. The following week she reported that she and her sister had refrained from making an issue of their brother's slowness going downstairs, and that he seemed more relaxed and no longer yelled at them. Thus, Susan had applied theoretical information about the syndrome to a specific problem in her daily life.

Siblings felt that the group sessions were most helpful in allowing them to talk about their brothers' problems. All indicated that they rarely talked to family members, friends, or individuals at school regarding their brother. Missie, age 12, reported that she frequently found herself blocking her brother from her mind when away from home. Others in the group said that they had had similar experiences, because it is easier to ignore the fact that their brother has problems than to share their concerns with others. When unpleasant incidents occurred, siblings shared information, feelings, or thoughts with their parents, but they did not feel free to fully express their feelings to other family members. Everyone in the group felt somewhat uncomfortable about explaining their brother's condition to friends beyond telling them that he was mentally retarded. When embarrassing situations occurred, e.g., their brother eating out of garbage cans or begging friends or fellow students for money, all of the siblings agreed that it was much better to walk away from the situation than to attempt an explanation about the syndrome.

Siblings, in general, felt that their brothers' behaviors had caused them considerable embarrassment and pain. In sharing experiences, they discovered many similarities. The siblings did not actually blame their parents for the behavior of their P-W syndrome brother, but they did think the parents were more lenient toward him. All of the siblings were afraid of destructive tantrums. All reported having to lock themselves in rooms to avoid being pursued by their P-W brother during a tantrum. These incidents had happened rarely. Each had a special way of handling his or her brother so that the tantrums did not get out of hand.

During the group sessions it was learned that: 1) understanding the condition does not always make it more bearable to live with, 2) siblings are isolated from situations in which they can ventilate feelings or thoughts about their P-W siblings, 3) many siblings reported a high frequency of wandering about the house during the night by their P-W brother, and 4) although parents are not always blamed for the behavior of their P-W individual, in general, siblings considered parents to be more lenient toward the P-W sibling than toward themselves.

Group meetings for siblings will continue to be scheduled to further explore this area of intervention. This will provide more data and allow siblings to assist in developing tools that are more useful than existing ones for treating the P-W population.

The author also has had experience with siblings in the 12- to 14-year-age range on an individual basis. Rebecca was 14 years old and according to her parents had been coping well with her older brother, John, who had P-W syndrome. In junior high school they were placed at the same school, he in a self-contained special education class and she in regular classes. Her brother soon became well known throughout the school for rummaging through garbage cans and eating the lunches of other people. These behaviors, difficult at home, became unbearable to her in the school setting. She was teased by other children in her classroom and was rejected by friends who had been close to her when they had been in elementary school. The mother learned that her daughter was finding it extremely difficult to cope with school when she began refusing to attend, claiming she was ill. Initially, intervention consisted of contacting school personnel and asking them to inform people at school about John's problems, and to assist the children in understanding what he was doing. This plan did not work because the junior high school personnel had only a limited amount of time to spend on the issue. The eventual solution was for the girl to change schools. As time went on, her mother explained the syndrome and the reasons for her brother's extreme behaviors. Consequently, she became comfortable bringing friends home and explaining her brother's temper tantrums and his eating behaviors, but she has not been able to resolve the issue outside of the home. Changing schools enabled her to keep a portion of her life separate from her brother's and greatly reduced the impact of his problems on her. The mother played a major role in the work of this P-W patient.

CONCLUSION

The work of the author with parents and siblings of P-W children has forced the use of a variety of innovative models to cope with the problems presented. Although family functioning is similar to that of families of mentally retarded children, the eating problems, unpredictable behavior, and poor health complicate intervention strategies. The limited ability of the P-W syndrome child to understand his or her hunger and unpredictable temper tantrums is frustrating for the family and for those trying to intervene. The goal is to assist parents in their daily dealings with their P-W children and to learn from them which interventions work.

The information gathered thus far indicates that families have many needs that are psychosocial or educational in nature. There is a critical need that health care personnel be better informed about the early symptoms of P-W syndrome. Parents must be given the facts about the suspected diagnosis of their child by sensitive professionals who can provide continuing support and care (see also Herrmann, Chapter 18, this volume). More dissemination of information is important since there are many health professionals who are unaware of P-W syndrome. Further research on this syndrome is another critical need (see Sulzbacher, Holm, & Pipes, Chapter 25, this volume). Various aspects of the syndrome (mental retardation, hypotonia, and metabolic differences) and the developmental changes of the child over time remain unexplained and often add confusion for parents, as well as limit what professionals are able to do to help. Resource development for P-W children is important since they are often left out of service programs because their needs are unique and they require constant attention. This means that the P-W child who creates a great amount of stress in the family has nowhere to go when the family needs some respite. In addition to meeting current needs, planning must include the transition to a group home or other permanent placement in adulthood.

In summary, ways to assist parents and siblings studied in the P-W Clinic at the University of Washington have been discussed. These methods need to be adapted to the syndrome and to the individual cases. Yet, the strength of the family is the key to any successful intervention. Therefore, assessing the needs of the family—parents and siblings—is critical in serving the P-W child.

REFERENCES

Dunn, H.G. The Prader-Labhart-Willi syndrome: Review of the literature and report of nine cases. *Acta Paediatrica Scandinavica*, 1968, Suppl. 186, 1-38.
Farber, B. Perceptions of crisis and related variables in the impact of a retarded child on the mother. *Journal of Health and Human Behavior*, 1960, *1*, 108-118.
Farber, B. *Mental retardation: Its social context and social consequences.* Boston: Houghton Mifflin Co., 1968.
Grossman, F. *Brothers and sisters of retarded children: An exploratory study.* Syracuse, N.Y.: Syracuse University Press, 1972.
Hall, B.D., & Smith, D.W. Prader-Willi syndrome: A resumé of 32 cases including an instance of affected first cousins, one of whom is of normal stature and intelligence, *The Journal of Pediatrics*, 1972, *81*, 286-293.
Holm, V.A., & Pipes, P.L. Food and children with Prader-Willi Syndrome. *American Journal of Diseases of Children*, 1976, *130*, 1063-1067.
Menolascino, F.J. A crisis model for helping parents cope more effectively. In *Challenges in mental retardation: Progressive ideology and services.* New York: Human Sciences Press, 1977.
Pipes, P.L., & Holm, V.A. Weight control of children with Prader-Willi syndrome. *Journal of The American Dietetic Association*, 1973, *62*, 520-524.
Rosen, L. Selected aspects in the development of the mother's understanding of her mentally retarded child. *American Journal of Mental Deficiency*, 1955, *59*, 522-528.
Wolfensberger, W. Counseling the parents of the retarded. In A.A. Baumeister (Ed.), *Mental Retardation: Appraisal, education, and rehabilitation.* Chicago: Aldine Publishing Co., 1967.

part IV

MEDICAL ASPECTS

chapter 20
MEDICAL MANAGEMENT OF PRADER-WILLI SYNDROME

Vanja A. Holm

In this chapter Dr. Holm discusses aspects of the management of Prader-Willi syndrome which primary care physicians need to be aware of.—*Eds.*

The signs and symptoms listed as clues to the diagnosis of Prader-Willi (P-W) syndrome (Holm, Chapter 3, this volume) are also medical problems that need management by physicians. Some of these are discussed in detail in the following chapters, and others, e.g., obesity, are covered extensively elsewhere. This chapter reviews the medical conditions that might need attention in patients with P-W syndrome, with emphasis on treatments not covered elsewhere.

HEALTH MAINTENANCE

Health maintenance is essential for P-W children. The infant with P-W syndrome—whether or not the condition has been diagnosed—soon accumulates such a long list of problems that health maintenance might be forgotten both by the family and by the physician. Handicapped children need immunization, preventive dental care, hearing and vision screening, tuberculin testing, and other standard preventive health measures at least as much as their normal siblings and peers. The person with P-W syndrome is prone to dental caries and the preventive measure of regular fluoride treatments during childhood will very likely minimize this problem. Eye problems are common in this condition; thus, repeated vision examinations are strongly indicated.

HYPOTONIA AND OTHER NEUROLOGICAL ABNORMALITIES

Physical therapy is recommended for the young hypotonic infant with P-W syndrome both by Zellweger (Chapter 5, this volume) and Carman (Chapter 24, this volume). The latter also describes some appropriate physical activities that can be carried out by the family. The physician will probably want to prescribe therapy for the hypotonia in infants and young children with P-W syndrome if therapists trained to work with young children are available in the community.

Hypotonia is a well recognized neurological hallmark of P-W syndrome. It is less well known that one often encounters other neurological abnormalities in this condition. Asymmetric reflex responses are fairly common. Ankle clonus might be elicited, unilaterally or bilaterally. Mild contractures, e.g., limitation of supination in one or both upper extremities, might be found. These abnormalities are usually subtle and easily overlooked. When noted, they should be observed over time. They usually prove to be static, and extensive neurological investigation, such as computerized tomography, is seldom indicated in P-W syndrome.

OBESITY

The management of obesity in P-W syndrome is discussed in several chapters in Part II of this book, and only aspects not covered elsewhere will be considered here.

Parents, patients, and physicians frequently consider appetite-suppressing medication as a temptingly simple solution to the hyperphagia in P-W syndrome. Many persons with this condition at sometime or another have been tried on dextroamphetamine before the use of this medication was banned by the FDA for this purpose. The suppressant effect on the appetite, in the few cases where this could be demonstrated, was invariably short-lived. Because of its ineffectiveness and potential danger (it suppresses growth and is prone to be misused), dextroamphetamine is not recommended for obesity management in P-W syndrome.

Many other medicines have been tried, often in desperation, in obesity management of P-W syndrome, including thyroid pills and diuretics. These medications do not reduce the abnormal accumulation of subcutaneous fat in P-W syndrome and should be used only on specific medical indications, i.e., hypothyroidism (highly unlikely) and congestive heart failure. To put it simply, no drug or combination of drugs cures the obesity in this syndrome, or cures any other kind of obesity.

Crash diets and fad diets are often tried. They are probably more dangerous in P-W syndrome than they are in persons with normal metabolic states and are certainly equally ineffective. Physicians should strongly advise P-W patients against any fast weight loss schemes, especially unsupervised diets that are nutritionally unbalanced. Special diets which have been medically prescribed and supervised have also been tried in this condition, e.g., the ketogenic diet (Nelson, Huse, Holman,

Kimbrough, Wahner, Callaway, & Hayles, Chapter 8, this volume) and the protein-sparing diet (Bistrian, Blackburn, & Stanbury, 1977). Neither has been shown to be effective over time in an outpatient setting. The only sound approach to obesity management is a well balanced diet with low caloric content (Pipes, Chapter 7, this volume). If obesity proves to be intractable and life-threatening, gastric bypass surgery could be considered in adolescents and young adults (Soper, Mason, Printen, & Zellweger, Chapter 9, this volume).

There remain a number of persons with P-W syndrome in whom gross obesity was not prevented and could not be controlled. Such individuals might be affected by any of the many known complications of obesity, e.g., the Pickwickian syndrome. The response to treatment of these disease states in P-W syndrome seems to be similar to other forms of obesity.

HYPOGONADISM

Hypogonadism is a collection of symptoms that present a variety of medical management problems in P-W syndrome depending on the age and sex of the patient. These are discussed separately.

Micropenis in Early Childhood

Most young boys with P-W syndrome have such a small penis that it becomes a cosmetic concern for psychological reasons. Parents are troubled, preschool teachers are surprised, and peers are contemptuous. After the boy is toilet-trained, small penile size usually prohibits urination in the accepted male standing-up position.

Treatment for micropenis with testosterone has been suggested by Guthrie, Smith, and Graham (1973). Two of their four patients had P-W syndrome. This and other treatments have been used successfully in young boys with P-W syndrome. It is preferable to start the treatment before the boy has become used to sitting down to urinate. Twenty-five milligrams of testosterone cypionate (depo-testosterone) is given intramuscularly every 3 weeks until an adequate penile length for childhood, 5 to 6 cm (Smith, 1976, p. 472), is obtained. From three to five injections are usually required. The cosmetic and functional result is satisfying to both the parents and the boys.

Undescended Testes

The testicles in P-W syndrome vary in size and location. Occasionally they are of appropriate prepubertal size and normal consistency in a boy who otherwise shows typical signs and symptoms of P-W syndrome (in these cases the penis is usually small). Sometimes testicular material, small in volume and with soft consistency, is present in the scrotal sac or the inguinal canal on one side or both. Most frequently the testes are undescended and their size and consistency are unknown.

Surgery to bring down undescended testes in normal boys is performed to preserve fertility, for psychological reasons, and because of the increased risk of malignancy in testes that remain undescended. Orchiopexy is performed on the assumption that the testes are normal. Potential for testicular growth and testosterone production in adolescence in males with P-W syndrome is variable. At this time prepubertal physical findings are not predictable. Therefore, the indications for surgery in boys with P-W syndrome have to be determined on an individual basis. Fertility is not an issue. The psychological impact of undescended testes might be. However, considering the overwhelming behavioral and social problems encountered during the later childhood years because of this condition, the possible problems secondary to undescended testes seem minimal by comparison. The increased malignancy risk needs to be considered, but it is not an issue during childhood. The conservative approach is to wait and see what happens in adolescence. Will the testes descend? Will they grow? How much testosterone will they produce, i.e., how complete will the development of secondary sexual characteristics be? In young adulthood, depending on the clinical situation, the testes might be brought down or removed, in which case testosterone replacement and prosthesis might be considered.

A more aggressive approach might be warranted in young boys in certain situations, for example, in a boy with one descended testis of near normal size and consistency. Testicular biopsy should be done during surgery to obtain information regarding possible fertility. In one such case encountered by the author, the histology was abnormal both in the descended and the undescended testes, but more markedly in the latter. If orchiopexy is contemplated on bilaterally undescended testes in childhood, it is advisable to obtain testosterone levels before and after priming with human chorionic gonadotropic to demonstrate that functional testicular material indeed is present before proceeding with the surgery.

Incomplete Adolescent Masculinization and Feminization

D.W. Smith, M.D. (personal communication) has suggested that endocrinological replacement therapy, as it has been used in Klinefelter and Turner syndromes, might be used for P-W syndrome patients. Similarly, R.H.A. Ruvalcaba, M.D. (personal communication) has said that testosterone was given to adult males and did not influence or complete the masculinization process, which indicates that it has to be given in adolescence to be effective. However, the parents and the boys are usually more concerned about the short stature than slow masculinization, if indeed that is present. Since precocious or otherwise disordered puberty might occur (Holm, Chapter 3, this volume), endocrinological evaluation is advisable before hormone treatment is considered. Females might be given replacement therapy if feminization (especially breast development) does not occur or stops prematurely. Short stature is usually of less concern in females. Again, this problem of incomplete feminization seems to have low priority both for the parents and the girls themselves. Intervention should be offered only when it is perceived as a problem.

SHORT STATURE

This problem is discussed in detail elsewhere (Nugent & Holm, Chapter 21, this volume). Oxandrolone treatment is being used in males, but must be considered experimental at this time

SCOLIOSIS AND OTHER ORTHOPEDIC PROBLEMS

Scoliosis in P-W syndrome and its treatment is discussed elsewhere in this volume (Laurnen, Chapter 23). Medical management of scoliosis is the same in P-W syndrome as that of idiopathic scoliosis in otherwise healthy adolescents. Similarly, treatment of congenital hip dislocation, common in P-W syndrome, and most other orthopedic conditions occurring in persons with the syndrome would not be different from treatment given to others. Two aspects warrant special mention, however.

Uneven Leg Length

Asymmetry in length of the lower extremities is not uncommon in the general population and is usually not treated unless it exceeds one-half inch. In standing, the leg length difference is compensated for by a mild functional spinal curve. In P-W syndrome, leg length difference appears to be surprisingly common. Considering the propensity to scoliosis in this population, a conservative approach would be to use a shoe lift to compensate for even a small leg length difference in growing children, although it is not known whether such a procedure will influence the development of a structural scoliosis.

Fractures

A small but significant number of patients with P-W syndrome sustain fractures after minor traumas. Therefore, in the P-W individual with a fracture the circumstance of the accident should be carefully assessed to determine whether this unusual degree of susceptibility is present. If so, special precautions might be necessary in the future. Grossly obese subjects have been known to become permanently wheelchair-bound following immobilization for medical reasons, a fact that needs to be considered in the treatment of fractures.

SKIN PROBLEMS

A variety of symptoms relating to the skin are present in P-W syndrome.

Skin Picking

Care givers often complain that persons with P-W syndrome dig at minor scrapes and insect bites or actually create sores on the intact skin. In such individuals one sees scars on easily accessible areas, especially the arms and hands. Large oral intake of vitamin B_1 (thiamine) is known to discourage mosquitoes and other biting insects and has been helpful in children plagued by insect bites that they pick. Otherwise, treatment is behavioral: the P-W person either must ignore the bite or use clothing that prevents access to most of the skin. Skin infections might become severe, especially when aggravated by poor circulation in the lower extremities in grossly obese subjects.

Decreased Pain Sensitivity

An unusually high tolerance for pain is noted in some P-W persons. Sensation is intact, but the awareness of pain seems diminished. This symptom is less common than skin picking, but those that show it usually also pick at their skin. Burns might result from lack of withdrawal from hot objects in persons with decreased awareness of pain. More important, such patients might not appreciate painful sensations from inner organs. A young man died of complications from a burst appendix without vomiting or complaining of pain, both of which are prominent symptoms of appendicitis. For unknown reasons many persons with P-W syndrome do not vomit. When caring for P-W persons, one therefore needs to be aware that some do not show the expected physiological responses to illness.

Bruising

Many P-W syndrome persons bruise easily. Parents of children with this syndrome have been referred to child protective services by uninformed teachers and neighbors who have noted many bruises and who are aware of the child's behavior problem. Thus, it is sometimes necessary for the child's physician to explain the susceptibility to bruising.

OTHER MEDICAL PROBLEMS

One might encounter a great many additional medical problems in the P-W syndrome patient. Treatment of most P-W persons is not different from that of the general population. This includes treatment for strabismus and seizure disorders. Diabetes mellitus is not as common in the syndrome as was previously thought. Food-related behavior problems might severely complicate the diet control necessary for the treatment of diabetes, which otherwise is not serious in this syndrome.

Finally, the use of behavior-modifying, mood-altering, antipsychotic, and sedative drugs in this syndrome has been suggested. No medication has been consistently successful in treatment of the behaviors encountered in P-W syndrome. Persons with classical schizophrenic symptomatology have responded to specific treatment for this condition. An occasional person with depression has responded to antidepressant drugs. Most medications used for behavioral control in P-W syndrome have been used in institutional settings and seem to be given more for the benefit of the staff than of the patients. If such drugs are used, careful documentation of their benefits should be a prerequisite for long term use.

REFERENCES

Bistrian, B.R., Blackburn, G.L., & Stanbury, J.B. Metabolic aspects of a protein-sparing modified fast in the dietary management of Prader-Willi obesity. *The New England Journal of Medicine,* 1977, *296,* 774-779.

Guthrie, R.D., Smith, D.W., & Graham, C.B. Testosterone treatment for micropenis during early childhood. *The Journal of Pediatrics,* 1973 *83,* 247-252.

Smith, D.W. *Recognizable patterns of human malformation: Genetic, embryologic and clinical aspects* (2nd ed.). Philadelphia: W.B. Saunders Co., 1976.

chapter 21
PHYSICAL GROWTH IN PRADER-WILLI SYNDROME

Jane K. Nugent and Vanja A. Holm

In this chapter Drs. Nugent and Holm discuss aspects of growth in Prader-Willi syndrome including: endocrine studies, birth size, bone age, weight gain, and height. They describe their use of oxandrolone to stimulate height growth, with successful results to date.—*Eds.*

Obesity is the most important feature of Prader-Willi (P-W) syndrome. Short stature is also common, though less emphasized than other physical stigmata. Hall and Smith (1972) have reported that 94% of these patients are of short stature. The etiology of the growth failure is poorly understood. The literature on growth in P-W syndrome consists of reports by a number of investigators from different research centers, using a variety of study protocols. The number of patients available to each investigator for study is small; therefore, the conclusions to be drawn from each study are limited.

At the Prader-Willi Syndrome Clinic of the Child Development and Mental Retardation Center, University of Washington, some 60 persons with this syndrome have been seen over the years, with an active clinic population at any one time of 20 to 30 patients. Heights and weights are obtained on each clinic visit by the same staff, using the same measurement devices. Growth data are plotted on each visit on the growth curves published by the National Center for Health Statistics (*NCHS growth curves for children: Birth-18 years, United States,* 1977). Weight data on patients are reported elsewhere in this volume (Pipes, Chapter 7). Their height growth is reported in this chapter. In clinic patients for whom appropriate data were available, growth in height has also been analyzed in relation to the heights of their parents. As reported in Parts II and III of this volume, dietary information and comprehensive learning and psychological evaluations were also recorded and followed regularly.

This chapter was prepared when Dr. Nugent was a Fellow in Pediatric Endocrinology at the University of Washington School of Medicine, Seattle (NICHD Training Grant HD-00404 (1977-1979)).

Additional information on growth was obtained from 98 questionnaires returned from all over the United States (Holm, Chapter 3, this volume). Data from reliable sources, such as physicians' records, accurate enough for the study of growth patterns, were used for comparison with growth patterns of normal children. Information on birth weights and lengths from these same questionnaires was also analyzed and compared to normal values.

This chapter includes a review of available endocrinological studies on growth in P-W syndrome, a report of findings on birth size, bone age, and weight status in untreated P-W syndrome, a summarization of data on height growth, which will be published in detail elsewhere, and, finally, provides suggestions for possible management of growth failure in the syndrome based on the experience of the authors.

ENDOCRINE STUDIES ON GROWTH IN P-W SYNDROME

The literature on the possible role of growth hormone in the short stature of the child with P-W syndrome is confusing. Normal growth hormone levels are noted in several case reports (Bier, 1970; Landwirth, Schwartz, & Grunt, 1968; Seyler, Arulanantham, & O'Connor, 1979). Dunn (1968) tested five out of nine patients with P-W syndrome and found their growth hormone levels to be normal. Hamilton, Scully, and Kliman (1972) noted that growth hormone was detectable (3 ng/dl) in the basal state and was normally elevated (to 11 and 20 ng/dl, respectively) in two patients tested after exposure to accepted hypoglycemic stimuli. They also confirmed observations made by previous investigators that thyroid function tests, as well as tests of adrenal axis and adrenocorticotropic hormone responses, were in the normal range. In 1974, Theodoridis, Brown, Chance, and Rudd reported normal growth hormone response to oral glucose stimulation in four out of six patients, but two patients clearly demonstrated subnormal values. Tolis, Lewis, Verdy, Friesen, Solomon, Pagalis, Pavlatos, Fessas and Rochefort (1974) studied two males and three females. They found adrenal and thyroid tests to be within normal limits and demonstrated that growth hormone levels were normal during a five-hour glucose tolerance test in which growth hormone levels were determined every 30 minutes (one was also normal after 500 mg of L-dopa and one after insulin-induced hypoglycemia). Parra, Cervantes, and Schultz (1973) have shown that plasma immunoreactive insulin was elevated and that growth hormone levels were blunted in response to oral glucose, protein glucose meal, and intravenous arginine in six children with P-W syndrome. However, these responses were almost identical to those of a control group of children with long-standing obesity, who were otherwise normal.

Though the aberrations in growth hormone release in relationship to glucose metabolism demonstrated by some authors may be significant, these studies do not demonstrate that growth hormone deficiency accounts for short stature in P-W syndrome. Properly controlled fasting stimulation tests are needed to demonstrate growth hormone deficiency. When such studies are done, results indicate that growth hormone levels are normal in this syndrome. The literature also contains ample evidence that other endocrine systems, i.e., thyroid, parathyroid, and adrenal axes, are normal. Hypothalamic hypogonadism is the only endocrine disorder demonstrated in P-W syndrome with consistency (Tze, Dunn, & Rothstein, Chapter 22, this volume).

BIRTH SIZE

Throughout the literature, the infant later diagnosed as having P-W syndrome is usually described as the product of a full term pregnancy, but with a low birth weight. Decreased fetal activity is almost always noted. Many infants present with breech and transverse lies, thought to be a result of the hypotonia usually observed after birth. Prader, Labhart, and Willi (1956) originally described these features, which have been corroborated by many.

Dunn (1968) studied nine patients. He described them as small hypotonic infants at birth, with a mean birth weight of 2,834 grams, in spite of most of them being postterm. Pearson, Steinbach, and Bier (1971) reported five patients, all but one weighing less than 2,500 grams at birth. Juul and Dupont (1967) summarized available case reports from the literature and found that birth weight was less than 3,000 grams in 24 out of 33 cases where it had been reported. Zellweger and Schneider (1968) reviewed their 14 cases and found that of the 10 males and four females, nine were products of a 40-week gestation, two of a 39-week gestation, two of a 38-week gestation, and one of a 43-week gestation. Only two patients weighed over 3,200 grams, seven between 3,000 grams and 3,200 grams, and five less than 3,000 grams. All infants were between 48 cm and 50 cm long, which is between the 25th and 50th percentile for length.

Birth weights of 25 patients seen at the Prader-Willi Syndrome Clinic at the University of Washington ranged from 4 pounds 5 ounces to 7 pounds 12 ounces. The mean birth weight was 6 pounds (2,700 grams), which is less than the 10th percentile according to the 1977 NCHS growth charts. Eighty-five percent of the babies were under 7 pounds (3,200 grams) and 50% were under 6 pounds (2,700 grams), which is striking considering that 90% of these infants were full term or the result of over a 38-week gestation. Many, however, presented in unusual positions such as breech, brow, or transverse lie, consequently leading to difficult deliveries.

Data on birth weights from the questionnaire study (Holm, Chapter 3, this volume) showed that in 53 males the mean birth weight was 2,750 grams (6 pounds, 2 ounces) and in 42 females it was 2,650 grams (5 pounds, 14 ounces). Mean birth length in 45 males for whom this information was provided was 50.8 cm (20 inches) and in 37 females it was 48.2 cm (19 3/8 inches). Twenty-two percent of 94 cases were breech presentations and 18% were delivered by cesarean section.

Thus, most persons with the syndrome start life with a birth weight that is small for gestational age, 2,750 grams for males, compared to a median birth weight of 3,400 grams for normal males, and 2,650 grams for females, compared to a median birth weight of 3,250 grams. Birth length is similar to that of normal neonates, 50.8 cm for males, compared to a median birth length of 49.9 cm for normal males, and 48.2 cm for females, compared to a median birth length of 49.3 cm.

BONE AGE

According to most reports, skeletal maturation of patients with P-W syndrome tends to fall behind chronological age (Hall & Smith, 1972). Dunn (1968) reported that six male patients less than 4 years of age had retarded bone ages, but that one female did not. He also noted a less significant or no delay in bone age as the males got older and normal bone age in a 13-year-old girl. Zellweger and Schneider (1968) found that 11 out of their 14 patients had bone ages more than 1 year below chronological age. Their patients were all less than 9 years old. Laurance (1967) reported data from nine patients. Four patients had normal bone ages, four showed skeletal retardation from 6 months to 2 years, and one had advanced bone age. Cohen and Gorlin (1969), Evans (1964), and Dubowitz (1967), among others, have reported retarded bone ages, especially in younger patients.

The bone age of patients in the P-W Syndrome Clinic at the University of Washington was determined by comparison of left-hand x-rays with those published by Greulich and Pyle (1959) and by comparison of multiple center analysis to the closest 6-month interval. Of the 19 patients who had had bone age determinations, seven (four males and three females) had bone ages equal to their chronological age. One female and two males had bone age retardation of less than 1 year. In three females and two males, bone age and height age were from 1 to 2 years behind their chronological age. Five male patients had advanced skeletal age, but all of these bone ages were still in the normal range in the adolescent years.

With this background one can conclude that bone age in P-W syndrome usually is within normal limits, i.e., within 2 years above or below chronological age. It tends to lag behind in childhood and might become advanced in the adolescent years. The implication for our overall understanding of P-W syndrome is unclear, but these findings seem compatible with hypothalamic hypogonadism. Nevertheless, evaluation of skeletal age in relationship to height age continues to be an essential tool in the clinical assessment of growth problems in the individual patient with P-W syndrome.

WEIGHT IN UNTREATED PERSONS WITH P-W SYNDROME

Obesity is a significant characteristic of P-W syndrome. In the experience of most authors, obesity has its onset during the preschool years. Cross-section data on weight from a questionnaire study (Holm, Chapter 3, this volume) was plotted on NCHS growth curves. Figure 21.1 depicts weight in 44 children, 24 males and 20 females, from birth to 36 months of age. As can be seen, all children with P-W syndrome suffer a period of failure to thrive in early infancy. By 6 months of age some children are above the 50th percentile and by 1 year some are already above the 95th percentile in weight. However, several children are still below the 5th percentile in weight when approaching their third birthday.

Weight data on the same population from the questionnaire study (Holm, chapter 3, this volume) from ages 3 to 23 years have been plotted in Figure 21.2. As can be seen, an occasional P-W child is still below the 50th percentile for weight by age five, but, without nutritional intervention, all are above the 50th percentile thereafter. A regression line was calculated from the data and is displayed in Figure 21.2. It indicates relentless weight gain in untreated P-W syndrome throughout early adulthood. This line of expected weight gain can be used to compare results of treatment in P-W syndrome, as has been done elsewhere in this volume (Pipes, Chapter 7; Soper, Mason, Printen, & Zellweger, Chapter 9).

Patients sometimes become immensely obese later in life (Figure 21.3). However, quantitative information about weight in adults with this syndrome is meager. In case reports, weights of 100 kg (220 pounds) and above and heights not much over 5 feet (152 cm) are noted (Bianchine, Stambler, & MacGregor, 1971; Reed, Ragsdale, Curtis, & Richards, 1968). If weight gain is not checked, the outcome might be early death, as described in several case reports (Jenab, Lade, Chiga, Diehl, 1959; Reed et al., 1968; Soper et al., Chapter 9). An unsuccessful nutrition management case (Holm & Pipes, 1976) died at 18 years weighing over 300 pounds; he was 163 cm (5 feet, 5 inches) tall.

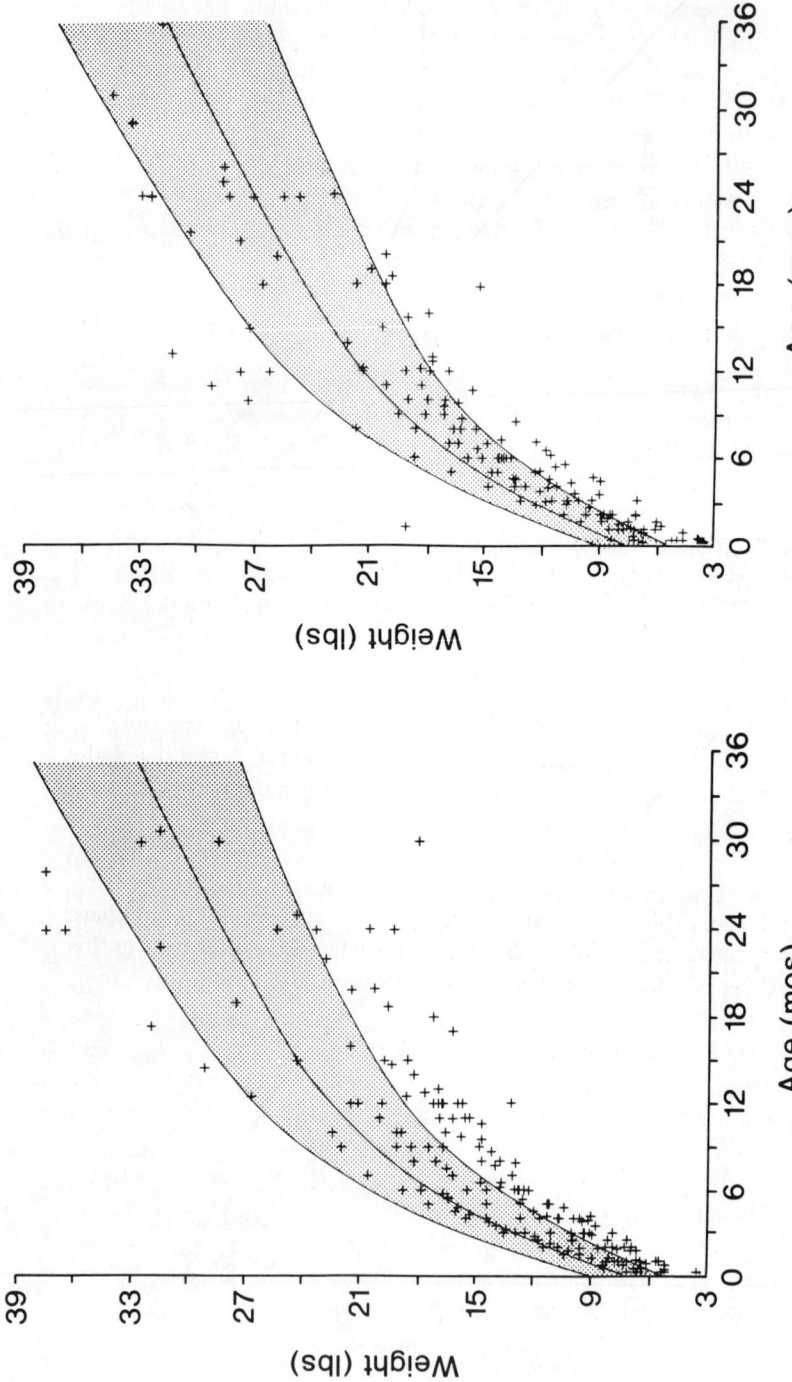

Figure 21.1. Weights of P-W syndrome patients from birth to 36 months. *A*, 24 males; *B*, 20 females.

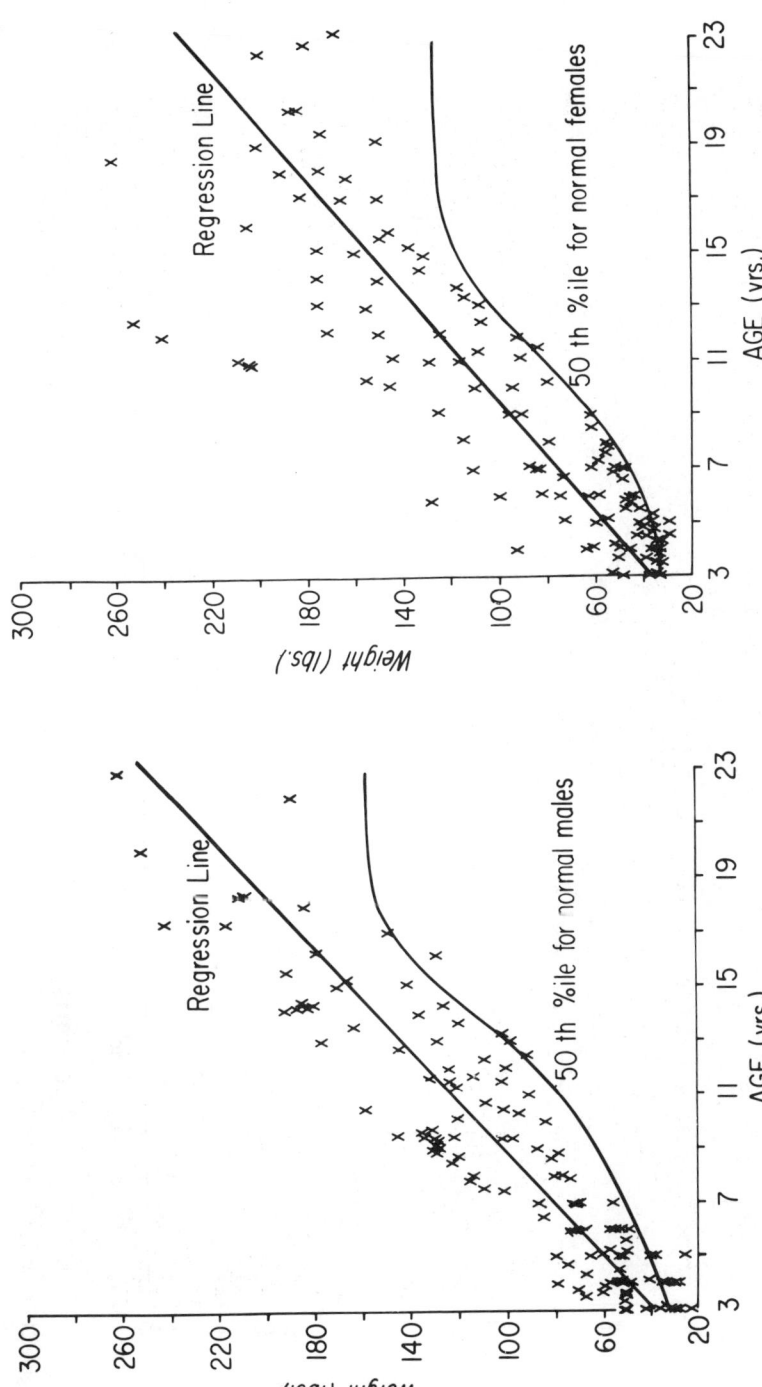

Figure 21.2. Weights of P-W syndrome patients from age 3 to 23 years. *A*, 24 males; *B*, 20 females.

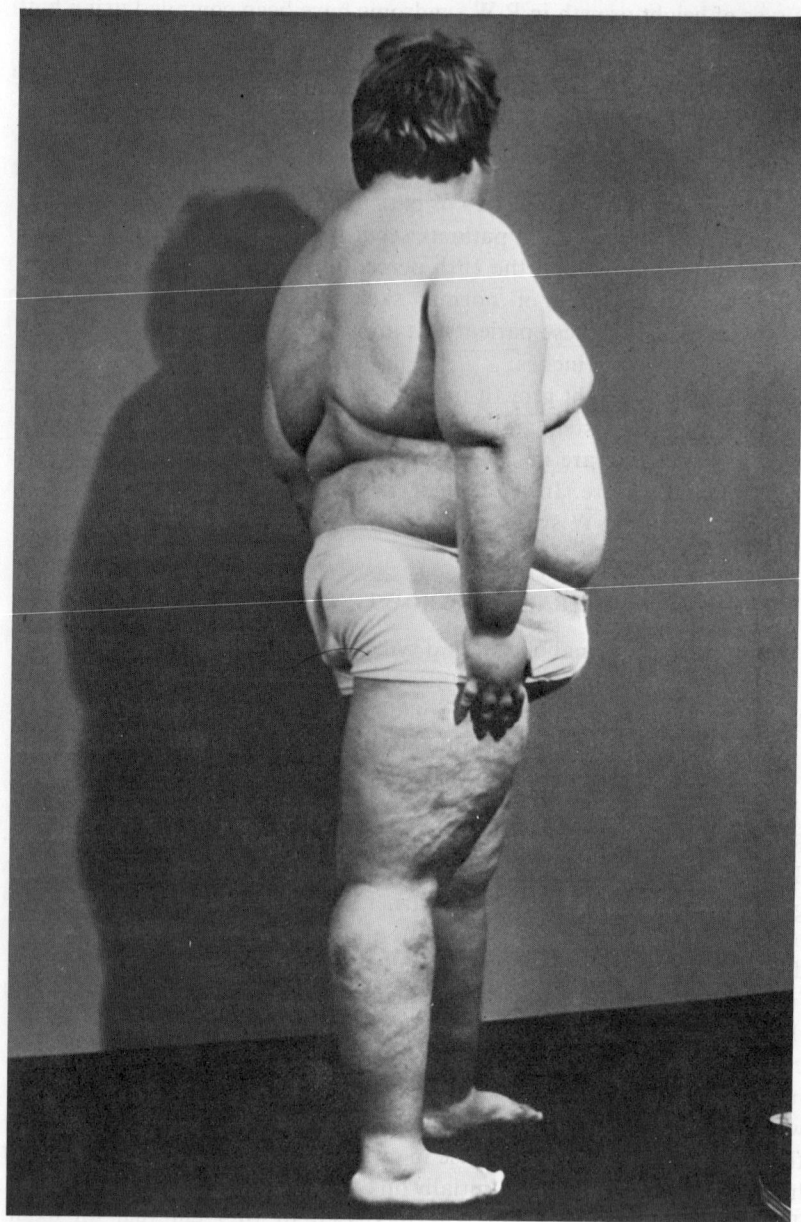

Figure 21.3. Untreated P-W syndrome obesity.

HEIGHT GROWTH IN P-W SYNDROME

Curves of height growth in P-W syndrome have been compiled using both data from the patients in the Prader-Willi Syndrome Clinic at the University of Washington and from the questionnaire study, which will be reported elsewhere. In summary, although these children start with normal birth length, as previously shown, by their third year most fall below the 25th percentile for linear height. Interestingly, it is also during the first 3 years of life that most P-W patients begin to gain weight rapidly. After 3 years of age, these patients seem to grow parallel to the normal curve but usually around the 10th percentile. Lack of a pubertal growth spurt is seen in spite of normal skeletal age and, therefore, open epiphyses. Most of these patients attain a final height between 4 feet, 10 inches and 5 feet, 3 inches.

Analysis of height growth in relation to mid-parental height according to Tanner, Goldstein and Whitehouse (1970) revealed that the majority of P-W patients are not experiencing growth patterns consistent with their familial stature. Instead, their growth is typical of the expectation for patients with P-W syndrome.

OXANDROLONE THERAPY OF GROWTH RETARDATION

Oxandrolone is an anabolic steroid synthesized by Pappo and Jung (1962) that is reported to have significant anabolic potency with low androgenic effect, and thus minimal stimulation of epiphyseal closure (Fox, Minot, & Liddle, 1962). This medication has been found to stimulate acceleration of linear growth in normal males with a diagnosis of maturational delay (Hopwood, Kelch, Zipf, & Hernandez, 1979; Moore, Tattoni, Limbeck, Ruvalcaba, Lindner, Gareis, Al-Agba, & Kelley, 1976). In 1977 Moore, Tattoni, Ruvalcaba, Limbeck, and Kelley reported that 25 females with gonadal dysgenesis (45 XO or Turner syndrome) gained a significant height advantage of 6.1 cm over the mean expected height in the syndrome after a course of oxandrolone therapy. These findings were confirmed by Urban, Lee, Dorst, Plotnick, and Migeon (1979), who reported that nine patients with gonadal dysgenesis experienced a significant increase in final height after receiving oxandrolone therapy for from 8 to 46 months. Raiti, Trias, Levitsky, and Grossman, (1973) treated one female with P-W syndrome with oxandrolone, growth hormone, and a combination of both. She had no increase in growth rate on growth hormone, but her growth velocity doubled initially on oxandrolone and the combination. The control rate of 5.8 cm/year increased to 10.9 cm/year on oxandrolone, and to 12.7 cm/year on the combination. However, because of decreasing response, her average growth velocity over the 3 years, 6 months of observation and treatment was only 0.5 cm/year, greater than the control rate. Many years of even this small growth advantage could significantly increase ultimate height attainment beyond the usual expectation for P-W syndrome, as has been reported in patients with gonadal dysgenesis.

There are several theoretical reasons for believing that oxandrolone might be effective in P-W syndrome: skeletal maturation is not advanced, patients might have androgen deficiency, and patients experience no pubertal growth spurt. It is therefore recommended that treatment with anabolic steroid be tried in the hope of achieving further growth in children with P-W syndrome. Such treatment should only be done as part of a controlled study, however. Preliminary observations of the authors, based on treating three boys with oxandrolone in early adolescence after growth arrest, indicate a similar response to that seen in patients with Turner syndrome (Moore et al., 1977). Therefore, it is suggested that earlier treatment, as in gonadal dysgenesis, at around 8 years of age, should also be considered in P-W syndrome, especially for boys. Our experience with one female patient treated at age 16 was less successful. Her voice began to change, which disturbed her more than her short stature, and she chose to discontinue the treatment. This suggests that greater caution should be exercised in treating P-W females with oxandrolone.

SUMMARY

Several broad conclusions about P-W syndrome can be drawn from the data presented in this chapter.

1. Children with P-W syndrome often present in unusual obstetrical positions attributable to hypotonia. They are usually full term and are born with normal birth length, but with birth weights below the 10th percentile for normal full term children. Thus, most newborns with P-W syndrome are small for gestational age.
2. Weight, if not controlled, increases relentlessly through adolescence and early adulthood and is indeed life-threatening.
3. Height growth percentile falls from normal at birth to below the 25th percentile by 3 years of age. After this age most P-W patients grow around the 10th percentile until puberty, when growth stops without a normal pubertal growth spurt. Most P-W syndrome children are short considering mid-parental height expectations, indicating that their linear growth is dictated by the syndrome, not their family height heritage. Ultimate height is around 5 feet in both males and females.
4. Accelerated skeletal maturation does not account for short stature and growth arrest.

5. Oxandrolone might stimulate growth in P-W syndrome patients. It could be tried starting around 8 years of age, but should be given only as part of a controlled study.

REFERENCES

Bianchine, J.W., Stambler, A.A., & MacGregor, M.I. The Prader-Willi syndrome with cardiorespiratory complications. *Birth Defects,* 1971, *7,* 301.
Bier, D.M. The Prader-Willi syndrome. *California Medicine,* 1970, *112,* 65-73.
Cohen, M., & Gorlin, R.J. The Prader-Willi syndrome. *American Journal of Diseases of Children,* 1969, *117,* 213-218.
Dubowitz, V. A syndrome of benign congenital hypotonia, gross obesity, delayed intellectual development, retarded bone age, and unusual facies. *Proceedings of the Royal Society of Medicine,* 1967, *60,* 1006-1008.
Dunn, H.G. The Prader-Labhart-Willi syndrome: Review of the literature and report of nine cases. *Acta Paediatrica Scandinavica,* 1968, Suppl. 186, 1-38.
Evans, P.R. Hypogenital dystrophy with diabetic tendency. *Guy's Hospital Reports,* 1964, *113,* 207-222.
Fox, M., Minot, A.S., & Liddle, G.W. Oxandrolone: Potent anabolic steroid of novel configuration. *Journal of Clinical Endocrinology and Metabolism,* 1962, *22,* 921-924.
Greulich, W.W., & Pyle, S.I. *Radiographic atlas of skeletal development of the hand and wrist* (2nd ed.). Stanford, Calif.: Stanford University Press, 1959.
Hall, B.D., & Smith, D.W. Prader-Willi syndrome: A resumé of 32 cases including an instance of affected first cousins, one of whom is of normal stature and intelligence. *The Journal of Pediatrics,* 1972, *81,* 286-293.
Hamilton, C.R., Jr., Scully, R.E., & Kliman, B. Hypogonadotropinism in Prader-Willi syndrome: Induction of puberty and spermatogenesis by clomiphene citrate. *The American Journal of Medicine,* 1972, *52,* 322-329.
Holm, V.A., & Pipes, P.L. Food and children with Prader-Willi syndrome. *American Journal of Diseases of Children,* 1976, *130,* 1063-1067.
Hopwood, J.J., Kelch, R.P., Zipf, W.B., & Hernandez, R.J. The effect of synthetic androgens on the hypothalamic-pituitary-gonadal axis in boys with constitutionally delayed growth. *The Journal of Pediatrics,* 1979, *94,* 657-662.
Jenab, M., Lade, R.I., Chiga, M., & Diehl, A.M. Cardiorespiratory syndrome of obesity in a child: Case report and necropsy findings. *Pediatrics,* 1959, *24,* 23-30.
Juul, J., & Dupont, A. Prader-Willi syndrome. *Journal of Mental Deficiency Research,* 1967, *11,* 12-22.
Landwirth, J., Schwartz, A.H., & Grunt, J.A. Prader-Willi syndrome. *American Journal of Diseases of Children,* 1968, *116,* 211-217.
Laurance, B.M. Hypotonia, mental retardation, obesity, and cryptorchidism associated with dwarfism and diabetes in children. *Archives of Diseases in Childhood,* 1967, *42,* 126-139.
Moore, D.C., Tattoni, D.S., Limbeck, G.A., Ruvalcaba, R.H.A., Lindner, D.S., Gareis, F.J., Al-Agba, S., & Kelley, V. Studies of anabolic steroids: Effect of prolonged oxandrolone administration on growth in children and adolescents with uncomplicated short stature. *Pediatrics,* 1976, *58,* 412-422.
Moore, D.C., Tattoni, D.S., Ruvalcaba, R.H.A., Limbeck, G.A., & Kelley, V. Studies of growth in children and adolescents with gonadal dysgenesis. *The Journal of Pediatrics,* 1977, *90,* 462-466.

NCHS growth curves for children: Birth-18 years, United States (DHEW Publication No. (PHS) 78-1650). Hyattsville, Md.: National Center for Health Statistics, 1977.

Pappo, R., & Jung, C.J. 2-oxasteroids: A new class of biologically active compounds. *Tetrahedron Letters,* 1962, *9,* 365.

Parra, A., Cervantes, C., & Schultz, R.B. Immunoreactive insulin and growth hormone responses in patients with Prader-Willi syndrome. *The Journal of Pediatrics,* 1973, *83,* 587-593.

Pearson, K.D., Steinbach, H.L., & Bier, D.M. Roentgenographic manifestations of the Prader-Willi syndrome. *Pediatric Radiology,* 1971, *100,* 369-377.

Prader, A., Labhart, A., & Willi, H. Ein Syndrom von Adipositas, Kleinwuchs, Kryptorchismus und Oligophrenie nach myantonieartigem Zustand im Neugeborenenalter. A syndrome of obesity, short stature, cryptorchidism, and oligophrenia, with amyotonia in the newborn period. *Scheizerische Medizinische Wochenschrift,* 1956, *86,* 1260-1261.

Raiti, S., Trias, E., Livitsky, L., & Grossman, M.S. Oxandrolone and human growth hormone. *American Journal of Diseases of Children,* 1973, *126,* 597-600.

Reed, W.B., Ragsdale, W., Jr., Curtis, A.C., & Richards, H.J. Acanthosis nigricans in association with various genodermatoses: With emphasis on lipodystrophic diabetes and Prader-Willi syndrome. *Acta Dermato-Venereologica,* 1968, *48,* 465-473.

Seyler, L.E., Arulanantham, K., & O'Connor, C.F. Hypergonadotropic-hypogonadism in the Prader-Labhart-Willi syndrome. *The Journal of Pediatrics,* 1979, *94,* 435-437.

Tanner, J.M., Goldstein, H., & Whitehouse, R.H. Standards for children's height at ages 2-9 years allowing for height of parents. *Archives of Disease in Childhood,* 1970, *45,* 755-762.

Theodoridis, C.G., Brown, G.A., Chance, G.W., & Rudd, B.T. Plasma growth hormone levels in children with the Prader-Willi syndrome. *Australian Paediatric Journal,* 1974, *7,* 24-27.

Tolis, G., Lewis, W., Verdy, M., Friesen, H.G., Solomon, S., Pagalis, G., Pavlatos, E., Fessas, P., & Rochefort, J.G. Anterior pituitary function in the Prader-Labhart-Willi (PLW) syndrome. *Journal of Clinical Endocrinology and Metabolism,* 1974, *39,* 1061-1066.

Urban, M.D., Lee, P.A., Dorst, J.P., Plotnick, L.P., & Migeon, C.J. Oxandrolone therapy in patients with Turner syndrome. *The Journal of Pediatrics,* 1979, *94,* 823-827.

Zellweger, H., & Schneider, H.J. Syndrome of hypotonia-hypomentia-hypogonadism-obesity (HHHO) or Prader-Willi syndrome. *American Journal of Diseases of Children,* 1968, *115,* 588-598.

chapter 22

ENDOCRINE PROFILES AND METABOLIC ASPECTS OF PRADER-WILLI SYNDROME

W. Jun Tze, Henry G. Dunn,
and Raphe L. Rothstein

Drs. Tze, Dunn, and Rothstein review available endocrinological data on Prader-Willi syndrome and conclude that the endocrine-related clinical features (obesity, hypogonadism, disorders in sexual development, and disorders in growth) are secondary to a central nervous system abnormality, probably located in the hypothalamus.—*Eds.*

A developmental defect of the hypothalamus is considered the probable abnormality responsible for the clinical manifestations of Prader-Willi (P-W) syndrome, including the endocrine disturbances. The advances in radioimmunoassay measurements and in the synthesis of hypothalamic-releasing hormones have greatly enhanced the ability to delineate the endocrine status of P-W syndrome patients. In this chapter endocrine functions in this syndrome are reviewed, and data related to the accompanying clinical features are discussed.

The outstanding clinical features of P-W syndrome related to endocrine dysfunction include obesity, small stature, hypogonadism, and aberrations of sexual development. Obesity is a constant feature, but no primary hormonal cause for the obesity has been identified. The secondary metabolic changes are found to be similar to those of individuals with simple obesity.

Short stature with mildly delayed bone age before the onset of puberty is common, in contrast to the findings in other obese children who generally have a tall stature and accelerated skeletal maturation. It has been noted that after the age of 11 years to 12 years and throughout puberty, the majority of P-W patients have normal or advanced bone age in relation to chronological age. This group of individuals tends to have a unique growth pattern that generally follows the third percentile growth curve until the age of 11 years to 12 years. Instead of an adolescent growth spurt, an abrupt falling-off in growth velocity is observed (Nugent & Holm, Chapter 21, this volume). This occurs despite the presence of a significant advancement in skeletal maturation. This premature closure of epiphyses from advanced bone age invariably leads to a short final height in adulthood.

The onset of puberty in P-W syndrome patients is variable. The majority show delayed puberty, but normal and early pubertal development are also encountered. Hypogonadotropic hypogonadism is a finding that would implicate a central cause for delayed puberty with lack of secondary sexual characteristics and primary amenorrhea. The gonadotropin level is reported to be normal in some P-W syndrome patients who develop precociously. This might be a result of premature activation of gonadotropin release during disturbances in hypothalamic function.

One of the more striking features noted in males at birth is hypogonadism, manifested by the presence of cryptorchidism and micropenis. In females, the diagnosis at birth is more difficult to establish on clinical grounds. Low gonadotropin levels suggest secondary hypogonadism, and advances in fetal endocrinology have led toward a better understanding of how gonadotropin deficiency can cause these abnormal findings. Sexual differentiation in male external genitalia begins from 6 weeks to 8 weeks of fetal life and is completed at about 12 weeks in utero. Physical changes are brought about by the secretion of testosterone and Müllerian duct inhibitory factors by the fetal testes. The secretion of testosterone is stimulated by circulating human chorionic gonadotropin (HCG) in the fetus. Growth of the penis and descent of the testes occur at a time when HCG levels have decreased and pituitary luteinizing hormone (LH) levels have risen. In the absence of pituitary LH, as observed in hypogonadotropic hypogonadism, cryptorchidism is a common occurrence. Depending on the severity of the gonadotropin deficiency, the penis will be smaller than normal because of lack of adequate testosterone stimulation in utero. Testicular biopsy in some patients has demonstrated immature tubules and arrested tubular development (Hamilton, Scully, & Kliman, 1972; Wannarachue, Ruvalcaba, & Kelly, 1975). Isolated cases of absent or abnormal testicular function and more recently the finding of abnormal spermatogonia in patients with P-W syndrome have been reported (Katcher, Bargman, Gilbert, & Opitz, 1977; Seyler, Arulanantham, & O'Connor, 1979).

GONADOTROPIN

Circulating pituitary gonadotropin levels are usually found to be subnormal in P-W syndrome patients. Kauli, Prager-Lewin, and Laron (1978) report that in four patients who showed marked delay or arrest of puberty, the basal levels were low or normal. In six patients who eventually developed normal puberty, both LH and follicle-stimulating hormone (FSH) were found to be within the normal range. McGuffin and Rogol (1975) reported low basal LH and FSH in two male P-W patients. Wannarachue and his colleagues (1975) similarly reported low basal LH in nine female subjects. Among the patients in the study, 10 out of 17 were found to have low basal gonadotropin levels.

With the recent availability of luteinizing hormone-releasing hormone (LH-RH), several studies have been undertaken to evaluate the integrity of the hypothalamic-pituitary-gonadal axis in these individuals. Kauli and his colleagues reported on 10 females and four males. Five P-W patients had delayed pubertal development, four patients were normal, and early pubertal development was observed in the remaining five patients. LH-RH tests were performed in 11 of these patients. In the four patients who developed normal puberty, the basal level and peak response of both LH and FSH were within normal ranges. LH and FSH responses to LH-RH were blunted in the five subjects who showed marked delay in puberty. Repeated stimulation with LH-RH led to an augmented LH response that suggested hypothalamic hypogonadotropinism in one case. Two of the male patients with bilateral cryptorchidism were found to have extremely blunted LH response to stimulation at 24 years and 25 years of age, respectively. Tolis, Lewis, Verdy, Friesen, Solomon, Pagalis, Pavlatos, Fessas, and Rochefort (1974) studied two male and three female P-W syndrome patients whose ages varied from 16 years to 20 years. One male had unilateral cryptorchidism and the other had bilateral cryptorchidism. Pubertal development was significantly delayed in both males and in one of the females. These patients all demonstrated a very blunted LH response. Following prolonged administration of LH-RH, increased LH response was elicited in these three patients, again suggesting a hypothalamic defect. A number of other scattered case reports have shown blunted responses of LH and FSH to LH-RH. The authors of this study have found blunted LH and FSH response to LH-RH stimulation in 10 out of 17 P-W syndrome patients tested. In two of these patients puberty did develop at a much later age and the previously blunted response reverted to normal. This finding suggests that the hypothalamic abnormality is not complete and spontaneous pubertal development may eventually take place. The finding of gonadotropin deficiency in this syndrome may be implicated as a cause for small genitalia and cryptorchidism.

Clomiphene citrate is a synthetic non-steroidal compound that prevents normal feedback inhibition of estrogen on the secretion of FSH and LH. McGuffin and Rogol (1975) studied LH-RH response in two females with P-W syndrome before and after clomiphene therapy. Before clomiphene therapy, the LH response to LH-RH was extremely blunted in these patients and the FSH response was normal in one patient and blunted in the other. Following clomiphene therapy, the LH response in the first patient reverted to normal, but its effect was lost 6 months after cessation of clomiphene therapy. In the second patient, LH response increased to a low normal range after clomiphene therapy, and the FSH response became normalized. In both patients estradiol rose to mid-cycle level following treatment. These data support the hypothesis that there is a hypothalamic abnormality in P-W syndrome.

Recently, Seyler and his colleagues (1979) reported a case of P-W syndrome with hypergonadotropic hypogonadism with small testes of less than 0.5 cm in size. Exaggerated LH and FSH response was found following LH-RH infusion. In addition, no testosterone response was observed after a course of HCG administration. These findings are consistent with primary hypogonadism or lack of testicular tissue. The high level of gonadotropin observed here can be explained by the lack of negative feedback signal to the hypothalamic pituitary axis.

PLASMA TESTOSTERONE, ESTRADIOL, AND URINARY ESTROGEN

Plasma testosterone levels are reported to be uniformly subnormal in male P-W syndrome patients. Plasma testosterone response to HCG stimulation has been variable. Morgner, Geisthövel, Niedergerker, and von zur Mühlen (1974) and Wannarachue and his colleagues (1975) report normal testosterone levels following a short course of HCG administration. However, Hamilton and co-workers (1972) and Seyler and colleagues (1979) report subnormal responses in patients in their studies. The authors of this study observed that one out of three male patients had a subnormal response to HCG stimulation, while the other two male patients showed a normal response. Hall and Smith (1972) report one case with a basal plasma testosterone level of 0.04 μg/100 ml, which rose markedly to 0.9 μg/100 ml (normal adult level, 0.28 to 1.4 μg/100 ml) after 1 month of HCG therapy. This level returned to pretreatment level at the end of 4 months.

Only limited information is available on serum estradiol in P-W syndrome. Tolis and his colleagues (1974) determined serum estradiol in three mature female patients to be 30, 40, and 62 pg/ml (basal estradiol is 40 to 120 pg/ml in normal adult females in the follicular phase). McGuffin and Rogol (1975) report that serum estradiol is 10 pg/ml and <10 pg/ml in their two adult female patients.

Urinary estrogen studies have been reported only in a limited number of young patients. MacMillan, Kim, and Weisskopf (1972) found total urinary estrogen levels of 7 and 10 μg/24 hours in young female patients of ages 6 and 11 years respectively. Urinary estrone, estradiol, and estriol in an 8-year-old female patient studied by Parkin (1973) and in a 14-year-old female patient studied by Wannarachue and his colleagues (1975) were 1.5, 2, 1.3 and 2, 1, and 8 µg/24 hours, respectively.

BLOOD AND URINE STEROID AND OTHER ADRENAL STUDIES

Basal plasma cortisol level was reported to be normal in two separate studies. The circadian rhythm of plasma cortisol was normal in all patients examined by Tolis and his colleagues (1974). Plasma cortisol level was appropriately elevated in response to hypoglycemic stress induced by acute insulin administration, suggesting a normal hypothalamic-pituitary-adrenal axis.

Basal levels of 24-hour urinary 17-ketosteroids (17KS) and 17-OH-cortico-steroids (17OHCS) were normal in P-W syndrome patients studied by Hamilton and colleagues (1972) and Tolis and colleagues (1974). Other studies including those by Hoefnagel, Costello, and Hatoum (1967), and Laurance (1967), and Wannarachue and colleagues (1975) report normal 24-hour urinary 17KS and 17 ketogenic steroids (17KGS) in a total of 20 P-W syndrome patients.

Metyrapone test was performed to evaluate the hypothalamic-pituitary-adrenal axis by measuring urinary 17KGS or 17OHCS response. Fourteen patients were reported to have normal steroid metabolite response to the metyrapone inhibition test (seven studies). Observation of six patients in our study yielded similar normal responses. In a study by Tolis and colleagues (1974), normal adrenal tetrahydro-11-deoxycortisol response was observed in all four patients following metyrapone administration.

Adrenocorticotropic hormone (ACTH) infusion test to evaluate adrenal function was performed by Landwirth, Schwartz, and Grunt (1968), by Lawrence (1967), and Wannarachue and his colleagues (1975). Normal urinary 17KS, 17KGS, and 17OHCS, as well as blood cortisol response following ACTH infusion, was observed. The eight patients in this study demonstrated normal adrenal function, including basal urinary steroids, circadian rhythm of serum cortisol, metyrapone test, and ACTH infusion. These findings support the reports of normal hypothalamic-pituitary-adrenal axis in P-W syndrome patients.

GROWTH HORMONE

Serum growth hormone (GH) is generally believed to be normal in P-W patients (10 studies), but response to evocative stimuli may be variable.

This is at least partly attributed to the metabolic changes that are secondary to obesity. The ingestion of glucose is followed by either a normal or low growth hormone profile in P-W patients studied. Parra, Cervantes, and Schultz (1973) observed no differences in GH levels among six P-W patients, six healthy individuals, and 12 obese, otherwise healthy, individuals, except at 4 hours when P-W patients and obese individuals had lower values than normal. Theodoridis, Albutt, and Chance (1971) compared the GH response of six P-W patients following oral glucose tolerance test (OGTT) with that of 13 non-obese children. Four of the six P-W patients gave maximum GH response within the range of response of the control group. The remaining two patients had significantly lower GH levels than the controls. Tolis and his colleagues (1974) also found a low GH response to OGTT in two out of five patients.

With insulin-induced hypoglycemia, normal GH responses were reported by Landwirth and colleagues (1968) and Seyler and colleagues (1979) in their respective patients. Tolis and colleagues (1974) found blunted GH response to insulin-induced hypoglycemia in one out of two patients. No GH response following insulin-induced hypoglycemia was noted in the study of McGuffin and Rogol (1975).

The findings concerning GH response to arginine infusion were again variable. MacMillan et al. (1972) reported that of two P-W patients, one had normal and the other a blunted GH response. Parra and colleagues (1973) observed that the GH response to arginine in a group of six P-W patients was similar to healthy and obese individuals.

When L-dopa was used as a stimulant, one normal and one subnormal response were observed by Brissenden and Levy (1973) in two male monozygotic P-W twins.

In the experience of the authors, GH response to various stimuli is rather variable. More than one-half the patients showed a subnormal response to at least one of the stimuli used, but in general no patient was found to have an abnormal response to all the stimuli employed in this group of patients. Hence, there is no confirmation of GH deficiency in P-W syndrome, and the short stature cannot be attributed to lack of GH.

PROLACTIN

Basal prolactin was found to be normal in five P-W syndrome patients studied by Tolis and colleagues (1974). The prolactin response to thyrotropin-releasing hormone (TRH) stimulus was also found to be normal. In five P-W syndrome patients from this study, all had normal basal prolactin level and in four patients the prolactin response to TRH was normal. Normal response was also elicited following the administration of chlorpromazine and L-dopa in these patients.

THYROID FUNCTION

Hamilton and co-workers (1972), Brissenden and Levy (1973), Tolis and colleagues (1974), McGuffin and Rogol (1975), and Wannarachue et al. (1975) have measured circulating thyroid hormones in P-W syndrome. The results of thyroid function studies including serum T_4, T_3, and T_3 resin uptake levels were found to be uniformly normal. Twenty-four-hour ^{131}I thyroid uptake was normal in two patients studied by Hamilton et al. (1972), and in one patient studied by Zarate, Soria, Canales, Kastin, Schally, and Guzman Toledano (1973/1974); it was also normal in three out of four patients of Tolis and colleagues (1974), while the fourth patient had a borderline uptake. Basal thyroid-stimulating hormone (TSH) levels and response to TRH stimulation were normal in two patients examined by Tolis and his colleagues (1974). Seven patients in our study showed normal basal TSH, T_3, T_4, and TSH response to TRH stimulation.

BLOOD CHEMISTRY AND URINE SPECIFIC GRAVITY

Serum lipid, cholesterol, triglycerides, and lipoprotein are generally found to be within the normal range in P-W syndrome patients. Theodoridis et al. (1971) found elevated levels of serum-free fatty acid (FFA) and triglycerides in seven children. Parra et al. (1973) report high fasting levels of FFA, similar to those of obese children. The range of FFA during OGTT and arginine infusion are in general similar to those of normal children.

Bier, Kaplan, and Havel (1977) studied fat mobilization and transport in six patients with P-W syndrome. The FFA concentrations were within the normal range for obese children. Measurements of the effect of norepinephrine, insulin, glucose, and 5-methylpyrazole-3-carboxylic acid on plasma levels of FFA, glycerol, and ketones provide no evidence for abnormal mobilization of fat from adipose tissue. Plasma lipids and post-heparin lipolytic activity showed no evidence of abnormal lipogenesis; this is consistent with normal uptake of fat and normal fatty acid composition of adipose tissue.

Serum electrolytes, calcium, phosphorus, alkaline phosphatase, and urea nitrogen were found to be normal in all P-W patients examined by the various investigators. Uric acid and urine specific gravity were included in measurements used in this study, and the findings were also normal.

GLUCOSE AND INSULIN LEVELS

Fasting blood glucose levels are generally reported to be normal in P-W syndrome, but hypoglycemic levels of 35 and 28 mg/dl following a period of fasting was reported by Brissenden and Levy (1973) in two male monozygotic twins. Basal serum insulin levels are normal or elevated, but significantly lower than those in simple obesity.

Historically, impaired carbohydrate tolerance was reported in P-W syndrome but the true incidence of diabetes is unknown. The carbohydrate intolerance seen as a result of our study resembles that of obese patients. Hall and Smith (1972) reviewed 30 cases of P-W syndrome, in which they found abnormal glucose tolerance in five out of 14 patients. One of these five patients developed non-ketotic diabetes mellitus that was treated with oral hypoglycemic agents for 4 years then followed by insulin therapy. This patient was massively obese, and blood glucose levels returned to normal following significant weight reduction. It would appear that the carbohydrate abnormality in this case was a result of obesity rather than the result of any underlying defect of this syndrome. Parra et al. (1973) studied six children with P-W syndrome and had findings similar to those seen in children with long-standing obesity, with minor differences. Fasting glucose levels and response to glucose tolerance tests were similar. However, insulin response differed in that the basal insulin level in P-W syndrome was similar to that of a normal child. Laurance (1967) and others report normal glucose response to OGTT in their P-W syndrome patients. Zellweger and Schneider (1968) report normal glucose tolerance tests in all but one out of 14 young P-W syndrome children with ages ranging from 1 year to 9 years. Laurance observed a diabetic type of glucose tolerance curve in only one out of nine P-W syndrome patients studied. Dunn (1968), in a very detailed report, observed that seven out of nine children had a normal glucose tolerance test at the time of first evaluation. Two of these seven patients subsequently developed an abnormality on repeat testing and one boy became frankly diabetic. McGuffin and Rogol (1975) report abnormal glucose response to OGTT in two P-W syndrome patients.

Bier et al. (1977) carried out studies using intravenous glucose tolerance test (IVGTT). The mean glucose assimilation coefficient (K value) of the four non-diabetic P-W syndrome patients was 1.9%/minute. One diabetic patient had a K value of 0.99%/minute. The insulin responses to IVGTT in three of the four non-diabetic P-W patients were characteristic for obese individuals. The other non-diabetic patient had an impaired insulin response to IVGTT challenge similar to that of the diabetic subjects. These data would suggest that insulin response to glucose stimulation is in the normal range, consistent with the patient's obesity. The delayed initial rise in insulin and late peak response found in maturity-onset diabetes has not been observed in these patients.

Based on the above information, glucose intolerance in P-W syndrome is variable and the incidence of diabetes mellitus seems to be less than suggested in early reports. Most of the abnormality in carbohydrate tolerance is not significantly different from that seen in other obese patients and in one case the diabetes actually improved with weight loss. In this study, impaired glucose tolerance and hyperinsulinism were found in several patients, but there were no clear-cut differences from obese children. Current evidence would suggest that success in weight reduction in P-W syndrome patients would abolish many of the abnormalities associated with carbohydrate tolerance.

SUMMARY

1. Generalized obesity has consistently been observed in patients with P-W syndrome. Evidence suggests abnormality in the regulaton of food intake rather than hormonal disorder as the cause. Hyperinsulinism, high fasting levels of free fatty acid, and triglyceride levels similar to those in obese individuals, were found in the majority of the patients.
2. Reduced final height is a consistent feature in P-W syndrome patients and the degree of short stature is variable. These patients lack the pubertal growth spurt. The abnormal growth pattern has no hormonal basis. Thus far, information on somatomedin levels in these patients is lacking. Thyroid and adrenal function are intact. Skeletal maturation process also shows heterogeneity because the skeletal age is usually retarded during early life, but a rapid advance seems to occur after 11 years to 12 years of age.
3. A wide variability in the pattern of sexual development is seen in P-W syndrome, but the majority of patients follow a course of delayed puberty with occasional cases of precocious puberty. In patients who eventually develop normal puberty, the basal levels and peak responses of both LH and FSH to LH-RH are within the range of those observed in normal controls. In some cases where there is marked delay or arrest of puberty, the basal levels are normal or low and the responses of LH and FSH to LH-RH are blunted.
4. Testosterone level is low in male patients. However, basal serum estradiol level in female patients was found to be normal in a few reported cases. Low basal LH and FSH and subnormal response to LH-RH stimulation are observed in the majority of male and female patients. Augmentation of LH and FSH response to LH-RH after a course of LH-RH administration has been achieved, suggesting that hypothalamic hypogonadotropinism is the cause of the hypogonadism. High dosage of clomiphene citrate has normalized the levels of LH, FSH, estradiol, and testosterone in P-W patients, and has normalized their response to LH-RH stimulation. HCG stimulation in these patients results in an increase in testosterone response in most cases studied. Isolated cases of hypergonadotropic hypogonadism have been reported.

5. Despite early belief that there is an increase in the incidence of diabetes mellitus in P-W syndrome patients, fasting blood sugar is normal, and the presence of glucose intolerance is often secondary to obesity. Basal insulin levels are generally slightly increased, but often normal and significantly less than those in obese control subjects. Hyperinsulin response to glucose challenge is equal to, or less than that seen in obese subjects.
6. Other hormonal and biochemical data are found to be normal in P-W syndrome patients. Prolactin responses to TRH, chlorpromazine, and L-dopa are normal. Serum calcium, phosphorus, electrolytes, CO_2, and urine specific gravity and osmolality are also within normal limits.

CONCLUSION

It is reasonable to conclude that obesity, hypogonadism, and disorders in growth and sexual development are secondary to a central nervous system abnormality, probably located in the hypothalamus. Endocrine dysfunction in P-W syndrome patients is restricted to hypothalamic hypogonadotropism. Other endocrine functions are normal except for an occasional blunted GH response to stimulation.

ACKNOWLEDGMENTS

The authors wish to express their thanks to Dr. Joseph Tai for his literature search and compilation of the data, to Carolyn Graves, B.N., and to Sally Dean for clerical assistance.

REFERENCES

Bier, D.M., Kaplan, S.L., & Havel, R.J. The Prader-Willi syndrome: Regulation of fat transport. *Diabetes*, 1977, *26*, 874-881.

Brissenden, J.E., & Levy, E.P. Prader-Willi syndrome in infant monozygotic twins: *American Journal of Diseases of Children*, 1973, *126*, 110-112.

Dunn, H.G. The Prader-Labhart-Willi syndrome: Review of the literature and report of nine cases. *Acta Paediatrica Scandinavica*, 1968, Suppl. 186, 1-38.

Hall, B.D., & Smith, D.W. Prader-Willi syndrome: A resumé of 32 cases including an instance of affected first cousins, one of whom is of normal stature and intelligence. *The Journal of Pediatrics*, 1972, *81*, 286-293.

Hamilton, C.R., Jr., Scully, R.E., & Kliman, B. Hypogonadotropinism in Prader-Willi syndrome: Induction of puberty and spermatogenesis by clomiphene citrate. *The American Journal of Medicine*, 1972, *52*, 322-329.

Hoefnagel, D., Costello, P.J., & Hatoum, K. Prader-Willi syndrome. *Journal of Mental Deficiency Research*, 1967, *11*, 1-11.

Katcher, M.L., Bargman, G.J., Gilbert, E.F., & Opitz, J.M. Absence of spermatogonia in the Prader-Willi syndrome. *European Journal of Pediatrics*, 1977, *124*, 257-260.
Kauli, R., Prager-Lewin, R., & Laron, Z. Pubertal development in the Prader-Labhart-Willi syndrome. *Acta Paediatrica Scandinavica*, 1978, *37*, 763-767.
Landwirth, J., Schwartz, A.H., & Grunt, J.A. Prader-Willi syndrome. *American Journal of Diseases of Children*, 1968, *116*, 211-217.
Laurance, B.M. Hypotonia, mental retardation, obesity and cryptorchidism associated with dwarfism and diabetes in children. *Archives of Disease in Childhood*, 1967, *42*, 126-139.
MacMillan, D.R., Kim, C.B., & Weisskopf, B. Syndrome of growth resistance, obesity, and intellectual impairment with precocious puberty. *Archives of Disease in Childhood*, 1972, *47*, 119-121.
McGuffin, W.L., & Rogol, A.D. Response to LH-RH and clomiphene citrate in two women with the Prader-Labhart-Willi syndrome. *Journal of Clinical Endocrinology and Metabolism*, 1975, *41*, 321-331.
Morgner, K.D., Geisthövel, W., Niedergerke, V., & von zur Mühlen, A. Hypogonadismus in folge Mangels an Luteotropin-Releasing-Hormon (LHRH) bei Prader-Labhart-Willi Syndrom. *Deutsche Medizinische Wochenschrift*, 1974, *99*, 1196-1198.
Parkin, J.M. Syndrome of growth resistance, obesity and intellectual impairment with precocious puberty. *Archives of Disease in Childhood*, 1973, *48*, 86-87.
Parra, A., Cervantes, C., & Schultz, R.B. Immunoreactive insulin and growth hormone responses in patients with Prader-Willi syndrome. *The Journal of Pediactrics*, 1973, *83*, 587-593.
Seyler, L.E., Arulanantham, K., & O'Connor, F.C. Hypergonadotropic hypogonadism in the Prader-Labhart-Willi syndrome. *The Journal of Pediatrics*, 1979, *94*, 435-437.
Theodoridis, C.G., Albutt, E.C., & Chance, G.W. Blood lipids in children with the Prader-Willi syndrome: A comparison with simple obesity. *Australian Journal of Paediatrics*, 1971, *7*, 24-27.
Tolis, G., Lewis, W., Verdy, M., Friesen, H.G., Solomon, S., Pagalis, G., Pavlatos, F., Fessas, P., & Rochefort, J.G. Anterior pituitary function in the Prader-Labhart-Willi (PLW) syndrome. *Journal of Clinical Endocrinology and Metabolism*, 1974, *39*, 1061-1066.
Wannarachue, N., Ruvalcaba, R.H.A., & Kelley, V.C. Hypogonadism in Prader-Willi syndrome. *American Journal of Mental Deficiency*, 1975, *79*, 592-603.
Zarate, A., Soria, J., Canales, E.S. Kastin, A.J., Schally, A.V., & Guzman Toledano, R. Pituitary response to synthetic luteinizing hormone-releasing hormone in Prader-Willi syndrome, prepubertal and pubertal children. *Neuroendocrinology*, 1973/1974, *13*, 321-326.
Zellweger, H., & Schneider, H.J. Syndrome of hypotonia, hypomentia, hypogonadism (HHHO) or Prader-Willi syndrome. *American Journal of Diseases of Children*, 1968, *115*, 588-598.

chapter 23
SCOLIOSIS IN PRADER-WILLI SYNDROME

Edwin L. Laurnen

The incidence of scoliosis in patients at the University of Washington Prader-Willi Syndrome Clinic is much higher than in previously published series, suggesting that it may be under-diagnosed. In this chapter Dr. Laurnen describes both the techniques for examination for scoliosis and appropriate therapy.—Eds.

Scoliosis is a lateral curvature of the spine. The reported incidence of scoliosis in the United States varies in different localities, but approximately 2% of normal adolescents have structural curvatures requiring treatment or continued observation. The incidence of scoliosis in Prader-Willi (P-W) syndrome has not been accurately determined. In most articles on this syndrome scoliosis either is not mentioned or is noted only occasionally. Typically, in Zellweger and Schneider's (1968) series of 14 patients, only one patient is said to have had scoliosis. The experience of a few authors would indicate that scoliosis might be more common. Laurance (1967) described nine patients, three with scoliosis. Pearson, Steinbach, and Bier (1971) published radiological findings in five patients with P-W syndrome of whom three had scoliosis. Reports by Gabilan and Royer (1968) and Smith, Neeman, Wulff, and Seely (1970) also indicate that scoliosis might be more common in patients with P-W syndrome than is implied by most case studies. To define further the incidence of scoliosis in P-W syndrome, patients with this condition attending the P-W Clinic at the Child Development and Mental Retardation Center at the University of Washington were evaluated for lateral spine curvatures by physical and radiological examination.

The result of this study has been reported elsewhere (Laurnen & Holm, 1980). In summary, in 30 patients 87% were found to have a structural scoliosis greater than 10°. The rest of the patients also had scoliosis, but of lesser magnitude, averaging 7°. Structural scoliosis was found in all age groups. There were cases of infantile (birth to 4 years), juvenile (4 to 10 years), adolescent (10 years to skeletal maturity), and adult scoliosis.

Analysis of the various curve patterns revealed essentially no difference in types and degrees of scoliosis in patients with P-W syndrome as compared to scoliosis in the general population.

Two cases required active treatment for progressive scoliosis. One 14-year-old patient was treated with Boston bracing and one 12-year-old patient needed surgical correction.

Thus, this study has indicated that scoliosis in P-W syndrome seems to occur early, sometimes before the onset of obesity, and is slowly progressive, and that two cases of young adolescents required active treatment. The cause of most cases of scoliosis, in P-W patients as well as the general population, remains unknown. The curves of adults averaged about 20°, suggesting that scoliosis in the majority of patients with P-W syndrome is not significantly progressive, although the curves all appear to be structural in character. Kyphosis, a convex spinal curve, sometimes called round-back or hunch-back, often seems to accompany scoliosis in the adult patient with P-W syndrome.

Patients with P-W syndrome should be evaluated routinely for scoliosis, employing the examination technique described by the Scoliosis Research Society (Note 1). Figures 23.1 and 23.2 show a P-W syndrome patient with scoliosis. Note that the patient should also be examined when bending forward with hands clasped together (Fig. 23.2). It is recommended that clinical examinations be conducted for scoliosis every 6 months for P-W syndrome patients, with x-ray examinations as indicated. Mild to moderate scoliosis is somewhat difficult to detect clinically because of the obesity and relatively short stature of individuals with P-W syndrome. It is therefore prudent to obtain baseline roentgenograms of the spine in such patients to document the presence or absence of scoliosis. These should be taken while the patient is standing. Figure 23.3 shows an x-ray film of the spine of the patient seen in Figures 23.1 and 23.2. Clinical scoliosis is more easily detected in patients who are satisfactorily managed on a dietary program of weight control.

Scoliosis may progress slowly, rapidly, or not at all. Early detection is essential for the best treatment results. Scoliosis can be treated by bracing for mild to moderate curves and by surgery for severe curves. Exercise alone has not been found to significantly correct a scoliosis deformity.

Bracing is reserved for curves that are progressive and approaching 20°. The main function of bracing is to stop progression of the deformity. Bracing is not expected to correct the lateral curvature to normal. Best results with bracing are found in mild to moderate curves between 20° and 40°. When bracing is instituted for a progressive curve, treatment is necessary until skeletal maturity, at which time the curvature appears to stabilize and progression is much less likely to continue. The brace is worn continuously day and night, with 1 hour out of the brace allowed for bathing. Regular follow-up of patients who are braced is necessary to ensure that the brace is fitting satisfactorily and that the curve is being supported by the brace without further progression. Bracing requires patient cooperation, which has been a problem in P-W syndrome. The treatment

Scoliosis 295

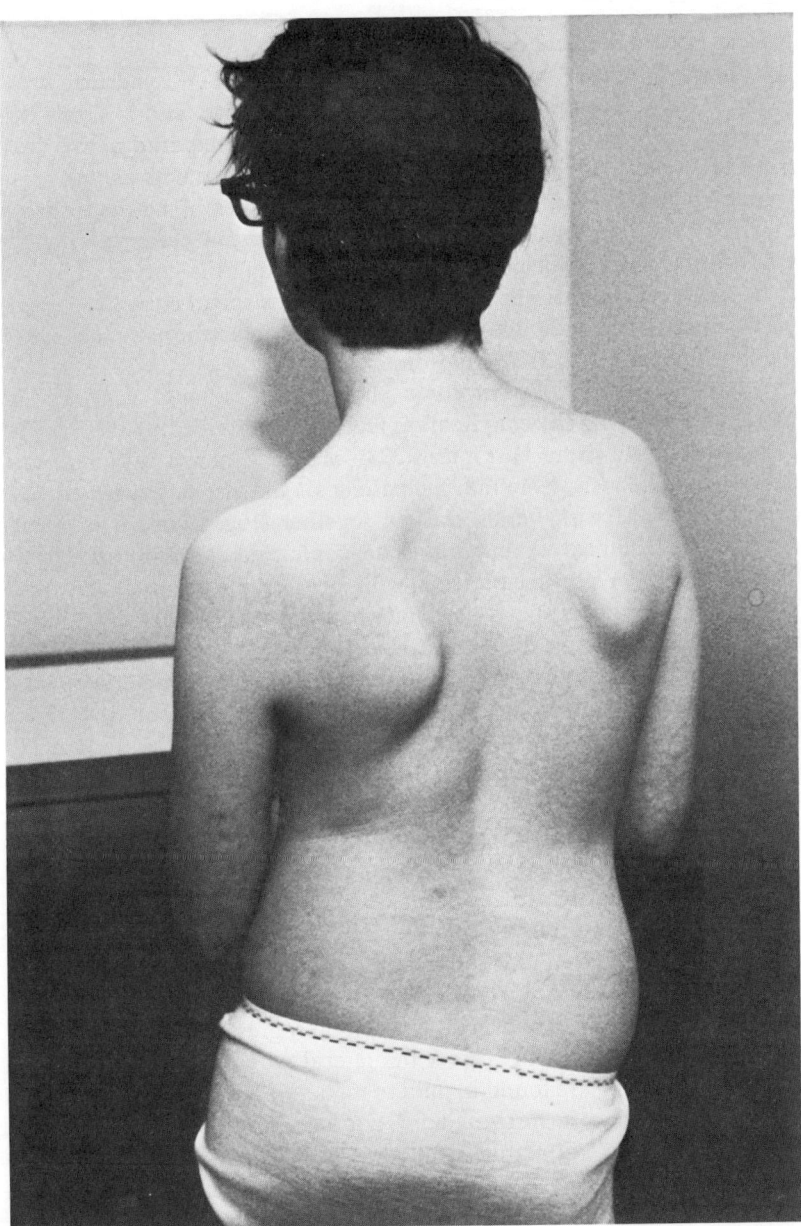

Figure 23.1. A P-W patient with scoliosis standing erect.

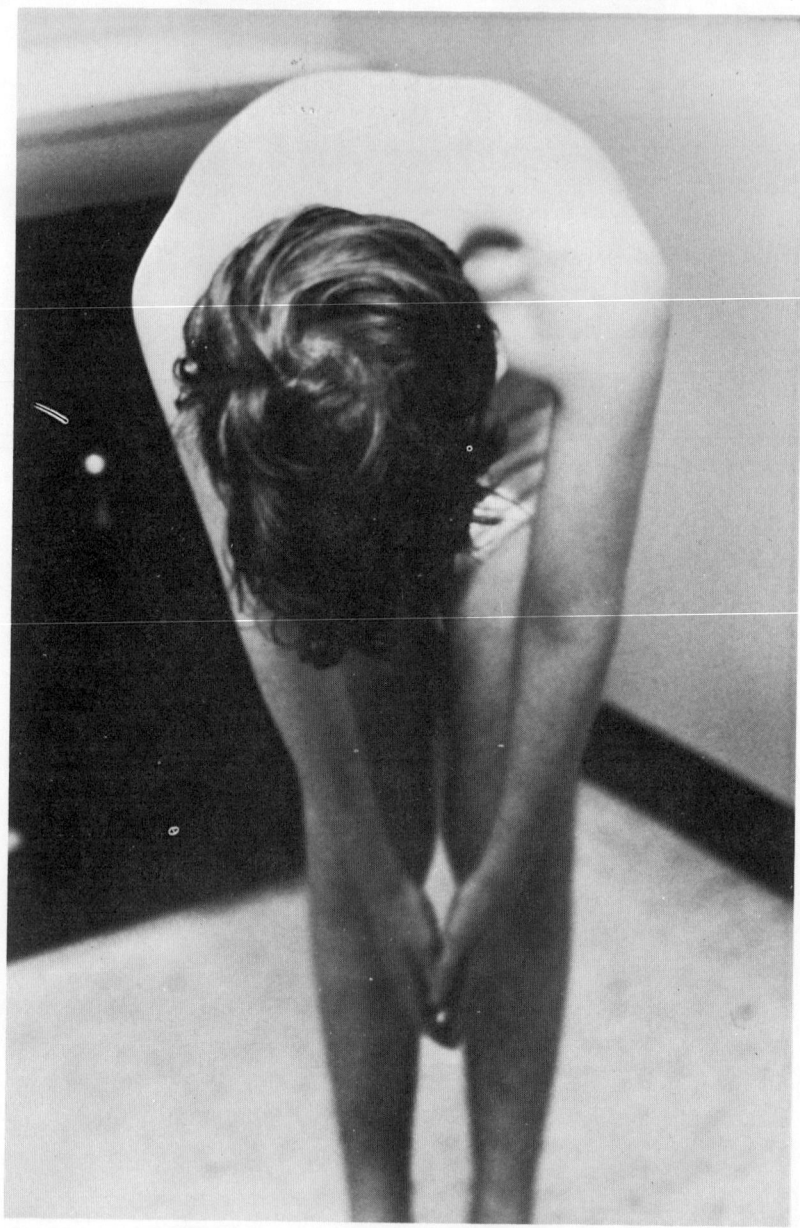

Figure 23.2. The patient shown in Figure 23.1 bending forward.

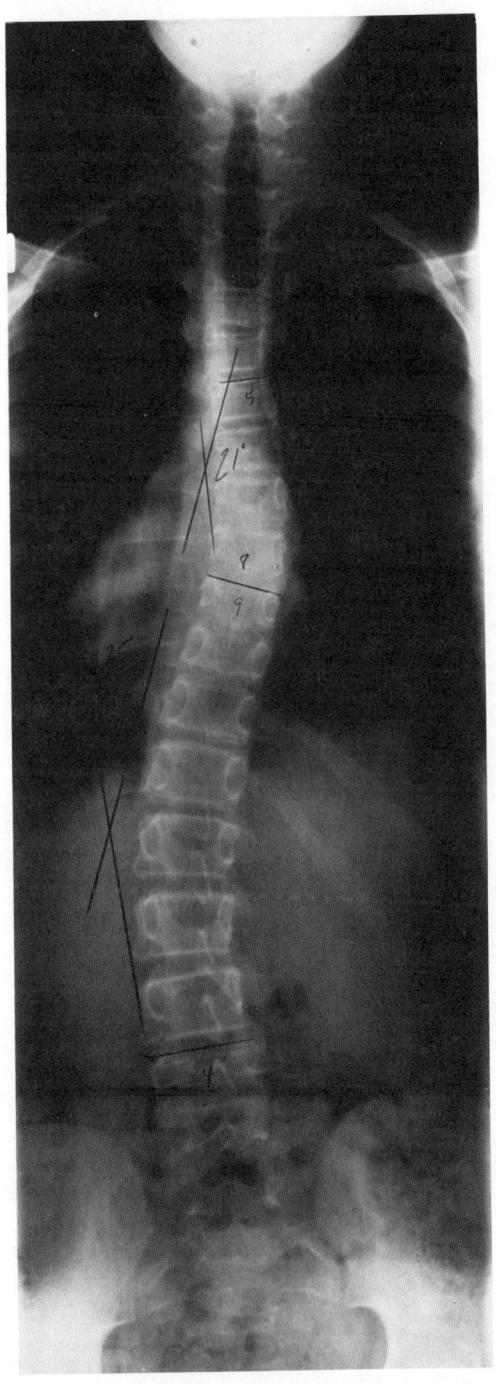

Figure 23.3. A spinal roentgenogram of the patient shown in Figures 23.1 and 23.2.

has been compromised because of refusal to wear the brace accompanied by temper outbursts.

Curvatures greater than 40° are often not satisfactorily controlled by bracing and many ultimately require surgical treatment. Surgery is indicated for those patients with curvatures of approximately 45° or greater, who do not respond satisfactorily to bracing. Surgery most commonly involves the use of Harrington rods for internal stabilization and for improvement of the curvature, combined with spinal fusion. After surgery the patients are supported with protective plaster body cast immobilization until the fusion becomes solid. Surgery is indicated in severe scoliosis to prevent continued progression of the deformity. Severe scoliosis curvatures interfere with cardiopulmonary function and are associated with degenerative arthritis in adulthood.

In summary, scoliosis is very common in P-W syndrome patients and seems to be independent of the degree of obesity. Eighty-seven percent of 30 patients with P-W syndrome were found to have structural scoliosis of 10° or greater. Analysis of the infantile, juvenile, adolescent, and adult subgroups would suggest that scoliosis is present from an early age and is only slowly progressive in most patients throughout adulthood. Some curves, however, are rapidly progressive, and patients with P-W syndrome should be evaluated for scoliosis regularly. If the curve is found to be progressive and approaching 20°, bracing is advisable to prevent further progression and, if successful, to avoid the necessity of surgical treatment.

REFERENCE NOTE

1. Scoliosis Research Society. *Scoliosis: A handbook for patients.* Chicago: Author, no date. (This pamphlet is available from the Scoliosis Research Society, 430 North Michigan Avenue, Chicago, Ill. 60611.)

REFERENCES

Gabilan, J.C., & Royer, P. Le syndrome de Prader, Labhart et Willi (étude de onze observations). *Archives Françaises de Pédiatrie*, 1968, *25*, 121-149.

Laurance, B.M. Hypotonia, mental retardation, obesity, and cryptorchidism associated with dwarfism and diabetes in children. *Archives of Disease in Childhood*, 1967, *42*, 126-139.

Laurnen, E.L., & Holm, V.A. Scoliosis in the Prader-Willi syndrome. *Orthopedic Transactions: Journal of Bone and Joint Surgery,* (Abstract) *4(1),* 37, Spring, 1980.

Pearson, K.D., Steinbach, H.L., & Bier, D.M. Roentgenographic manifestations of the Prader-Willi syndrome. *Radiology*, 1971, *100*, 369-377.

Smith, J.D., Neeman, J., Wulff, J., & Seely, J.R. Clinical-metabolic study of the Prader-Willi syndrome. *The Journal of the Oklahoma State Medical Association*, 1970, *63*, 234-238.

Zellweger, H., & Schneider, H.J. Syndrome of hypotonia-hypomentia-hypogonadism-obesity (HHHO) or Prader-Willi syndrome. *American Journal of Diseases of Children*, 1968, *115*, 588-598.

chapter 24
PHYSICAL EXERCISE FOR CHILDREN AND ADULTS WITH PRADER-WILLI SYNDROME

Paula M. Carman

> In this chapter Ms. Carman discusses the exercise needs of infants, children, and adults with Prader-Willi syndrome, including those with scoliosis. Suggestions for appropriate exercise for each age group are included.—*Eds.*

Hypotonia, weak muscles, and delayed motor skills are consistently noted in children with Prader-Willi (P-W) syndrome. Although there are references in the literature to delayed developmental milestones such as sitting and walking (Dunn, 1968; Holm, Chapter 3, this volume), there has been no documentation of motor skills in older children. Gross motor and fine motor skill levels in 25 children diagnosed with P-W syndrome were evaluated by the author at the Child Development and Mental Retardation Center, University of Washington, between 1974 and 1977. The age range was from 22 months to 17 years, average age 8 years. All showed significant gross motor skill delays, without apparent relationship to obesity. Gross motor and fine motor quotients (GMQ, FMQ) were computed by dividing the skill level by the chronological age. The average GMQ was 0.4 (0.2 to 0.65) and the average FMQ was 0.6 (0.33 to 0.89). If skills had been appropriate for age level, without delays, the GMQ and FMQ would be 1.0. A child of 10 years whose gross motor skills are at the 5-year level would receive a GMQ of 0.5. Most of these children avoided active physical exertion in their play. The relationship between weight management and physical proficiency in this syndrome is not currently known. An analysis of body fat and gross motor performance in 56 normal adults revealed that obesity had a negative effect on three components of movement: dynamic strength, gross body coordination, and stamina (Brady, Knight, & Berghage, 1977). Experience with several weight-controlled children at the University of Washington's P-W Syndrome Clinic indicates that increased gross motor activities with peers, especially biking and running, follow weight loss.

Persons with P-W syndrome also show qualitative deficits in their motor skills. Balance reactions are usually poor and protective arm extension responses may be slow. The desire to move and to explore the environment is curtailed by insecurity and a low energy level. Muscle strength and coordination are diminished by inactivity, setting up a cycle that perpetuates itself. The cycle can be broken by teaching activities in small enough steps so that they can be accomplished successfully.

Muscle tone becomes more normal as P-W children get older, but the need for special assistance in planning physical activities continues. Considerations that influence choice of activities include: degree of obesity, stamina, strength, coordination, level of understanding instructions, individual interests, and medical considerations. For example, some individuals with P-W syndrome have been reported to have osteoporotic bones, which would make them susceptible to fractures (Pearson, Steinbach, & Bier, 1971). In the author's experience with 30 children, one child sustained fractures from minor accidents (e.g., falling onto the floor after tripping). This suggests caution in choice of activities, but no avoidance of activity. Normal calcification of bones is stimulated by weight-bearing activity and depressed by inactivity.

Consultation with an occupational therapist or physical therapist to set up a specific therapy program would probably be useful for persons at any age who have P-W syndrome, but is most important for the young child. Improvement of basic skills at an early age helps the children's self-confidence and enables greater participation in recreational activities as they get older. Such participation promotes social skills and peer acceptance, and improves coordination, strength, and endurance. Physical exercise can also help control obesity. This chapter outlines by age groups, appropriate activities that have been found most helpful to persons with P-W syndrome. Since scoliosis (lateral curvature of the spine) occurs in a significant number of persons with P-W syndrome, a discussion of exercise for that condition is included.

THE INFANT

Hypotonic babies need some support for protection when held, but they must also be encouraged to use their muscles. For example, when a baby has trunk control adequate for sitting upright on an adult's knee, with support only at the hips, he should be encouraged to sit that way rather than to lean back against the adult while sitting. It is most effective to turn the child to face the adult and carry on some pleasant social exchange. In this way there is nothing convenient to lean against, yet the child can feel secure if held at the hips or thighs by the caregiver.

Because the head falls back as the P-W syndrome child is pulled to a sitting position during the early months, head control needs to be practiced under less strenuous conditions to gradually improve neck and trunk strength. At first, balancing the head in the upright position is important. As the head becomes more stable, the body can be tilted backward, forward, and laterally just enough so that the child is able to maintain the head upright. The degree of body tilt is increased as skill improves. Development of head control is important for enabling the young child to develop further motor skills and to visually explore the environment. A physical therapist or occupational therapist might be helpful in demonstrating other appropriate activities for an individual infant.

Hypotonic babies are often content to remain lying on their backs for long periods of time. We have noted that as a result persons with P-W syndrome often have skull asymmetry with one side of the occiput (back part of the head) flattened, reflecting their preferred head position in infancy. Frequent changes of position will prevent this, will be mentally stimulating, and will promote better motor development as well. Lying on the side provides complete support and positions the arms together to promote hand use. Lying on the stomach encourages development of head extension and strengthens the trunk muscles. When a child has difficulty raising the head from this position, a wedge, cylindrical cushion, or rolled-up towel placed under the chest and shoulders will usually make the position more acceptable. An infant seat provides head and trunk support while allowing the child to play with his hands and to explore the environment visually. Ribbons, utensils, bells, toys, and other common objects suspended in front of the child will offer stimulation for reaching and manipulating with the hands.

Movement has been shown to increase the rate of motor development. Studies have been done with both normal and developmentally delayed children with low muscle tone receiving specific movement stimulation. Motor skills, which were tested pre- and posttreatment and compared to a control group, showed improvement from treatment (Clark, Kreutzberg, & Chee, 1977; Kantner, Clark, Allen, & Chase, 1976). Examples of movement that would be appropriate for movement stimulation for babies with P-W syndrome include: slowly rolling the child, carefully bouncing the child on a knee, slow rocking, and swinging the child while holding the trunk firmly under the arms. An occupational or physical therapist may be able to provide more specific suggestions and precautions for an individual child. Usually these activities are enjoyed and elicit positive reactions. Signs of discomfort or distress should be heeded by stopping the activity and trying it again more briefly or less intensely at another time. Strong negative reactions, such as prolonged discomfort or disorientation, indicate that the activity should be avoided completely. Movement can be uncomfortable when a child is not feeling well. Walkers and jumpers are best avoided unless used with discretion and at the suggestion of a therapist. Although they can increase strength and muscle tone, abnormal motor patterns may develop that interfere with posture and balance in subtle ways. Studies of normal children have shown that walkers are of questionable value. Kauffman & Ridenour (1977) have reported that the mechanics of locomotion of infants was modified negatively by use of a walker, although the long term effects on movement seemed minimal. It can be assumed that a child with low muscle tone would more readily develop undesirable movement or posture when using a walker and would be less likely to achieve normal muscular coordination. It is far better for a child to lie on his stomach where the activity around him will encourage head raising and eventual reaching, rolling, and crawling. Placing toys a little beyond reach in front or to the side encourages movement. The distance can be increased as the child demonstrates progress.

THE PRESCHOOL CHILD

Movement builds strength. Normal preschool-age children are spontaneously active much of the time, but the hypotonic P-W child often needs extra incentives or attention to get started. Swimming is an activity that encourages involvement and can be started at a young age. Just playing with water stimulates movement: at the beach, in a pool, or in the yard playing with a sprinkler or garden hose.

The prone (stomach-down) position should continue to be encouraged for play activities with small toys; this position strengthens the upper trunk and shoulder muscles. Kneeling is another position in which the child may be encouraged to play near a low table, for strengthening hip muscles and practice of balance.

Sitting up from the supine position (lying on back) with assistance from someone holding the hands may be practiced as soon as neck strength is adequate for raising the head.

Chair-type swings, hammocks, or swings with strap seats (that hug the hips as a person sits down) may be used initially with very little motion, increasing the motion as the child becomes more comfortable. This type of movement can be very powerful in its effect and should not be overdone. The child's facial expressions and verbal requests will indicate whether the movement should be stopped.

Rolling across a carpeted floor, on the grass, or on a blanket is also a stimulating activity for preschoolers. Holding onto a bean bag or ball with two hands held above the head while rolling is a challenging change that can be suggested when rolling becomes easy.

Somersaults forward and backward usually require assistance for some time, but they help the child become more flexible with practice.

Balance will benefit from activities that stimulate the child's muscles in a variety of positions. When a child is sitting on an adult's lap with support at the hips, displacing him laterally will challenge the trunk muscles to maintain the upright position. The adult can easily do this by raising the heel of one foot, and thus the knee, which tilts the child as he straddles both adult knees. The hands and knees position can also be encouraged with the rocker board, for development of balance in a more stable position. Standing on a rocking board or a twister board also stimulates balance; hand support is needed at first, but can be gradually withdrawn as confidence improves.

Playing with a ball is another activity that encourages active participation on the part of the P-W child. Practice can begin as soon as the child is stable in independent sitting. While a ball is rolled toward the child, an adult sits behind to help with the motions of catching and pushing or throwing the ball back. As the child improves with practice, balls of different sizes can be used. A larger ball encourages use of two hands; a small ball only requires one hand and is more difficult to catch, but easier to throw.

When the child is walking well, catching and throwing a ball can be practiced in the upright position. Starting with a large ball (4 to 8 inches) that requires use of two hands, the ball is tossed from a short distance, almost dropping it onto the child's outstretched arms. As the distance is increased, the ball can be bounced. It should arrive at the child's chest level, with care being taken not to hit the face.

Walking in the neighborhood and in parks builds strength and endurance in young children with P-W syndrome. Running for part of the distance stimulates the cardiovascular system. It helps children to have a goal when running, such as a tree or street corner, and to gradually increase the distance. Discussing observations of flowers, trees, and animals makes the expeditions more interesting. When a stroller is used for long walks, the child can push it until it is time to get in.

Tot trikes, which are pushed with the feet on the floor, prepare the child for pedaling a tricycle, which helps to build strength and coordination of leg muscles. The presence of other young children who enjoy riding tricycles motivates participation.

Tasks to develop fine motor skills at preschool ages can be done with playdough, construction toys (blocks and legos), puzzles, and crayons. Exploration and discussion of texture, size, weight, firmness, and other qualities of basic materials (wood, plastic, and metal) will heighten awareness and increase learning.

Use of a scooter board can be started during the preschool years and continued in the early school years. The board can be made by attaching four ball-type swivel casters to a board measuring a maximum of 12 by 14 inches. A child can use it while lying face down or sitting. On a level surface, children can propel themselves with their hands or hold onto a rope pulled by someone else (Figure 24.1). Inclined surfaces provide an exciting ride, but require a safe, level run-out space. If several scooter boards are available, other children may participate. When this happens, many new ideas evolve from the children, such as spinning in one place, running through an obstacle course, swishing under a suspended blanket, or running into a pile of leaves or cushions. It is important that everyone involved know that these boards are not safe to stand on. Unlike skateboards they can move in all directions because of the swivel wheels.

THE SCHOOL-AGE CHILD

Children with P-W syndrome should be encouraged to participate in physical education classes, although the program may require modification so that the child does not experience frequent failure or become frustrated. A few exercises at the beginning of class time could be chosen with the needs of the P-W child in mind and would be useful for all the children involved. Track and field sports and swimming can be organized to improve skill through self-competition for time or endurance. Relays are good for group participation and competition, with decreased importance placed on individual performance. In team activities in which children are grouped according to ability, success becomes possible and there is motivation to try harder. There are many activities that stress participation rather than winning and losing, which would be appropriate for children with P-W syndrome, such as the group games described in *The New Games Book* (Fluegelman, 1976).

Social groups that hike, swim, camp, and do craft activities are good for promoting exercise and friendships (Scouts, Boys' Club/Girl's Club, YWCA/YMCA, etc.). Many of these groups offer recreation programs for special populations. Many city or county park departments also have special programs that are supervised, structured, and designed to meet individual needs. The Special Olympics program (which is usually coordinated through local park and recreation programs) offers instruction and supervised practice in specific sports such as track and field and swimming, culminating in a large competitive event. Every child receives some kind of award for effort and participation. Several of the children at the P-W Syndrome Clinic have won awards, made friends, and gained satisfaction through participation in the Special Olympics running and swimming events. One of these children is shown in Figure 24.2.

Tricycle and bicycle riding play an important role for social interaction in most neighborhoods at preschool and school ages. Many children in the P-W Syndrome Clinic have learned to ride bicycles, but usually not before the age of 8 or 10 years. Training wheels were often necessary for an

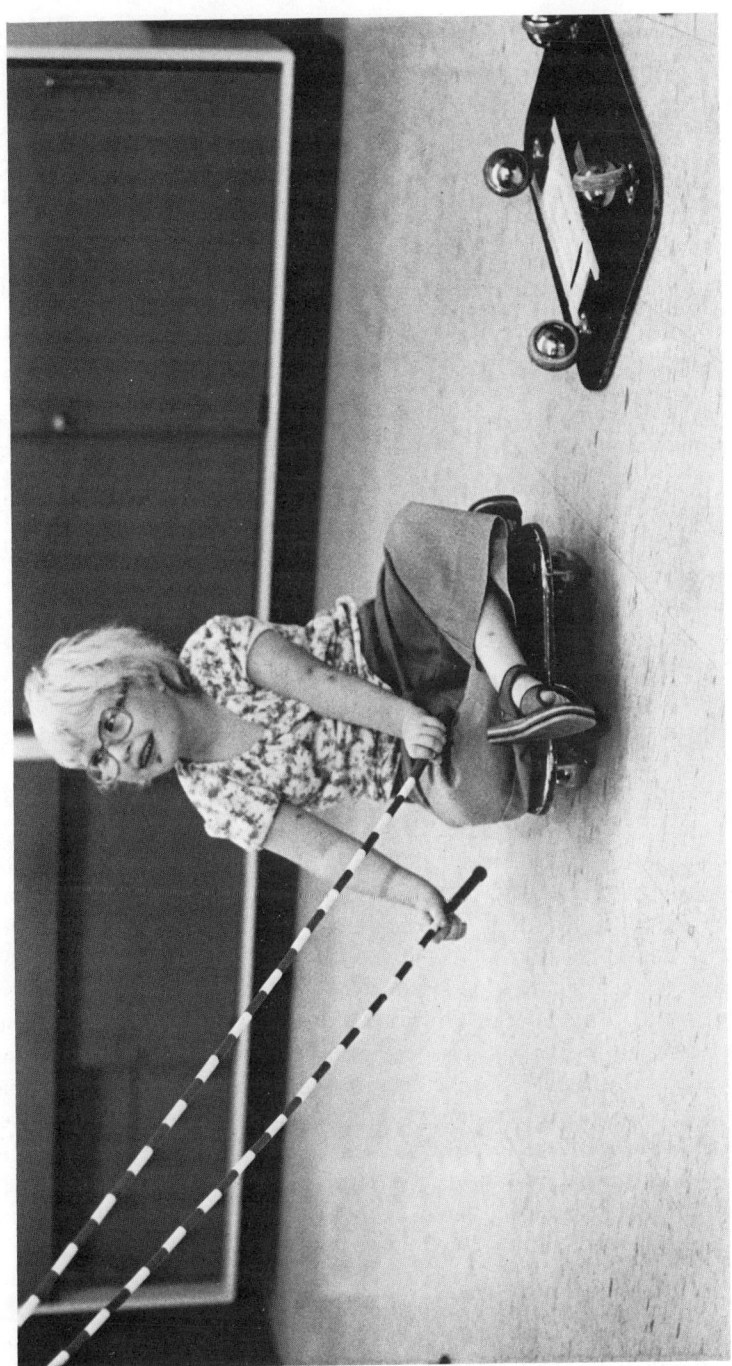

Figure 24.1 A P-W syndrome child enjoying a scooter board.

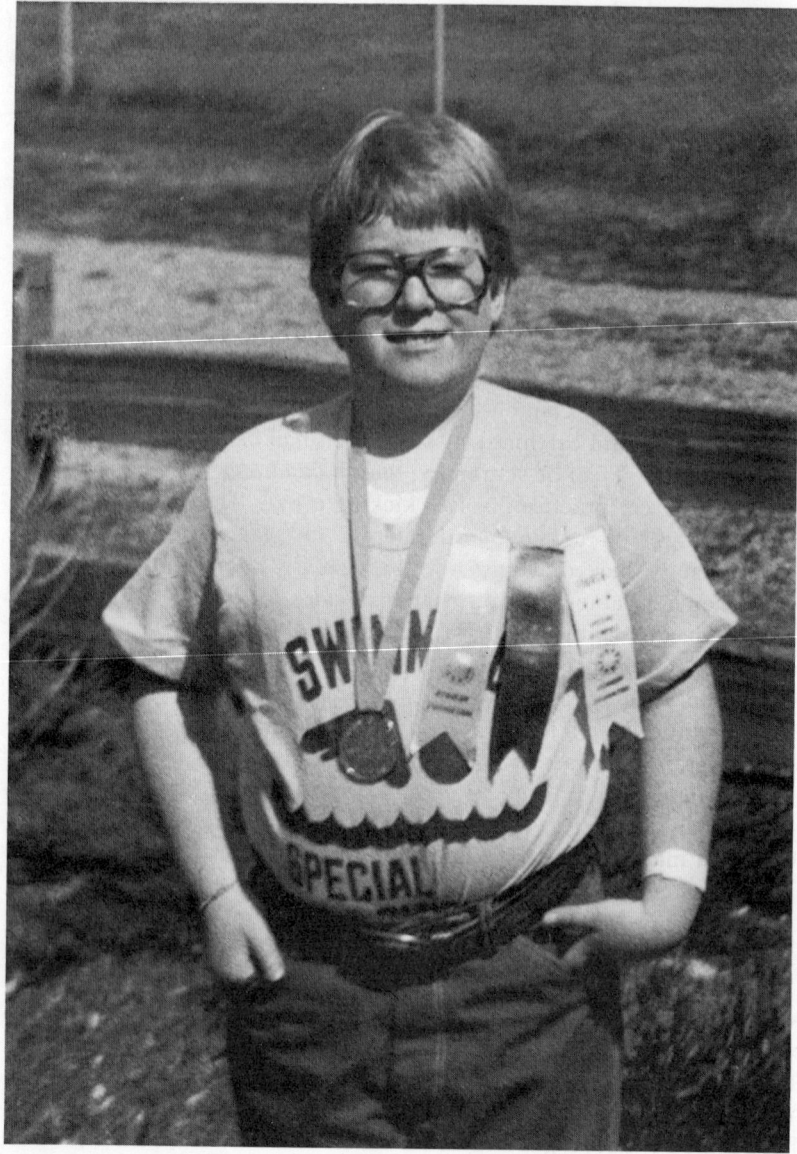

Figure 24.2 P-W syndrome did not stop this young man from winning awards for swimming in the Special Olympics.

extended period of time; as the child's confidence increased they were elevated about an inch before complete removal. Large tricycles may be more realistic than bicycles for many children, depending on developmental maturity.

Ball games become important social activities during the school years. Team sports such as basketball and baseball may or may not be feasible for children with P-W syndrome, depending on the degree of competition. Practice activities for either sport are common in most neighborhoods and learning the basic skills involved will promote interaction with other children. For basketball this means learning to bounce the ball, throwing and catching with another person, and shooting the ball toward a basketball hoop. The hoop can be positioned lower than regulation height so that the child can experience success. In baseball the basic skills include learning to catch a ball with and without a mitt and learning to throw the ball to another person. Throwing the ball against the wall and catching it can also be a game for one person with several variations (with or without a bounce, clap once or twice before catching, turn around between throwing and catching). A suspended ball can be used to practice batting. At first it can be stationary; later it can be swung by another person. Basic soccer practice involves kicking a ball. This can be practiced between two or more people to develop motor planning and balance, or the ball can be kicked against a wall repeatedly by one person.

Other enjoyable activities that promote coordination and strength and have been used by some P-W syndrome patients in our clinic include: rowing or paddling a boat, hiking, jogging (see Figure 24.3), dancing, badminton, croquet, and bowling. Some families in the clinic own horses that are gentle enough for their children to ride safely. Some riding stables have programs for special populations, but the individual's weight and ability to mount and dismount should be considered. Exercise machines such as standing cycles and rowing boats are not as much fun as the real thing, but may be more practical for some individuals who have no other source of exercise.

THE ADULT

Most of the activities mentioned in the section on school-age children may be used for exercise by the P-W adult. The choice depends on many factors including health, energy level, interests, ability, availability, and cost. Adults may learn to make an exercise program part of the daily routine. They could be encouraged to listen to music while exercising, to do the exercises with a friend, or to use a timer. Recording on a calendar the length of time spent exercising can make the calendar a quiet reminder to do some form of exercise daily.

Directions for basic exercises follow:

1. Sit-ups
    a. Start in sitting position on floor, knees bent and together; slowly go backward part of the way toward the supine position; then

raise the back. As strength improves, regular sit-ups, going all the way to the floor, can be done.
  b. With a partner, take turns going back and coming up (one goes down as the other comes up, like a see-saw).
2. Sit on the floor with legs straight; shift weight and lift one hip up; then shift to the alternate side and lift the other hip; try moving forward or backward while shifting weight.
3. Lie on stomach and raise head, with arms outstretched, and legs (if possible) up from the surface. Hold the "flying" position as long as possible, or move arms and legs as if swimming.

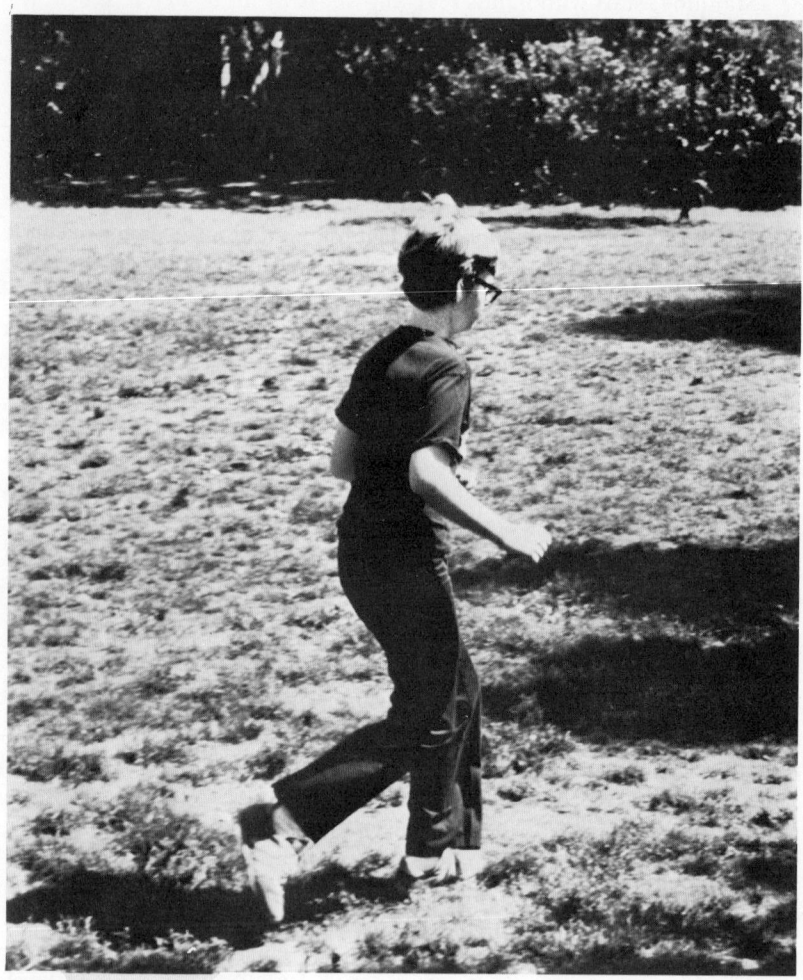

Figure 24.3 Jogging is part of this young P-W syndrome person's successful weight control program.

4. Lying on back, touch knee to nose. Alternate legs, returning head and leg to the floor each time before starting the next one.
5. Lying on back, knees bent, feet on floor, pull stomach in while inhaling breath deeply; relax with exhalation.
6. Lying on back, knees bent, feet on floor, move both knees laterally to touch the floor on the right side. Return to starting position; then move both knees to the other side. (The lower torso and legs are twisting while the upper torso and arms remain stationary.)
7. Standing, feet apart, stretch arms up high; tilt arms and trunk to one, then to the other side, stretching arms up as high as possible each time they are returned upright. Repeat the sequence.
8. Standing, start with hands reaching above head; bend and reach, trying to touch left heel with both hands. Reach up again before bending to touch right heel. Repeat sequence.

It is important to continue an exercise program. A regularly scheduled group activity, especially if it is enjoyable, will make this more likely. Community resources should be investigated for activity programs for adults and special populations. Aerobic dancing is a new form of exercise that could be scaled down slightly or just followed at one's own pace. This could also be done at home once some basic movements are learned. Activity programs for adults can also be organized with the help of the city or county park departments, the Association for Retarded Citizens, the YWCA/YMCA, community colleges, sheltered workshops, or group home associations.

Exercise can be built into the daily routine, such as walking to visit friends, and using the stairs instead of elevators. One of the adolescents in the clinic earned money by walking a neighbor's dog, which enhanced the motivation to exercise on a regular basis.

SCOLIOSIS

Scoliosis has been identified in a high percentage of individuals with P-W syndrome in our clinic and seems to be more common in the syndrome than was previously thought (Laurnen, Chapter 23, this volume). Although the cause of the spinal curvature is not known, low muscle tone and muscle weakness may be factors. The role of exercise in treatment of scoliosis is debated. A recent study of the effects of exercise on minimal idiopathic scoliosis (5°-20° curvature) did not show a significant difference in outcome between an exercise group and a retrospective control group (Stone, Beckman, Hall, Guess, & Brooks, 1979). It should be noted, however, that the amount and frequency of exercise was minimal, per week. There was no mention of abnormal muscle tone or strength. In P-W syndrome, the value of exercise for mild scoliosis deserves study because of the initial muscle weakness.

If the curve is greater than 20°, exercise alone cannot control the progression of curvature, and supportive bracing is commonly prescribed (James, 1976; Stone et al., 1979). To prevent loss of muscle strength during the period of supportive bracing, specific exercises are recommended (Blount & Moe, 1973). Use of an appropriate brace without exercise therapy is reported to produce slower and less satisfactory results; inactive patients frequently showed initial improvement, which was then lost until an exercise program was started.

Hypertonic hamstring muscles, leg length differences, and sensory differences may contribute to the cause of scoliosis in normal children. It is not known whether these factors contribute to scoliosis in P-W syndrome, but medical evaluations should be made with these possibilities in mind. Pearson et al. (1971) noted that differences in leg lengths were present in several of their P-W syndrome patients. Similar observations have been made in our clinic.

The exercise program used for scoliosis would be appropriate for any adult or child with weak abdominal muscles who is willing to exercise, regardless of whether or not a scoliosis has been identified. They are also appropriate for people with lordosis (sway back), which has frequently been noted in P-W syndrome patients at the clinic.

The pelvic tilt position is maintained during all exercises for scoliosis or lordosis. The easiest way to learn the pelvic tilt position is to assume the quadruped (hands and knees) position, then pull the stomach in and tighten the buttocks until the back is slightly rounded. One should hold the position to a count of 10, then relax and let the trunk sag to appreciate the position opposite, pelvic tilt. Guidance from a therapist will ensure understanding of the correct procedure. Physical guidance in assuming the correct position may be needed at first so that is can be felt; a mirror may also be useful for visual understanding of this movement.

Another way to practice the pelvic tilt is to stand with the back against a door frame, knees bent, and feet close to the door frame. Then the gluteal muscles (buttocks) and the abdominal muscles (stomach) should be tightened to flatten the small of the back against the door frame. This position should be held as long as possible. When the position is learned, the individual should try to walk and stand with tensed abdominal and gluteal muscles, with increasing duration and frequency.

One exercise that can be practiced while maintaining pelvic tilt in the quadruped position follows: Lift one limb at a time and hold it out even with body, balancing on three limbs. When the arm is held up and forward, the weight is on the other arm and the two knees; the back should be held flat. Alternate holding up each limb, balancing on the others.

Other strengthening and flexibility exercises commonly recommended for persons with scoliosis are described by Blount and Moe

(1973). Exercises to be done within the brace must be individually prescribed and taught.

CONCLUSION

The suggestions outlined in this chapter provide a starting point for planning exercise for P-W persons of different ages, including those with scoliosis. An individualized program can be designed by an occupational or physical therapist and is especially important for the young hypotonic child. An appropriately planned program of physical exercise can contribute significantly to the physical and emotional well-being of the person with P-W syndrome.

REFERENCES

Blount, W.D., & Moe, J.H. *The Milwaukee brace*. Baltimore: Williams & Wilkins Co., 1973

Brady, J.I., Knight, D.R., & Berghage, T.E. Relationship between measures of body fat and gross motor proficiency. *Journal of Applied Psychology*, 1977, *62*, 224-229.

Clark, D.L., Kreutzberg, J.R., & Chee, F.K.W. Vestibular stimulation influence on motor development in infants. *Science*, 1977, *196*, 1228-1229.

Dunn, H.G. The Prader-Labhart-Willi syndrome: Review of the literature and report of nine cases. *Acta Paediatrica Scandinavica*, 1968, Suppl. 186, 1-38.

Fluegelman, A. (Ed.). *The new games book/New Games Foundation*. New York: Doubleday & Co., 1976.

James, J.I.P. *Scoliosis*. New York: Churchill Livingstone, 1976.

Kantner, R.M., Clark, D.L., Allen, L.C., & Chase, M.F. Effects of vestibular stimulation on nystagmus response and motor performance in the developmentally delayed infant. *Physical Therapy*, 1976, *56*, 414-421.

Kauffman, I.B., & Ridenour, M. Influence of an infant walker on onset and quality of walking pattern of locomotion: An electromyographic investigation. *Perceptual and Motor Skills*, 1977, *45*, 1323-1329.

Pearson, K.D., Steinbach, H.L., & Bier, D.M. Roentgenographic manifestations of the Prader-Willi syndrome. *Pediatric Radiology*, 1971, *100*, 369-377.

Stone, B., Beckman, C., Hall, V., Guess, V., & Brooks, H.L. The effect of an exercise program on change in curve in adolescents with minimal idiopathic scoliosis. *Physical Therapy*, 1979, *59*, 759-763.

chapter 25
THE PRADER-WILLI SYNDROME
Directions in Future Research

Stephen Sulzbacher, Vanja A. Holm, and Peggy L. Pipes

> In this chapter the implications of some previous chapters and some unpublished research reports for future research on Prader-Willi syndrome are discussed. —Eds.

It should be apparent from the preceding chapters that significant advances have occurred in the understanding and treatment of Prader-Willi (P-W) syndrome and that the prospects for even greater understanding and better treatments for this disorder are reasonably good. This volume summarizes a quarter of a century of pioneering clinical research on P-W syndrome. The knowledge acquired has often been the result of serendipitous findings, duly recorded and analyzed. What is called for now is more systematic application of the scientific method to discover the mechanisms responsible for the developmental deviations seen in P-W syndrome.

Medical research reported and discussed in this volume raises many new questions. One example is the finding of Schwartz, Brunzell, and Bierman (Chapter 10, this volume) of high lipoprotein lipase levels in adults with this condition. Is this consistent in P-W syndrome persons of all ages? If so, is it already present during the early failure to thrive period? Could this finding be used as a diagnostic marker? How might the high level of lipoprotein lipase be causally related to the syndrome?

In conditions like P-W syndrome where the basic etiology remains unknown, even seemingly unlikely clues should be pursued. For example, one of the authors (V.A.H.) investigated the hypothesis that a zinc deficit could explain the manifestations of P-W syndrome (Holm & Worthington, Note 1). Zinc content of hair samples in 10 boys, 5 to 11 years of age, with an unequivocal diagnosis of P-W syndrome, was compared to that of 11 control subjects of the same age and sex living in the same geographical area (Seattle). The mean zinc content of the hair from the boys with P-W syndrome was 775.30 ppm ($\pm$197.57 SD; range 289–1000). In the controls, it was 837.37 ppm ($\pm$103.16 SD; range 660–935). Of course, this difference is not statistically significant. Unfortunately, negative research results seldom appear in the scientific literature. Publication of negative results obtained in pursuing interesting scientific questions might prevent others from conducting similar unproductive studies, or might encourage replication with different methods that might yield positive results.

Clinical observations have for a long time implicated a hypothalamic defect as the cause of P-W syndrome. Recent studies reported in this book tend to support this contention (Tze, Dunn, & Rothstein, Chapter 22; Warren & Hunt, Chapter 12). However, the results of studies of the hypothalamic-pituitary axis have been variable. Many questions have yet to be answered. What are the clinical differences between persons with abnormal versus normal response? What are the prognostic and therapeutic implications of these studies in P-W syndrome? Could they be used in individuals to predict sexual development in adolescence? Could they be used as guidance for hormonal replacement? Another area of research discussed in a previous chapter is oxandrolone (Nugent & Holm, Chapter 21). The efficacy of this drug in promoting growth in P-W syndrome needs further exploration. Additional medical research that might be useful includes further neuropathological investigations of the hypothalamic area. To date only a few cases have been studied using conventional methods. Neuroendocrinological studies, for example on endorphine, seem to be promising avenues for research. There are also reports of chromosomal abnormalities in the literature that further research could clarify. Epidemiological research is sorely needed to pinpoint the prevalence of this condition.

Pharmacological studies should also be carried out. Although the effectiveness of the hypocaloric regimen has been proved, the constant surveillance necessary for P-W individuals to adhere to such a regimen is usually resented and is often a factor in the etiology of a variety of behavior problems. If drugs to control the insatiable appetite could be found, dietary management as well the daily lives of P-W syndrome individuals and of their families would be simplified. Additional pharmacological research on new behavior-modifying drugs is also indicated for this patient population, particularly for temper tantrums and episodes of anxiety in the adult.

There are several nutritional questions to which attention should be directed. Do nutritional deficiencies result from the long term use of the severely restricted low calorie diet? What is the explanation for the excessive weight gain on a comparatively low energy intake? How does constant hunger and food-getting affect other behaviors?

A nutritional study recently completed at the University of Washington (Otto, Note 2) investigated the effects of sugar ingestion on activity level and learning. The impetus for the study came from reports by several parents that whenever their P-W syndrome children consumed large quantities of sugar, their behavior deteriorated for anywhere from several hours to several days. Hyperactivity, crankiness, and temper outbursts were typically mentioned. One parent insisted that a single stolen candy bar would cause the behavior. A method devised by Swanson. Kinsbourne, Roberts, and Zucker (1978) for evaluating medication effects in hyperactive children was used in this study. Nine P-W children, including those whose parents felt they were sensitive to sugar, were tested on two measures of activity and a paired-associates learning task. There were 3 testing days in this double-blind trial: one for sugar (3g/kg of body weight), one for saccharin of equivalent sweetness, and one for polycose (a carbohydrate equivalent in calories to the sugar). The effects of sugar on any of the measures could not be detected. However, it was learned from blood glucose tests taken as part of the study that sugar is metabolized by P-W individuals at a rate that is within normal limits. Further metabolic research is definitely indicated.

The research of Warren and Hunt (Chapter 12, this volume) is another example of the scientific approach to problem solving. They reasoned inductively from the clinical evidence of the appetite and weight regulation disorder and from the rage reactions that the hypothalmus was involved. Relating this finding to theories about hypothalamic functioning, they deduced that there should also be short term memory difficulties. Their research confirmed that hypothesis. Such research, relating findings from individuals with P-W syndrome to other bodies of knowledge, should have highest priority.

More clinical research is needed to find better ways of teaching P-W individuals to monitor their own weight and to obtain more information on how they can adjust better to late adolescence and adulthood in the community. Pioneering efforts at establishing group homes specifically for those with P-W syndrome have shown some success in managing weight while providing some normal community experiences. Similar results have been obtained with some P-W persons in group homes serving a general population of developmentally disabled people. The value of peer support groups for those with P-W syndrome also needs further exploration. The concept of a systematic tenant support service for developmentally disabled persons living on their own is being tried in the Seattle area and holds promise of being a useful adjunct for community living for those with P-W syndrome.

Finally, a need for refinement of educational techniques is seen, particularly at the middle school and high school levels, to maximize skill acquisition and social learning which could lead to more productive and satisfying lives. The school curriculum for P-W persons at the elementary level need not be much different from that provided for other learning-disabled children. There are some special problems requiring more individualized programming in shopping, meal and menu planning, and community mobility for P-W persons who are trying to avoid situations in which they would be tempted to steal or consume food. These issues have been discussed by Sulzbacher, Crnic, and Snow (Chapter 11, this volume), but more research is needed to find more effective ways of teaching. There is also little known about the efficacy of various counseling or psychotherapy techniques with the P-W adult. Many parents and professionals are convinced that more could be discovered about subtle cognitive processing differences occurring in P-W syndrome. A better understanding of these suspected deficits could lead to specific psychotherapeutic and educational remedies.

Throughout history scientists have frequently been able to gain a better understanding of a widespread phenomenon, like obesity, from the intensive study of the special case, like P-W syndrome. It should be obvious that intensive research on P-W syndrome can yield information about obesity, hormone function, and brain function, which could benefit many more people than the relatively small number afflicted with this disorder. In other words, we are now at the point where basic research on phenomena related to P-W syndrome holds promise for significant advancement of knowledge in general.

It is hoped that the next 25 years are as productive and beneficial as the previous quarter century has been in improving the prospects for a better life for individuals with Prader-Willi syndrome.

REFERENCE NOTES

1. Holm, V.A., & Worthington, B. *Zinc in the Prader-Willi Syndrome*. Unpublished manuscript, University of Washington, 1979.
2. Otto, P. *Sucrose-induced behavior changes in children with Prader-Willi syndrome*. Unpublished M.S. thesis, University of Washington, 1980.

REFERENCE

Swanson, J., Kinsbourne, M., Roberts, W., & Zucker, K. Time-response analysis of the effect of stimulant medication on the learning ability of children referred for hyperactivity. *Pediatrics,* 1978, *61,* 22-29.

THE PRADER-WILLI SYNDROME
An Annotated Bibliography

Afifi, A.K. Histology and cytology of muscle in Prader-Willi syndrome. *Developmental Medicine and Child Neurology*, 1969, *11*, 363-364.
A brief summary of an article published elsewhere (Afifi & Zellweger, 1969). Medical Aspects.

Afifi, A.K., & Zellweger, H. Pathology of muscular hypotonia in the Prader-Willi syndrome: Light and electron microscopic study. *Journal of the Neurological Sciences*, 1969, *9*, 49-61.
Muscle biopsies on seven cases of P-W syndrome, clinically described elsewhere (Zellweger & Schneider, 1968), are reported to show essentially normal light microscopy, as has been reported by others. Studies of neuromuscular function in P-W syndrome up to the time of this report are summarized in a table. This is the first electron microscopy report on the appearance of muscles in P-W syndrome. Five illustrations show ultrastructural changes that could be compatible with myopathy, neuropathy, or muscular immobility and disuse. The authors discuss the etiology of hypotonia in P-W syndrome and seem to favor the last explanation in view of the normality of other neuromuscular studies done by themselves and others. Medical Aspects.

Altman, K., Bondy, A., & Hirsch, G. Behavioral treatment of obesity in patients with Prader-Willi syndrome. *Journal of Behavioral Medicine*, 1978, *1*, 403-412.
A detailed description of how to set up and maintain a behavior modification program for weight loss for an inpatient and an outpatient with P-W syndrome. Both subjects lost significant amounts of weight. The results of the study are amplified by Hirsch and Altman (Chapter 15, this volume). Obesity Control, Behavioral Aspects.

Anand, S.K., Kogut, M.D., & Liberman, E. Persistent hypernatremia due to abnormal thirst mechanism in a 13-year-old child with nephrogenic diabetes insipidus. *The Journal of Pediatrics*, 1972, *81*, 1097-1105.
This article reports on a 13-year-old boy said to show the "clinical features" of P-W syndrome, but many aspects are atypical: hypotonia was not marked, there is no mention of behavioral problems, caloric intake was excessive for P-W syndrome, and the photograph fails to demonstrate typical facial features, small hands and feet, and the subcutaneous fat distribution usually seen in this condition. Medical Aspects.

Beange, H., & Caradus, V. The Prader-Willi syndrome. *Australian Journal of Mental Retardation,* 1974, *3,* 9-11.
Presentation of 15 cases of P-W syndrome from Australia, with a brief literature review. Case Reports.

Bianchine, J.W., Stambler, A.A., & MacGregor, M.I. The Prader-Willi syndrome with cardiorespiratory complications. *Birth Defects,* 1971, *7,* 301.
A young adult female with P-W syndrome and Pickwickian syndrome is described. Blood gas and pulmonary function studies at 348 and 296 pounds showed alveolar hypoventilation with carbon dioxide retention and restrictive ventilatory defect, the latter unchanged by weight reduction. Medical Aspects, Case Report.

Bier, D.M. Medical staff conference: The Prader-Willi syndrome. *California Medicine,* 1970, *112,* 65-73.
A case of a 21-year-old Mexican-American male with P-W syndrome is described. Features of the syndrome are reviewed. Case Reports, Review Article.

Bier, D.M., Kaplan, S.L., & Havel, R.J. The Prader-Willi syndrome: Regulation of fat transport. *Diabetes,* 1977, *26,* 874-881.
This paper describes studies to determine whether abnormalities in fasting lipogenesis cause obesity in P-W syndrome. Six patients, age 7 years, 10 months to 22 years, 8 months, were studied, one of whom had insulin-dependent diabetes. Fasting glucose was normal in the other five patients. The diabetic subject had fasting glucose levels of 124 to 145 mg/dl. Insulin responses to stimulation with glucose were in the normal range but consistent with the patients' obesity. Plasma-free fatty acids (FFA) were within the normal range. Plasma glycerol levels were high compared to the FFA values. All but the patient with diabetes had a normal response of FFA and brisk reductions of acetoacetate and β-hydroxybutyrate during intravenous glucose tolerance tests. Lipolytic response to norepinephrine stimulation was not impaired. Lipoprotein electrophoretic patterns were normal in every patient as were electron microscopic examinations of adipose tissue. These results do not support the hypothesis that individuals with P-W syndrome have depressed hormone-stimulated lipolysis. Endocrinology, Obesity Control.

Bistrian, B.R., Blackburn, G.L., & Stanbury, J.B. Metabolic aspects of a protein-sparing modified fast in the dietary management of Prader-Willi obesity. *The New England Journal of Medicine,* 1977, *296,* 774-779.
Four individuals with P-W syndrome, 12 to 24 years of age, were treated in a metabolic unit with a protein-sparing modified fast. One individual continued the diet and weight loss as an outpatient. Two did not lose as rapidly as outpatients; their weight leveled off before achieving desired weight and they later gained weight. One individual was unable to main-

tain the protein-sparing diet or weight loss as an outpatient. Endocrinology, Obesity Control.

Bolaños, F., López-Amor, E., Vásquez, G., Lisker, R., & Morato, T. Hypothalamic-pituitary gonadal function in two siblings with Prader-Willi syndrome. *Revista de Investigacion Clinica,* 1974, *26,* 53-62.

A sister and brother (22 and 19 years old, respectively), from a consanguineous marriage, with symptoms of P-W syndrome are described and the results of the studies of their hypothalamic-pituitary-gonadal axes are given. (Spanish, English summary.) Case Reports, Endocrinology, Etiology.

Bottel, H. The eating disease. *Good Housekeeping,* May 1977, p. 176.

This is a discussion of P-W syndrome in the popular press, mentioning the advantages, for the P-W child, of early diagnosis and weight control.

Brissenden, J.E., & Levy, E.P. Prader-Willi syndrome in infant monozygotic twins. *American Journal of Diseases of Children,* 1973, *126,* 110-112.

Typical features of P-W syndrome are described in twin brothers with a 98% probability of being monozygous. Etiology, Case Reports.

Bühler, E.M., Rossier, R., Bodis, I., Vulliet, V., Bühler, U.K., & Stalder, G. Chromosomal translocation in a mentally deficient child with cryptorchidism. *Acta Paediatrica,* 1963, *52,* 177-182.

A 6-year-old boy with chromosomal abnormality and symptoms of P-W syndrome is described. This case was confirmed as P-W syndrome in a subsequent publication (Fraccaro et al., 1977). Etiology, Diagnosis.

Clarren, S.K., & Smith, D.W. Prader-Willi syndrome: Variable severity and recurrence risk. *American Journal of Diseases of Children,* 1977, *131,* 798-800.

This review of family histories of 39 cases of P-W syndrome suggests low recurrence risk within a family. Diagnostic difficulties are discussed, with the suggestion that a spectrum of effect and severity exists in addition to the "classical" P-W syndrome cases. A hypothetical model of the cause of the disorder is presented. Diagnosis, Etiology.

Cohen, M.M., Jr., & Gorlin, R.J. The Prader-Willi syndrome. *American Journal of Diseases of Children.* 1969, *117,* 213-218.

Two boys with P-W syndrome are described, one with unusual dermatoglyphic patterns. Case Reports, Medical Aspects.

Constant craving for food causes health problems. *JAMA: The Journal of the American Medical Association,* 1976, *235,* 245-246.

A short news item about P-W syndrome in a professional journal. Medical Aspects, Obesity Control, Behavioral Aspects.

Coplin, S.S., Hine, J., & Gormican A. Out-patient dietary management in the Prader-Willi syndrome. *Journal of the American Dietetic Association,* 1976, *68,* 330-334.

A 6-month study of the dietary management of children with P-W syndrome treated for obesity with a conventional hypocaloric regimen as outpatients was conducted. Three of eight children showed a weight loss after 6 months. The subjects required fewer calories than age group peers of the same height and weight. Frequent home visits and telephone follow-up by the dietitian provided the parents with motivation and dietary insights. Obesity Control.

DeFraites, E.B., Thurmon, T.F., & Farhadian, H. Familial Prader-Willi syndrome. *Birth defects: Original article series,* 1975, *11* (4), 123-126.

Five cases of P-W syndrome in an inbred Louisiana family are described. The findings are presented as suggestive of autosomal recessive inheritance patterns. Following the paper, other researchers discussed the diagnosis of P-W syndrome and questioned it in all but the proband. Etiology.

Down, J.L.H. On polysarcia and its treatment. In *On some of the mental affections of childhood and youth.* London: J.H. Churchill, 1887.

As pointed out by McKusick (1978), this is probably the first description of a person with P-W syndrome in the medical literature. When Dr. Down first saw this girl in 1850 at age 13 years, she was "of feeble mind," 4 feet, 4 inches tall and weighed 113 lbs. She is said to have had a voracious appetite. She had not menstruated by 25 years of age, remained the same height, and weighed 210 lbs. She also is said to have had small hands and feet.

Dubowitz, V. A syndrome of benign congenital hypotonia, gross obesity, delayed intellectual development, retarded bone age, and unusual facies. *Proceedings of the Royal Society of Medicine,* 1967, *60,* 1006-1008.

Two cases (one boy and one girl) are described in detail. The author mentions that he has observed a decline in IQ over the years and considers the syndrome fairly common. Case Reports.

Dubowitz, V. *The floppy infant.* 2nd Ed. Clinics in Developmental Medicine No. 76. London: Spastics International Medical Publications/William Heinemann, 1980.

This discussion of hypotonia mentions P-W syndrome several times. The detailed discussion of P-W syndrome on pages 126-131 includes two case reports with photographs of the same male from infancy to age 8 and same female from infancy to age 15 years. Case Reports, Review Article, Diagnosis.

Dunn, H.G. The Prader-Labhart-Willi syndrome: Review of the literature and report of nine cases. *Acta Paediatrica Scandinavica,* 1968, Suppl. 186, 1-38.

Nine cases from Vancouver, B.C., including two females. Extensive literature review; 77 references. The author reports observations of declining IQ and many medical studies, including one pneumoencephalogram. Three of eight chromosome studies are described as abnormal, one with an XYY karyotype. Case Reports, Review Article, Medical Aspects, Endocrinology.

Dunn, H.G., Ford, D.K., Auersperg, N., & Miller, J.R. Benign congenital hypotonia with chromosomal anomaly. *Pediatrics*, 1961, *28*, 578–591.
One case report, not recognized as P-W syndrome at the time of writing. At the 73rd meeting of the American Pediatric Society in Atlantic City, N.J., 1963, the authors reported that this was a case of P-W syndrome. The patient had an extra chromosome in the 21–22 group. Case Reports, Etiology.

Emberger, J.M., Rodière, M., Astruc, J., & Brunel, D. Syndrome de Prader-Willi et translocation 15-15. *Annales de Génétique*, 1977, *20*, 297–300.
A female with P-W syndrome and chromosome 15 abnormality is described (see also Fraccaro et al., 1977). (French, English summary). Etiology, Diagnosis, Case Reports.

Endo, M., Tasaka, Y., Matsuura, N., & Matsuda, I. Laurance-Moon-Biedl syndrome (?) and Prader-Willi syndrome (?) in a single family. *European Journal of Pediatrics*, 1976, *123*, 269–276.
This article describes a sister and brother with mental retardation, hypogonadism, obesity, and abnormal blood sugar regulation. The sister seems to have most of the additional features typical of P-W syndrome and the boy has additional findings suggesting the Laurence-Moon-Biedl syndrome. Endocrinological studies carried out were otherwise unremarkable. The authors speculate about possible explanations. Etiology, Endocrinology.

Evans, P.R. Hypogenital dystrophy with diabetic tendency. *Guy's Hospital Reports*, 1964, *113*, 207–222.
Eight cases from England, all boys. Case Reports.

Fiser, R.H., Jr., Bray, G.A., Carrel, R.E., Stites, L.J., Cohen, A.H., Swerdloff, R.S., Odell, W.D., & Fisher, D.A. Evidence for hypothalamic-pituitary dysfunction in the Prader-Willi syndrome. *Pediatric Research*, 1974, *8*, 368.
Brief abstract describing two cases of P-W syndrome, 15 and 22 years of age, studied endocrinologically and at autopsy. The results suggest a functional hypothalamic abnormality. Endocrinology, Pathology.

Forssman, H., & Hagberg, B. Prader-Willi syndrome in boy of ten with prediabetes. *Acta Paediatrica*, 1964, *53*, 70–78.
One case report from Sweden of a 10-year-old boy with P-W syndrome. Case Reports.

Foster, S.C. Prader-Willi syndrome: Report of cases. *Journal of the American Dental Association*, 1971, *83*, 634–638.

The dental findings in two cases of P-W syndrome are described, emphasizing enamel hypoplasia, one of several dental aberrations described in this syndrome. Medical Aspects.

Fraccaro, M., Zuffardi, O., Buhler, E.M., & Jurik, L.P. 15/15 translocation in Prader-Willi syndrome. *Journal of Medical Genetics,* 1977, *14,* 275-278.

This study shows that some P-W syndrome cases may be a result of a chromosome 15 abnormality, but that other cases clearly are not. The authors suggest that there may be two or more different disorders with similar phenotypes (see also Bühler et al., 1963). Etiology, Diagnosis.

Frenk, E., & Calame, A. Hypopigmentation oculo-cutanée familiale à transmission dominante due à un trouble de la formation des mélanosomes. *Schweizerische Medizinische Wochenschrift,* 1977, *107,* 1964-1968.

This study is primarily about a family with a dominant genetic pigmentation disorder, but presents a case study of one member of the family who also has P-W syndrome. The authors conclude that the two disorders are an unrelated coincidence. (French, English summary). Case Reports, Etiology, Medical Aspects.

Gabilan, J.C., & Royer, P. Le syndrome de Prader, Labhardt et Willi (étude de onze observations). *Archives Françaises de Pédiatrie,* 1968, *25,* 121-149.

Eleven cases of P-W syndrome are described in detail, with two cases in the same family (a sister and a brother) and another case from a consanguineous marriage. Abnormal EEGs are reported in two cases. Five testicular biopsies were within normal limits for age. Orthopedic abnormalities (scoliosis, lordosis, coxa valga, hip dislocation, and epiphysiolysis) are described in detail and illustrated with roentgenograms. (French). Case Reports, Medical Aspects, Etiology, Review Article.

Gellis, S.S., & Feingold, M. (Eds.). *Atlas of mental retardation syndromes.* Washington, D.C.: U.S. Government Printing Office/U.S. Department of Health, Education, & Welfare, 1968.

A picture book of syndromes which includes color plates of P-W syndrome. Diagnosis.

Gorlin, R.J., Pindborg, J.J., & Cohen, M.M., Jr. Prader-Willi syndrome. In *Syndromes of the head and neck* (2nd ed.). New York: McGraw-Hill Book Co., 1976.

This well known textbook of syndromes involving facial structures has a brief chapter reviewing P-W syndrome. One paragraph outlines the oral manifestations that have been described in the literature. Medical Aspects, Diagnosis.

Gotlin, R., Dubois, R., Mace, J., & Myer, W. Carbohydrate metabolism in the Prader-Willi syndrome. *Clinical Research,* 1972, *20,* 274.

Four individuals with P-W syndrome were studied to determine whether obesity in this syndrome differs metabolically from other exogenous obesity. Peroral intestinal biopsies were performed on two subjects after a 48 to 56-hour fast and 96 hours of high carbohydrate feeding to determine pyruvate kinase activity. All subjects had insulin and glucose rises in response to IV glucagon after a 5-hour fast and manifested ketosis and a rise in free fatty acids after a 48 to 56-hour fast. Jejunal mucosal pyruvate kinase levels rose normally with carbohydrate feedings in one subject. The obesity in these individuals did not differ metabolically from other exogenous obesity. Endocrinology, Medical Aspects.

Guanti, G. A new case of rearrangement of chromosome 15 associated with Prader-Willi syndrome. *Clinical Genetics*, 1980, *17*, 423-427.
A 3½-year-old boy with typical findings of P-W syndrome had a chromosomal abnormality consisting of a translocation between the short arm of chromosome 9 and the long arm of chromosome 15. Case Report. Etiology.

Guthrie, R.D., Smith, D.W., & Graham, C.B. Testosterone treatment for micropenis during early childhood. *The Journal of Pediatrics*, 1973, *83*, 247-252.
Successful treatment of four patients with testosterone to increase penis size is described. Two of the four boys had P-W syndrome. Endocrinology.

Haberfellner, H., Glatzl, J., & Unterkircher, R. Prader-Willi Labhart-Syndrom im Säuglingsalter. *Pädiatrie und Pädologie*, 1974, *9*, 123-129.
This is a case study of an infant with P-W syndrome. An abnormality of chromosome 16 was found in the patient and his mother, but the father and two sisters showed normal chromosomal patterns. A deficit of IgA was also detected by immunoelectrophoresis. However, the patient died of bronchiolitis several months later (no autopsy was performed) and thus no further tests were run. (German, English summary), Case Reports, Endocrinology, Etiology.

Hall, B.D., & Smith, D.W. Prader-Willi syndrome. A resumé of 32 cases including an instance of affected first cousins, one of whom is of normal stature and intelligence. *Pediatrics*, 1972, *81*, 286-293.
A figure illustrates the mean percent occurrence of abnormalities in P-W syndrome. The authors discuss possible pathogenesis, and speculate that P-W syndrome is due to a localized developmental defect in the hypothalamic region. Review Article, Etiology, Diagnosis.

Hamilton, C.R., Jr., Scully, R.E., & Kliman, B. Hypogonadotropinism in Prader-Willi syndrome: Induction of puberty and spermatogenesis by clomiphene citrate. *The American Journal of Medicine*, 1972, *52*, 322-329.

Three case reports of males, who were studied at ages 19, 20, and 23 years, respectively, showing hypogonadotropic hypogonadism. Testicular biopsies performed in two patients were abnormal. One case (age 23) was treated with clomiphene citrate for 40 days. The authors state that plasma luteinizing hormone (LH), testosterone, and urinary gonadotropin levels rose to the normal range, that normal spermatogenesis was present on repeat testicular biopsy, and that physical signs of puberty became evident. They suggest that clomiphene citrate may be an effective treatment for male hypogonadism in P-W syndrome. No report confirming these observations has yet appeared in the medical literature. Endocrinology, Case Reports.

Hawkey, C.J., & Smithies, A. The Prader-Willi syndrome with a 15/15 translocation. *Journal of Medical Genetics*, 1976, *13*, 152-163.

A case is presented with P-W syndrome and abnormal chromosome 15. The authors reviewed 170 published cases and found 10 other abnormalities in 61 cases reporting chromosome analyses, and speculate on possible involvement of such abnormality in the pathogenesis of P-W syndrome (see also Fraccaro et al., 1977). Case Reports, Etiology, Diagnosis.

Heiman, M.F. The management of obesity in the post-adolescent developmentally disabled client with Prader-Willi syndrome. *Adolescence*, 1978, *13*, 291-296.

This is a brief description of a behavior modification program for two adolescents in an institution. Case Reports, Behavioral Aspects, Obesity Control.

Hoefnagel, D., Costello, P.J., & Hatoum, K. Prader-Willi syndrome. *Journal of Mental Deficiency Research*, 1967, *11*, 1-11.

Three cases of P-W syndrome, all boys, are described with a review of the literature up to that time. Symptoms from before birth through adulthood are presented in a table. Case Reports.

Holm, V.A., & Pipes, P.L. Food and children with Prader-Willi syndrome. *American Journal of Diseases of Children*, 1976, *130*, 1063-1067.

Data on growth, energy intake, and food behavior are presented on 14 children with P-W syndrome. Reasonably successful weight control programs were effected for 12 of the children. The children required fewer calories than their age group peers. Reported behaviors include sneaking food, gorging, obsession with food, and eating unappealing products. All families made special provisions for handling food and behavior. (See also Pipes & Holm, 1973.) Behavioral Aspects, Obesity Control.

Holm, V.A., & Pipes, P.L. On the management of the Prader-Willi syndrome. *The Journal of Pediatrics*, 1977, *91*, 355-356.

Letter to the editor regarding an article by Orenstein et al. (1977) that emphasizes the need for obesity prevention and nutritional management of this syndrome as opposed to progesterone treatment. Obesity Control.

Holmes, L.B. (Ed.). *Mental retardation: An atlas of diseases with associated physical abnormalities.* New York: Macmillan, 1972.

This large atlas of mental retardation syndromes has comprehensive illustrated text describing P-W and other syndromes. Diagnosis.

Holt, S.B. Dermatoglyphics in Prader-Willi syndrome. *Journal of Mental Deficiency Research,* 1975, *19,* 245-258.

Dermatoglyphic patterns in 13 patients with P-W syndrome were studied and reported not to differ from those of normal subjects. Medical Aspects.

Hooft, C., Delire, C., & Casneuf, J. Le syndrome de Prader-Labhardt-Willi-Fanconi: Etude clinique, endocrinologique et cytogénétique. *Acta Paediatrica Belgica,* 1966, *20,* 27-50.

Four cases less than 5 years of age are described. One had a pneumoencephalogram showing ventricle dilation and probable cortical atrophy. (French, English summary). Case Reports, Medical Aspects.

Hypotonia and obesity syndrome. *British Medical Journal,* September 16, 1967, p. 694.

Editorial pointing out the importance of including P-W syndrome in the differential diagnosis of neonatal hypotonia. Medical Aspects.

Ikeda, K., Asaka, A., Inouye, E., Kaihara, H., & Kinoshita, K. Monozygotic twins concordant for Prader-Willi syndrome. *Japanese Journal of Human Genetics,* 1973, *18,* 220-225.

Twelve-year-old monozygotic twin males with P-W syndrome are described. (English). Case Reports.

Jancar, J. Prader-Willi syndrome (hypotonia, obesity, hypogonadism, growth and mental retardation). *Journal of Mental Deficiency Research,* 1971, *15,* 20-29.

Five cases of P-W syndrome are described. Two of these occurred in brothers, but the description and pictures of these include several atypical features. Case Reports.

Jeffcoate, W.J., Laurance, B.M., Edwards, C.R.W., & Besser, G.M. Endocrine function in the Prader-Willi syndrome. *Clinical Endocrinology,* 1980, *12,* 81-89.

Five males ages 10 to 26 and three females ages 15 to 21 years were studied endocrinologically. The results suggest to the authors that, in addition to a hypothalamic defect, there is also a primary gonadal disorder present in P-W syndrome. Endocrinology.

Jenab, M., Lade, R.I., Chiga, M., & Diehl, A.M. Cardiorespiratory syndrome of obesity in a child: Case report and necropsy findings. *Pediatrics,* 1959, *24,* 23-30.

This is an early case report that was not recognized as P-W syndrome at the time of writing, but the findings are typical and it is generally accepted as a case of P-W syndrome. It was the first pathological report published. Case Reports, Pathology.

Johnston, J.G., & Robertson, W.O. Fatal ingestion of table salt by an adult. *The Western Journal of Medicine,* 1977, *126,* 141-143.

A 45-year-old woman with P-W syndrome died from salt poisoning after having consumed four cups of jam supplemented by 3 to 4 heaping tablespoons of salt, conceivably under the impression it was sugar. Insatiable appetite is blamed for the ingestion. It is noted that she did not vomit. Case Reports, Behavioral Aspects, Pathology.

Juul, J., & Dupont, A. Prader-Willi syndrome. *Journal of Mental Deficiency Research,* 1967, *11,* 12-22.

One male P-W syndrome patient from a Danish institution, 43 years old (oldest published case report) is described. Case Reports.

Kadrnka-Lovrencic, M., Oberiter, V., Reiner-Banovac, Z., Schmutzer, L.J., Resetic, J., & Najman, E.

Prader-Labhart-Willi syndrome: A contribution to the problem of pituitary responsiveness to luteinizing hormone-releasing hormone. *Acta Medica Iugoslavica,* 1974, *23,* 369-381.

Case report of a 7-year-old girl with P-W syndrome from Yugoslavia who was studied with luteinizing hormone-releasing hormone (LH-RH) with response of FSH but no increase in LH. (Long English abstract). Endocrinology.

Katcher, M.L., Bargman, G.J., Gilbert, E.F., & Opitz, J.M. Absence of spermatogonia in the Prader-Willi syndrome. *European Journal of Pediatrics,* 1977, *124,* 257-260.

Testicular biopsy results are reported for an 8½-year-old boy with P-W syndrome. They showed absence of germ cells and normal Sertoli cells, similar to findings in post-pubertal cases of P-W syndrome reported by others.

Kauli, R., Prager-Lewin, R., & Laron, Z. Pubertal development in the Prader-Labhart-Willi syndrome. *Acta Paediatrica Scandinavica,* 1978, *67,* 763-767.

This is a report on sexual development of 14 patients, 10 females and four males, showing a wide variability: delayed puberty in five, normal puberty in four (including one male who is said to have "normal sexual activity"), and sexual precocity in five (one "true" precocious puberty and four incomplete puberties with early pubarche). Five patients, including three with early pubarche, showed pubertal arrest. Luteinizing hormone-releasing hormone (LH-RH) was given to 11 patients. Six patients with normal or eventually normal sexual development responded in the normal range. In those with delay or arrest of puberty the LH and FSH responses to LH-RH were blunted. The authors conclude that there is a variability in the localization and extent of the hypothalamic lesion in P-W syndrome. Endocrinology.

Knorr, D. Pubertas tarda—Pubertätsadipositas-Hypogonadismus: Diagnostische und therapeutische Probleme. *Zeitschrift für Allgemeinmedizin,* 1977, *53,* 1470-1475.

The paper describes diagnosis and suggested treatments for several disorders involving hypogonadism and obesity. Distinctive features of P-W syndrome, Laurence-Moon-Biedl syndrome, Cushing syndrome, and others are illustrated. Only one paragraph discusses features of P-W syndrome. (German). Diagnosis.

Kollrack, H.W., & Wolff, D. Paranoid-halluzinatorische Psychose bei Prader-Labhart-Willi-Fanconi-Syndrome. *Acta Paedopsychiatrica,* 1966, *33,* 309-314.

A case report on a 20-year-old P-W patient (IQ of 47) who had two brief psychotic episodes 10 months apart. During these episodes he was anxious, agitated, and suspicious, and he hallucinated and manifested paranoid ideas. Librium was prescribed during one episode. Except for these two episodes this patient, who lived with his family, was described as docile and helpful at home. (German, English summary). Case Reports, Behavioral Aspects.

Kucerova, M., Strakova, M., & Polivkova, Z. The Prader-Willi syndrome with a 15/3 translocation. *Journal of Medical Genetics,* 1979, *16,* 234-235.

Brief case report of a 5-year-old boy with P-W syndrome and a monosomy of the short arm and partial monosomy of the long arm of chromosome 15 and probably also monosomy of a small part of the short arm of chromosome 3. Etiology, Case Report.

Kyriakides, M., Silverstone, T., Jeffcoate, W., & Laurance, B. Effect of naloxone on hyperphagia in Prader-Willi syndrome. *Lancet,* 1980, *1*(8173), 876-877 (letter to the editor).

Naloxone is known to control hyperphagia in genetically obese mice and rats by interfering with hypothalamic β-endorphine activity. Three adults with P-W syndrome were given 0.8 and 1.6 mg subcutaneously, with a saline placebo under double blind conditions. Naloxone, especially at the higher dose of 1.6 mg, reduced food intake in two male patients whose baseline food intake had been very high, but not in the one female patient (see also Sullivan, 1980, and McCloy, 1980). Obesity Control.

Landwirth, J., Schwartz, A.H., & Grunt, J.A. Prader-Willi syndrome. *American Journal of Diseases of Children,* 1968, *116,* 211-217.

An early case report of a 17-year-old boy with P-W syndrome. Case Reports.

Laurance, B.M. Hypotonia, mental retardation, obesity, and cryptorchidism associated with dwarfism and diabetes in children. *Archives of Disease in Childhood,* 1967, *42,* 126-139.
Nine cases from England, two of whom were females. The first four cases were reported at the 32nd Annual Meeting of the British Paediatric Association in Cambridge, 1961, and represent some of the first cases from England. EEGs, muscle studies, dermatoglyphic and chromosome studies were all normal. One testicular biopsy (illustration) is described as normal. There were three cases of scoliosis. Case Reports, Medical Aspects.

Laxova, R., Gilderdale, S., & Ridler, M.A.C. An aetiological study of 53 female patients from a subnormality hospital and of their offspring. *Journal of Mental Deficiency Research,* 1973, *17,* 193-225.
Two of the 53 patients in this study had diagnoses of "probably mild" P-W syndrome and had one and four offspring, respectively. The single child was reported to have an IQ of 90. Of the four siblings, two died of congestive heart failure in infancy, one was reported normal, and one died at 35 years with an IQ of 75 and a questionable diagnosis of P-W syndrome. The cause of death was septicemia associated with diabetes. Because P-W syndrome subjects are described only incidentally in an epidemiological study of inheritability of mental retardation, the cases are not described in sufficient detail to confirm diagnosis. These surprising findings should not be taken as conclusive evidence of fertility in P-W syndrome nor as evidence of the condition being inheritable. Since nearly all reported cases of P-W syndrome are sterile, the findings in this study, if confirmed, would be an important addition to our knowledge of P-W syndrome. Etiology.

Lucas, M. Translocation between both members of chromosome pair number 15 causing recurrent abortions. *Annals of Human Genetics,* 1969, *32,* 347-352.
This study does not mention P-W syndrome. A phenotypically normal woman who had 13 aborted pregnacies is presented. The woman was found to have a translocation involving chromosome pair number 15. The implications for P-W syndrome are that such translocations are found in some P-W persons and this case documents that an apparently normal woman can carry and transmit this error. Etiology.

McCloy, R.F., & McCloy, J. Naloxone and Prader-Willi syndrome. *Lancet,* 1980, *1*(8183), 1418 (letter to the editor).
This letter to the editor is in response to Kyriakides et al. (1980). The authors state that the suggestive appetite-decreasing effect of naloxone in P-W syndrome might be mediated by enkephalin receptors in the gut and enkephalinergic neurones in the vagus (see also Sullivan, 1980). Obesity Control.

Mace, J., Gotlin, R.W., & Dubois, R. Pathogenesis of obesity in Prader-Willi syndrome. *The Journal of Pediatrics*, 1974, *84*, 927-928.
Letter to the editor commenting on the article by Parra et al. (1973). The authors point out they also have shown that P-W syndrome children and normal obese children have similar response patterns (Gotlin et al., 1972). Endocrinology.

McGuffin, W.L., Jr., & Rogol, A.D. Response to LH-RH and clomiphene citrate in two women with the Prader-Labhart-Willi syndrome. *Journal of Clinical Endocrinology and Metabolism*, 1975, *41*, 325-331.
Case reports of two females, studied at ages 25 and 20 years. Response to luteinizing hormone-releasing hormone (LH-RH) showed heterogeneity (one was prepubertal, one was low normal). After clomiphene citrate a normal adult response of gonadotropins to LH-RH was obtained in both women. No changes in secondary sexual characteristics were noted; neither patient menstruated. Endocrinology, Case Reports.

McKusick, V.A. Prader-Willi syndrome. In *Mendelian inheritance in man* (5th ed.). Baltimore and London: Johns Hopkins Press, 1978.
This standard genetic compendium erroneously lists P-W syndrome under recessively inherited disorders. The references are up-to-date. McKusick points out that Down described a patient who appears to have had P-W syndrome in 1887.

MacMillan, D.R., Kim, C.B., & Weisskopf, B. Syndrome of growth resistance, obesity, and intellectual impairment with precocious puberty. *Archives of Disease in Childhood*, 1972, *47*, 119-121.
Two girls, 6 years, 4 months and 11 years, 5 months, are described with most of the typical findings of P-W syndrome. Both showed precocious but incomplete sexual development. The authors consider these girls to have a variant of P-W syndrome. Endocrinology, Case Reports.

Michaelsen, K.F., Lundsteen, C., & Hansen, F.J. Prader-Willi syndrome and chromosomal mosaicism 46XY/47XY+ mar in two cases. *Clinical Genetics*, 1979, *16*, 147-150.
A 2-year, 8-month-old boy and a 7-year, 10-month-old boy with P-W syndrome are described. Routine chromosome preparations showed both boys to be mosaic for an additional small acentric fragment of uncertain origin. Case Report. Etiology.

Michel, G., Chaussain, J.-L, & Job, J.-C. Les explorations endocriniennes dans le syndrome de Prader, Labhardt et Willi. *Archives Françaises de Pédiatrie*, 1976, *33*, 467-476.
Tests of anterior pituitary function and insulin secretion in nine P-W syndrome children revealed findings like those commonly found in subjects who are obese, cryptorchid, or both. Tests did not support the hypothesis of a primary hypothalamic-pituitary defect. (French, English summary). Endocrinology.

Monnens, L., & Kenis, H. Enkele onderzoekingen bij een patient met het syndroom van Prader-Willi. *Maandschrift vor Kindergeneeskunde,* 1965, *33,* 482-498.
A case report from the Netherlands. No prediabetic symptoms were found. (Dutch, English summary). Case Reports, Endocrinology.

Morgner, K.D., Geisthovel, W., Neidergerke, U., & von zur Mühlen, A. Hypogonadismus infolge Mangels an Luteotropin-Releasing Hormon (LH-RH) bei Prader-Labhart-Willi-Syndrom. *Deutsche Medizinische Wochenschrift,* 1974, *99,* 1196-1198.
A case report of endocrine studies of a 15-year-old boy with P-W syndrome. A deficiency in luteotropin-releasing hormone (LH-RH) was discovered. Other tests, including testosterone and insulin, were within normal limits. (German, English summary). Endocrinology, Case Reports.

Neason, S. *Prader-Willi syndrome: A handbook for parents.* Longlake, Minn.: Prader-Willi Syndrome Association, 1978.
Recommended reading for parents of P-W syndrome children. (This booklet may be ordered from: The Prader-Willi Syndrome Association, 5515 Malibu Drive, Edina, MN 55436.)

Nelson, R.A., Hayles, A.B., Novak, L.P., Margie, J.D , & Vernet, J. Abstract. *American Journal of Clinical Nutrition,* 1970, *23,* 667.
This abstract reviews data on three children with P-W syndrome, 4 to 14 years of age, treated with a 1,020 calorie ketogenic diet. All mothers noted a decrease in appetite. In two children the percentage of fat decreased and lean body mass increased. Obesity Control, Endocrinology.

Norman, D.M. Prader-Willi syndrome in a black: First case report. *The Journal of the American Osteopathic Association,* 1979, *79*(1), 89-90.
This is a case report of a 15-year-old black boy who has the typical findings of P-W syndrome. However, it is not the first case reported in a black person. See Vukcevich et al., 1973. Case Report.

Orenstein, D.M., Boat, T.F., Stern, R.C., Doershuk, C.F., & Light, M.S. Progesterone treatment of the obesity hypoventilation syndrome in a child. *The Journal of Pediatrics,* 1977, *90,* 477-479.
A case of a 4½-year-old girl with P-W syndrome is described. She demonstrated the obesity hypoventilation syndrome for which she was apparently successfully treated with progesterone. (See also Holm & Pipes, 1977).

Palmer, S.K., & Atlee, J.L., III. Anesthetic management of the Prader-Willi syndrome. *Anesthesiology,* 1976, *44,* 161-163.
Anesthetic management of an 8½-year-old boy with P-W syndrome during surgical correction of undescended testes is described. The authors point out that the hypotonia and decreased muscle mass should be considered in choice of anesthetic agents (possible problems with

muscle relaxants) and stress the need for glucose injection to prevent hypoglycemia to which they think P-W syndrome people are susceptible. Brief review of the syndrome's typical features. Medical Aspects, Case Reports.

Parkin, J.M. Syndrome of growth resistance, obesity and intellectual impairment with precocious puberty. *Archives of Disease in Childhool,* 1973, *48*, 86-87.

This is a letter to the editor responding to the article by MacMillan, Kim, and Weisskopf (1972) on precocious puberty in P-W syndrome. The author reports one girl who developed breast and pubic hair at age 7½ years and menarche at 8¼ years, accompanied by a growth spurt and advancement in bone age. Case Reports, Endocrinology.

Parra, A., Cervantes, C., & Schultz, R.B. Immunoreactive insulin and growth hormone responses in patients with Prader-Willi syndrome. *The Journal of Pediatrics,* 1973, *83*, 587-593.

Six children, one girl and five boys, with P-W syndrome (ages 5 years, 8 months to 10 years, 8 months) were studied with provocative tests. The responses (hyperinsulinemia and blunted growth hormone level) were similar to those of obese, but otherwise normal, children and were felt to represent an adaptive change to the obese state. Normal plasma glucose levels were demonstrated. Free fatty acid responses were similar to those of normal or obese children. No characteristic biochemical profile of P-W syndrome was demonstrated (see also Mace et al., 1974). Endocrinology.

Pathak, A.K., & Sharma, N.L. Syndrome of retarded growth, obesity, muscular hypotonia and mental deficiency (Prader-Willi syndrome): Report of a case. *Indian Journal of Pediatrics,* 1968, *35*, 447-449.

The parents were consanguineous and had an older child (also a girl) who died at 18 months of a "similar illness." Case Reports.

Pearson, K.D., Steinbach, H.L., & Bier, D.M. Roentgenographic manifestations of Prader-Willi syndrome. *Pediatric Radiology,* 1971, *100*, 369-377.

Five case reports of males with P-W syndrome ranging in age from 8 to 23 years are presented, with special emphasis on radiological findings. Sutural abnormalities and a sella turcica with a small lateral area are described in the skull roentgenograms. Scoliosis, coxa valga, extremities (especially femora) of unequal length, small hands and feet, thin corticus in the metacarpals and normal bone age are described. Case Reports, Medical Aspects.

Pipes, P.L., & Holm, V.A. Weight control of children with Prader-Willi syndrome. *Journal of The American Dietetic Association,* 1973, *62*, 520-524.

Experience with the dietary management of four children with P-W syndrome for whom obesity was prevented or controlled is presented.

Effective programs required individualization of the diet prescription, control of the food environment, careful education of parents, teachers, and others in the child's environment concerning the prescribed diet, frequent monitoring of the child's growth, energy, and nutrient intake, and adjustments in the diet prescription as the children grew older and taller. (See also Holm & Pipes, 1976). Case Reports, Obesity Control.

Prader, A., Labhart, A., & Willi, H. Ein Syndrom von Adipositas, Kleinwuchs, Kryptochismus und Oligophrenie nach myatonieartigem Zustand in Neugeborenenalter. *Schweizerische Medizinische Wochenschrift*, 1956, *86*, 1260–1261.

A report of a new syndrome observed in five males and four females ranging in age from 5 to 23 years. This is the first report in the literature that describes the syndrome subsequently named Prader-Willi syndrome. It is impressive that the authors' seven-paragraph description of the features of the syndrome is still considered essentially correct today. The report also distinguishes this syndrome from other similar syndromes, like Frohlich's and Laurence-Moon-Biedl. (German). Etiology, Diagnosis, Medical Aspects.

Prader, A., Labhart, A., Willi, H., & Fanconi, G. Ein Syndrom von Adipositas, Kleinwuchs, Kryptorchismus und Idiotie bei Kindern und Erwachsenen, die als Neugeborene ein myatonie-artiges Bild geboten haben. *Proceedings of the VIII International Congress on Pediatrics, Copenhagen, 1956*.

A pioneering report similar to Prader et al. (1956) above.

Prader, A., & Willi, H. Das Syndrom von Imbezillität, Adipositas, Muskelhypotonie, Hypogenitalismus, Hypogonadismus und Diabetes mellitus mit "Myatonie"—Anamnese. *Second International Congress on Mental Retardation, Vienna, 1961*. Basel and New York: S. Karger, 1963.

A more detailed report following up on the original 1956 paper that presented nine cases. The authors note that others in Switzerland and elsewhere have observed the syndrome after being alerted by the original paper. Diabetes mellitus and mental retardation are added to the clinical picture and further distinctions are made from other syndromes of hypotonia, such as Werdnig-Hoffmann disease. The authors also discuss the possibility that the syndrome might be the result of chromosome defect, but state that they have no proof. (German). Etiology, Diagnosis, Medical Aspects.

Raiti, S., Trias, E., Livitsky, L., & Grossman, M.S. Oxandrolone and human growth hormone. *American Journal of Diseases of Children*, 1973, *126*, 597–600.

Eight children with growth retardation, one of whom had P-W syndrome, were treated with human growth hormone alone, oxandrolone (Anavar) alone, and combined therapy. The P-W syndrome patient was a 10½-year-old girl. She showed no acceleration of growth from human growth hormone but doubled her prestudy growth rate on oxandrolone (Anavar). Her response to combined therapy was even better. The P-W syndrome patient showed marked acceleration in bone age during the whole treatment period (2.2 years/year of study), which was felt to be detrimental. She was also receiving levothyroxine throughout the study, and it is not known which one of the three hormones caused the acceleration in bone age. Endocrinology.

Reed, W.B., Ragsdale, W., Jr., Curtis, A.C., & Richards, H.J. Acanthosis nigricans in association with various genodermatoses: With emphasis on lipodystrophic diabetes and Prader-Willi syndrome. *Acta Dermato-Venereologica,* 1968, *48,* 465-473.

The authors state that three of 12 patients with P-W syndrome had mild acanthosis nigricans and multiple excoriations. One case report with autopsy findings is included. The same patient has previously been reported by Hoefnagel et al. (1967). Case Reports, Pathology.

Ridler, M.A.C., Garrod, O., & Berg, J.M. A case of Prader-Willi syndrome in a girl with a small extra chromosome. *Acta Paediatrica Scandinavica,* 1971, *60,* 222-226.

A case study of a P-W syndrome female with chromosome abnormalities is presented. Members of her family were also screened, but no chromosomal abnormalities were found. Case Reports, Etiology.

Rudd, B.T., Rayner, P.H.W., Smith, M.R., Holder, G., Jivani, S.K.M., & Theodoridis, C.G. Effect of human chorionic gonadotropin on plasma and urine testosterone in boys with delayed puberty. *Archives of Disease in Childhood,* 1973, *48,* 590-595.

Plasma and urine testosterone levels following treatment with human chorionic gonadotropin (HCG) were measured in 29 boys with delayed puberty, four of whom had P-W syndrome. Three of the four showed an inadequate response. Endocrinology.

Sánchez Villares, E., Martín Esteban, M., & Durantez Mayo, O. Amiotonía congénita con síndrome de Prader-Willi incompleto. *Boletín de la Sociedad Castellano-Astur-Leonesa de Pediatría,* 1964, *5,* 191-208.

A case report from Spain. The patient was a 4½-year-old male suffering from either Oppenheim's disease, Werdnig-Hoffmann disease, or Prader-Willi syndrome. (Spanish, English summary). Case Reports.

Savir, A., Dickerman, Z., Karp, M., & Laron, Z. Diabetic retinopathy in an adolescent with Prader-Labhart-Willi syndrome. *Archives of Disease in Childhood,* 1974, *49,* 963-964.

This finding has not been described by anybody else. Medical Aspects.

Schaison, G., Nathan, C., & Gilbert-Dreyfus. Un cas féminin de syndrome de Prader et Willi: Exploration à l'âge post-pubertaire. *Annales d'Endocrinologie,* 1973, *34,* 286-288.

An endocrine study of one female P-W syndrome patient. The authors found low levels of estradiol, LH, and FSH. Endocrinology.

Schneider, H.J., & Zellweger, H. Forme fruste of the Prader-Willi syndrome (HHHO) and balanced D/E translocation. *Helvetica Paediatrica Acta,* 1968, *2,* 128-136.

The authors present two cases of incomplete expression of the P-W syndrome symptom complex and suggest that the various chromosomal abnormalities found in some P-W persons may actually code for different disorders with the same or similar phenotypic expression. Etiology.

Schwartz, R.S., Brunzell, J.D., & Bierman, E.L. Elevated adipose tissue lipoprotein lipase in the pathogenesis of obesity Prader-Willi syndrome. *Transactions of the Association of American Physicians,* 1979, *92,* 89-95.

This article is reprinted as Chapter 10 in this book. Medical Aspects.

See, C. For some children life is one endless meal. *Today's Health,* January 1976, pp. 15-17; 50-51.

A popular account of P-W syndrome. Major emphasis is placed on unusual behaviors and their emotional impact in some families.

Seligman, J. The child glutton. *Newsweek,* October 13, 1975, p. 69.

A brief account of P-W syndrome for the non-professional reader.

Seyler, L.E., Arulanantham, K., & O'Connor, C.F. Hypergonadotropic hypogonadism in the Prader-Labhart-Willi syndrome. *The Journal of Pediatrics,* 1979, *94,* 435-437.

One 16-year-old male with typical features of P-W syndrome was functionally agonadal: testes were clinically absent, biopsy of a hypotrophic testicle in the inguinal canal at age 8 showed absence of normal histological findings, and no testosterone response to human chorionic gonadotropin could be demonstrated. Response to luteinizing hormone-releasing hormone (LH-RH) indicated a matured hypothalamic pituitary axis. These finds are in contrast to those reported by others in P-W males, who for the most part found incomplete hypothalamic maturation with potentially functional gonads. Endocrinology.

Smith, D.W. *Recognizable patterns of human malformation: Genetic, embryologic, and clinical aspects* (2nd ed.). Philadelphia: W.B. Saunders Co., 1976.

This classic reference book in dysmorphology (syndrome identification) is regularly updated as new information accumulates. It is a source for concise information (and pictures) on P-W syndrome. A unique aspect of this book is that it can be used to review the differential diagnosis of syndromes associated with obesity, hypotonia, hypogonadism, or other specific symptoms. Diagnosis.

Smith, J.D., Neeman, J., Wulff, J., & Seely, J.R. Clinical metabolic study of the Prader-Willi syndrome. *Journal of the Oklahoma State Medical Association,* 1970, *63,* 234–238.

Seven girls with P-W syndrome ages 5 to 19 years are described. Six had precocious puberty. Endocrine studies showed variable results. The authors emphasize abnormalities in carbohydrate-insulin regulation in their P-W subjects, even though there is little difference between these and normal obese controls. Endocrinology.

Soper, R.T., Mason, E.E., Printen, K.J., & Zellweger, H. Gastric bypass for morbid obesity in children and adolescents. *Journal of Pediatric Surgery,* 1975, *10,* 51–58.

The authors describe twenty-five children, 18 normal and seven with P-W syndrome, for whom surgical treatment of obesity was attempted. Twenty-two underwent gastric bypass, three gastroplasty. Six of the children with P-W syndrome lost weight postoperatively. Weight loss leveled off earlier in the P-W children, and they tended to resume weight gain, but at a slower rate. Medical Aspects, Obesity Control.

Spencer, D.A. Prader-Willi syndrome. *The Lancet,* 1968, *2,* 571.

In a letter to the editor the author noted that he had found three cases of P-W syndrome in three hospitals serving 840,000 persons and pointed out that the "mental state" in the syndrome had not been adequately described up to that time.

Steiner, H. Das Prader-Labhart-Willi-Syndrom: Eine morphologische Analyse. *Virchows Archiv Abteilung A Pathologische Antomie,* 1968, *345,* 205–227.

Autopsy findings on two P-W syndrome males, 28 and 23 years of age, and testicular biopsy from a patient of 15 years, 3 months are described in detail with 15 pictures of histological preparations. Testicular atrophy in varying degrees was found in all three cases. Persistence of thymus was noted in one case and lack of glycogen in liver and myocardiun in another. (German, English summary). Medical Aspects.

Stolecke, H., ter Huerne, C., & Tiling, E. Prader-Labhart-Willi-Syndrom: Klinische und psychopathologische Untersuchungsergebnisse bei 4 eigenen Patienten. *Monatsschrift fur Kinderheilkunde,* 1974, *122,* 10–17.

Diagnostic and treatment histories of four cases. (German, English summary). Case Reports, Endocrinology, Behavioral Aspects.

Sullivan, S.N. Naloxone and Prader-Willi syndrome. *Lancet,* 1980, *1*(8178), 1140 (letter to the editor). In response to Kyriakides et al.'s (1980) letter to the editor, Dr. Sullivan suggests that naloxone might decrease appetite in persons with P-W syndrome (if it indeed does) by delaying gastric emptying time (also see McCloy & McCloy, 1980). Obesity Control.

Tangsrud, S.E. Prader-Willi-Labhart syndrom. *Tidsskrift for Den norske laegeforening*, 1978, *16*, 839–840.
Two cases (one girl and one boy) are described. (Norwegian). Case Reports.

Theodoridis, C.G., Brown, G.A., Chance, G.W., & Rudd, B.T. Plasma growth hormone levels in children with the Prader-Willi syndrome. *Australian Paediatric Journal*, 1971, *7*, 24–27.
Growth hormone levels following 6-hour glucose tolerance tests in two girls and four boys with P-W syndrome, age range 7 years, 8 months to 14 years, 10 months, were compared to those of a control group of 13 non-obese normal children. Mean fasting growth hormone levels were lower in P-W children than in controls, but not significantly so. The maximum growth hormone responses of four of the six P-W children were within the normal range, but were clearly subnormal. Endocrinology.

Tolis, G., Lewis, W., Verdy, M., Friesen, H.G., Solomon, S., Pagalis, G., Pavlatos, E., Fessas, P., & Rochefort, J.G. Anterior pituitary function in the Prader-Labhart-Willi (PLW) syndrome. *Journal of Clinical Endocrinology and Metabolism*, 1974, *39*, 1061–1066.
Five patients, two males and three females, ages 16 to 22 years were studied. Results suggest that the functioning of the hypothalamic-pituitary-gonadotropin axis in P-W syndrome varies considerably. Endocrinology.

Vanelli, M., Chaussain, J.-L., Vassal, J., & Job, J.-C. L'insuffisance du développement de la verge (micropenis): Données étiologiques dans une serie de 25 cas. *Archives Françaises de Pédiatrie*, 1979, *36*, 471–478.
This is an endocrinological study of 25 boys with micropenis, two of whom had P-W syndrome. It demonstrates hypothalmic-pituitary deficiency in the P-W subjects as well as in 10 other boys. (French, English summary). Endocrinology.

Uehling, D. Cryptorchidism in the Prader-Willi syndrome. *The Journal of Urology*, 1980, *124*, 103–104.
The records of 30 male children with P-W syndrome were reviewed. Seventy percent had at least one undescended testis; in 45%, both were undescended. Twenty-two percent (4 of 18) followed up over a period of time had late spontaneous testicular descent. Orchiopexy is discouraged in this syndrome. Instead, watchful waiting or possibly exogenous gonadotropins are recommended. Medical Aspects.

Vukcevich, W.M., Adler, R.I., Hornblass, A.H., & Gombos, G.M. Cataracts with obesity, small stature, oligophrenia, and acromicria (Prader-Labhart-Willi syndrome). *American Journal of Ophthalmology*, 1973, *75*, 258–260.

This is a case report of an 11-year-old boy with P-W syndrome and cataracts. There are some unusual features in this case: a heart murmur and enlarged heart (thought to be caused by a ventricular septal defect or mitral insufficiency) were noted. The height (55 inches at 10 years) is above average and the facial features, as shown in accompanying photographs, do not seem typical for this syndrome. This is the only case reported in a black person. Ophthalmological findings (cataracts and nystagmus) have not previously been described in this syndrome. Case Reports, Medical Aspects.

Wannarachue, N., Ruvalcaba, R.H.A., & Kelley, V.C. Hypogonadism in Prader-Willi syndrome. *American Journal of Mental Deficiency*, 1975, *79*, 592-603.
Sexual development in nine female and two male subjects with P-W syndrome ranging in age from 10.5 to 44.6 years is reviewed. Both the process of development and degree of sexual maturity were variable, but were abnormal in all subjects. Testicular biopsies in the two males (both adults) showed abnormalities in germinal epithelium. Endocrinology.

Widhalm, K., & Deutsch, J. Behandlung der exzessiven Adipositas am Beispiel des Prader-Willi-Labhart-Syndroms. *Pädiatrie und Pädologie*, 1976, *11*, 297-304.
The authors successfully treated a 14-year-old P-W syndrome boy (weight, 93.45 kg; height, 143 cm) for obesity. Inpatient and outpatient diet therapy and outpatient psychological care resulted in a weight loss of 26 kg in 18 months. (German, English summary). Case Reports, Obesity Control, Behavioral Aspects.

Wisniewski, L.P., Witt, M.E., Ginsberg-Fellner, F., Wilner, J., & Desnick, R.J. Prader-Willi syndrome and a bisatellited derivative of chromosome 15. *Clinical Genetics*, 1980, *18*, 42-47.
A case of a 17-year-old boy with most of the typical findings of P-W syndrome is reported. Cytogenetic studies showed a small extra chromosome which is interpreted to be an inverted duplication of the short arm of chromosome 15. Case Report. Etiology.

Zárate, A., Soria, J., Canales, E.S., Kastin, A.J., Schally, A.V., & Guzmán Toledano, R. Pituitary response to synthetic luteinizing hormone-releasing hormone in Prader-Willi syndrome, prepubertal and pubertal children. *Neuroendocrinology*, 1973/1974, *13*, 321-326.
One case report of a girl with P-W syndrome who was 7 years of age when luteinizing hormone-releasing hormone (LH-RH) was given. She showed no response and the authors suggest that P-W syndrome is caused by a hypothalamic lesion associated with limited pituitary responses. Endocrinology, Case Report.

Zellweger, H. The HHHO or Prader-Willi syndrome. *Birth defects: Original article series,* 1969, *5*(2), 15-17.

This is a brief description of P-W syndrome based on the author's review article (Zellweger & Schneider, 1968). Review Article.

Zellweger, H., & Schneider, H.J. Syndrome of hypotonia-hypomentia-hypogonadism-obesity (HHHO) or Prader-Willi syndrome. *American Journal of Diseases of Children,* 1968, *115,* 588-598.

Two case reports, a review of 12 additional cases, and 79 cases from the literature are presented in this early review article that contains more behavioral descriptions than most early articles on this syndrome. Case Reports, Review Article, Behavioral Aspects, Medical Aspects.

Zellweger, H.U., Smith, J.W., & Cusminsky, M. Muscular hypotonia in infancy: Diagnosis and differentiation. *Revue Canadienne de Biologie,* 1962, *21,* 599-612.

This article reviews the differential diagnosis in muscular hypotonia in infancy. P-W syndrome is highlighted as a conclusion with one case report. Case Report.

Zuffardi, O., Buhler, E.M., & Fraccaro, M. Chromosome 15 and Prader-Willi syndrome. *Clinical Genetics,* 1978, *14,* 315-316. Brief abstract reviewing the authors' experience and information available in the literature on abnormalities of chromosome 15 and P-W syndrome. Etiology.

INDEX

Abnormalities of P-W syndrome, 47–53
  of CNS performance, 47–49
  of growth, 47
  of morphogenesis, 49–51
Academic achievement, 32
Acanthosis nigricans, 33
Acromicria, 7, 33, 49, 58, 70
Adipose tissue, 1, 105–106
  composition, 105, 114–117
  lipoprotein lipase, 30, 114–117, 137–143, 313
    ideal body weight and, 139–141
    methods and results, 138–143
    predisposing factor in development of obesity, 140
Adiposogenital dystrophy, 4, 6
Adolescence
  abnormal growth pattern, 281–282
  behavioral and cognitive disabilities, 155–157
  food behavior problems, 98
  lack of preadolescent growth spurt, 33
  running away from home, 157
  sexual development problems, 29, 264–265
Adrenocorticotropic hormone (ACTH) infusion test, 285
Adults
  exercise program, 307–309
  weight gain, 273, 275
Aggressiveness, 215, 217
Alström syndrome, 84
Anemia, 132
Aphasia, 31
Appetites, voracious, 5, 314
Apraxia, 31
  speech and language disorders, 182
Arginine infusions, 286
Atonic diplegia, 63
Autosomal dominant mutations, 83, 86

Bardet-Biedl syndrome, 51
Behavior characteristics, 44, 48
Behavior modification programs, 8, 66, 187
Behavioral and cognitive disabilities, 79, 147–159

cognitive disabilities, 147–148
treatment tactics, 148–159, 185–199
  0- to 3-year-old child, 148–149
  3- to 6-year-old child, 149–151
  6- to 12-year-old child, 151–154
  12- to 17-year-old adolescent, 155–157
  young adults, 157–159
  use of reinforcements, 151–152, 185
Behavioral approach to treatment, 185–199
  exercise programs, 191
  food selection, 191
  meal program, 187–189
    violations and contingencies, 190–191
  method, 187–192
  not appropriate for children, 197
  self-help skills, 195
  treatment elements, 187–192
  weight reduction programs, 185–199, 201–213
Behavioral problems relating to food, 34, 98, 217
  effect on family members, 233–235
  institutionalized, 215–218
  temper tantrums, 7, 34, 152, 219–228
  See also Food-related behavior
Bibliography, annotated, 317–336
Birth defects, 46–47
  deformations and malformations, 46
  factors causing, 46
Blood and urine studies, 285, 287
Body composition, effect of ketogenic diet, 105–108, 110–114
Bone age, 7, 79–81, 82, 272–273
Boys with P-W syndrome, 5, 7
Brain injuries, 6
Bruising, susceptibility to, 267
Bureau of Community Health Services (BCHS), 17, 19

Caloric intake, 30
Carbohydrate tolerance, impaired, 288–289
Cardiopulmonary problems, 60, 198
Caregivers, role of, 245
Carpenter syndrome, 51

Case studies, 5
  clinical experiences with 23 cases, 69–88
CDMRC, *see* Child Development and Mental Retardation Center
Central nervous system (CNS) disorders, 47
  abnormalities of performance, 47–49
  localized defect in development, 50
  research needs, 52–53
  symptoms essential for diagnosis, 31–33
Charcot-Marie-Tooth disease, 61–62
Child Development and Mental Retardation Center (CDMRC), University of Washington, 7, 9, 18
  interdisciplinary management, 9–10
  University Affiliated Facilities, 18–19
Children and infants
  abnormal birth and delivery, 28, 34
  birth defects, 46–47
  birth size, 271–272
  exercises for, 300–307
    preschool children, 302–304
    school-age children, 304–307
  fetal movements, 5, 74
  floppy infants, 246
  hypotonia and failure to thrive, 6, 7, 30–31, 246–247
  neonatal intensive care units, 22–23
  treatment tactics, 148–154
    0- to 3-year-old child, 148–149
    3- to 6-year-old child, 149–151
    6- to 12-year-old child, 151–154
Children's Bureau, 19
Cholesterol, 287
  ketogenic diet and, 109, 113
Chromosomal abnormalities, 6, 46, 51, 69
Clinical experience with 23 cases, 69–88
  behavior problems, 79
  birth history, 74
  bone age, 79–80
  dermatoglyphic patterns, 75–78
  development and growth, 75
  fetal movements, 74
  maternal age, 71
  mental development, 79
  neurological findings, 79
  parity, 74
  paternal age, 71–73
  physical findings, 75
Clinical Research Unit (CRU) of Camarillo State Hospital-UCLA, 186
Clinics for P-W syndrome patients, 9–10
Clomiphene citrate, 283–284
Cognitive deficits, 10, 161–177
  letter comparison tasks, 173–176
  picture recognition tasks, 161–169
  short term memory scanning, 169–173
Cognitive development, 147–148
Cognitive processing, 161–177
Cortisol levels, 285
Coxa valga, 6
Cryptorchidism, 5, 7, 282, 283

Dental problems, 6, 261
Dermatoglyphic patterns, 75–78, 85
Developmental disabilities, 9
  federal programs for, 17–24
Developmental milestone, 31
  delayed in infancy, 6–9
  See also Growth and development
Dextroamphetamine, 262
Diabetes mellitus, 5, 35, 121, 267
  incidence of, 27, 288
  unusual in P-W syndrome, 35–36
Diagnosis of P-W syndrome, 4–7, 27–44
  age at time of, 28, 230
  differential, 6–7, 59–65
  Down syndrome, 27
  early, 237
  evaluation, 51
  first phase, 55–69
    differential diagnosis, 59–65
    symptoms, 56–58
  guidelines, 27
  historical perspectives, 1–7
  infantile hypotonia, 28–29, 55–69
  mental retardation, 31–33
  parental response, 246–249
    need for more information on P-W syndrome, 247, 257
  in patients not currently obese, 27, 30–31
  physical stigmata, 27, 70, 75–78

questionnaire study, 28, 37–44
second phase, 57
symptoms essential for, 28–33
  dysfunctional CNS performance, 31–33
  dysmorphic facial features, 33
  hypogonadism, 29–30
  infantile hypotonia, 28–29, 55–69
  obesity, 30–31
  short stature, 33
symptoms in 50% to 90% of cases, 33–34
  behavioral problems relating to food, 34
  inability to vomit, 34
  scoliosis, 34
  skin problems, 33
  small hands and feet, 33
  strabismus, 34
symptoms in 10% to 50% of cases, 34–35
  abnormal birth, 34
  decreased pain sensitivity, 35
  myopia, 35
  speech articulation problems, 35
symptoms with less than 10% occurrence, 35
  congenital hip dislocation, 35
  diabetes mellitus, 35
  large head, 35
  seizure disorders, 35
workup, 51–52
Diarrhea following intestinal bypass, 122–123
Dietary management
  behavior modification programs, 8, 66, 185–199
  in children, 91–103
  control of insatiable appetite, 5, 314
  controls over access to food, 8
  crash and fad diets, 262
  dietary fiber foods, 118–119
  early intervention most effective, 92–97, 102
  energy needs of P-W patients, 7, 92–93
  environmental controls, 8, 91, 93
  establishing feeding program, 66
  exchange system, 93, 97
  family cooperation, 8, 66, 97–99
  first phase, 66
  individualized programs, 91, 93–97
  ketogenic diet, 91–92, 105–120

changes in body composition, 110–114
cholesterol and triglyceride levels, 109
disadvantages, 114
effect of exercise, 106–108
hyperphagia control and, 114
long term results, 108–114
uric acid excretion, 113
urinary nitrogen excretion, 109
weight loss, 110–113
limited success in treating obesity, 122
low calorie diet with behavioral controls, 7–8, 91–103, 263
maintenance of programmed weight loss, 201–203
  caloric restriction, 201–202, 213
  contingency contracting, 201–202, 205, 209–210
  during vacations, 210
  family support, 210–211
  punishment for food stealing, 203, 210
  results, 206–208
  self-monitoring, 201–203, 208–209
  weight loss program, 203, 211
methods, 91–92
nutritional management, 91–103
portion control, 97
protein-sparing modified fast, 91–92, 263
self-monitoring, 8, 201–203, 208–209, 315
short term weight losses, 201, 211
weight control programs, 95–97
  See also Nutritional management
Disabled Children's Program, 21–22
Down syndrome, 4, 62–63
  diagnosis, 27

Eating habits, 7–8, 39
  See also Dietary management; Food-related behavior
Educational programs, 10, 13, 32
  for adolescents, 155–157
  3- to 6-year-old children, 149–151
  6- to 12-year-old children, 151–154
  extracurricular activities, 153–154
  individualized, 155

Educational programs—*continued*
  language and social skills, 149–150
  learning disabled children, 315–316
  physical education, 154
  social relationships, 152–153
  special education eligibility, 151
Emotional lability, 148
Endocrine and metabolic aspects, 56, 281–291
  blood and urine studies, 285, 287
  estradiol and urinary estrogen, 284
  glucose and insulin levels, 287–288
  gonadotropin, 282–284
  on growth, 270–271
  growth hormone, 285–286
  plasma testosterone, 284
  prolactin, 286
  thyroid function studies, 287
Endorphine, 314
Energy needs of P-W patients, 7, 92–93
  weight gain on low energy intake, 314
Environmental controls, 8, 91, 93
Epiphysiolysis, 6
Estradiol, 284
Estrogen, urinary studies, 284–285
Etiology and pathogenesis, 45–53
  abnormalities of growth and development, 45
  hypothalamic dysfunction, 45, 49, 314
  implications for diagnosis, 51–52
  implications for patient care, 52
  implications for research, 52–53
  origins of birth defects, 46–47
Exercises, 154, 299–311
  for adults, 307–309
  for infants, 300–302
  physical education programs, 154, 300
  P-W group response to, 107–108
  preschool children, 302–304
  relaxation training, 220–221
  school-age training, 304–307
  for scoliosis, 309–311
  swimming, 302, 304
  team activities, 304
Extracurricular activities, 153–154
Eye problems, 261
Eyes, almond-shaped, 5, 33

Facial features in P-W syndrome, 33, 49
Facilities and services for P-W persons, 13
"Failure to thrive" stage, 7, 30–31, 121
Family relationships, 10–12
  assessing needs of family, 245–257
  behavior modification program supported by, 66
  conflicts, 249–251
  family syndrome, 84
  genetic counseling, 52
  guilt feelings, 247, 252
  handbook for, 11
  history, 37–38
  implications for individual and family, 229–244
  intervention strategies for, 245–257
  non-medical resources, 229, 237
  parental needs, 246–253
  sharing experiences with other parents, 10–13, 296
  parental response to diagnosis, 246–249
  questionnaire sent to, 230, 239–244
    burden to parents, 232
    burden to P-W syndrome person, 231–232
    evaluation of responses, 230–239
    impact on family finances, 232–233
    impact on family living, 233–234
    lack of knowledge and understanding of P-W syndrome, 235
    obesity and behavioral problems, 231–232
    P-W syndrome as social disorder, 236–237
    problem of delayed diagnosis, 230
  reality stress, 251–253
  religious support, 251
  siblings, 253–256
  group sessions for, 254–256
  social work intervention, 245–257
  support and guidance in carrying out nutritional management, 93, 102, 210–211
  value conflicts, 249–251

Fat and fatty acids, 287
  abnormality in body fat composition, 114–117
  in adipose tissue, 114–117, 121
  polyunsaturated, 115–116
Features of P-W syndrome, 1, 4–6, 281
  frequency of, 78
  in 17th century portraits, 1–4
Federal programs, 17–24
  funding for workshops, 17
  Genetic Diseases Act, 20–21
  historical background, 17–19
  interagency collaboration, 21–22
  neonatal intensive care units, 22–23
  Office of Maternal and Child Health, 19–23
  Supplemental Security Income-Disabled Children's Program, 21–22
  University Affiliated Facilities (UAFs), 18–19
Fetal movements, diminished, 5, 74
First phase of P-W syndrome, 55–68
  differential diagnosis, 59–65
    cerebral hypotonias, 62–65
    lower motor unit conditions, 59–62
    spinal cord lesions, 62
  symptoms, 56–58
  treatment, 65–66
    control of body temperature, 65
    physiotherapy, 65
Food-related behavior, 6, 34, 97–102, 217
  in adolescence, 98
  foraging for food, 7, 11, 34, 97, 99, 236, 251, 255–256, 316
  gorging food, 7, 34
  hoarding food, 217
  punishment for food stealing, 203, 210, 217, 236
  stress faced by parents, 251–252
Fractures after minimal trauma, 35, 265–266, 300
Frölich's syndrome, 4–6

Gastric bypass surgery and gastroplasty, 7, 123–133, 263
Gathered View, The (newsletter), 11

Genetic counseling, 20–21, 30, 52
Genetic Diseases Act, 20–21
Glucose and insulin levels, 287–288
Glycogenosis, neuromuscular (type II), 60
Gonadal dysgenesis, 277–278
Gonadotropin levels, 282–284
Group homes, 13, 157–159, 235–236, 257, 315
Growth and development, 39–40, 45, 75–77, 269–280
  abnormalities of CNS performance, 47–49
  abnormalities of growth, 47
  abnormalities of morphogenesis, 49–51
  birth size, 271–272
  bone age, 272–273
  endocrine studies, 270–271
  etiology of growth failure, 269–270
  height growth, 269, 273–277
  lack of pubertal growth, 277, 289
  linear growth, 76–77
  malformations, 49–51
  oxandrolone therapy, 277–278
  patterns of altered, 46–51
  weight data, 269
  weight in untreated persons with P-W syndrome, 273
Growth hormone deficiency, 270–271
  response in P-W syndrome, 285–286

Handicapped children
  federal programs for, 17–24
  special education classes, 32
Hands and feet, small, 5, 33
Head, large head circumference, 6, 35
Health, Education, and Welfare (HEW) Department, 17
Health maintenance, 261
Hemorrhages, intracranial, 6
Hereditary nature of P-W syndrome, 6, 30, 45, 83, 86
  autosomal dominant mutation, 83, 86
  risk of recurrence, 45, 52
HHHO (hypotonia-hypomentia-hypogonadism-obesity), 56

HHO (hypotonia-hypomentia and
    obesity) syndrome, 56
Hip dislocation, 6, 35, 265
Historical background, 1-15, 55-56
    diagnosis, 5-7
    interdisciplinary management, 9-10
    National Prader-Willi Syndrome
        Workshop, 12-13
    obesity control, 7-8
    paintings by Juan Carreño de Miranda, 1-4
    Prader-Willi Syndrome Association,
        11-12
    research needs, 10, 313-316
Human chorionic gonadotropin
    (HCG), 282, 284
Hyperphagia, 4, 34, 115
    fatty acid structure and, 117-119
    ketogenic diet and control of, 114,
        117-119
    symptoms, 34
Hypogenitalism, 7
Hypoglycemia, insulin-induced, 286
Hypogonadism, 6, 49, 263-265, 282
    essential symptom, 29-30
    first phase, 58
    hypothalamic, 271, 272
    incomplete adolescent masculinization and feminization, 264-265
    in males at birth, 31, 282
    micropenis in early childhood, 263
    undescended testes, 263-264
Hypothalamus, 30
    abnormalities, 56
    elevated adipose tissue lipoprotein lipase, 141-142
    developmental defect responsible
        for P-W syndrome, 6, 45,
        48-50, 56, 271-272, 281, 314
Hypothyroidism, 262
Hypotonias, 6, 48
    cerebral or supranuclear, 55, 62-65
        atonic diplegia, 63
        congenital or early onset myotonic dystrophy, 63-64
        Down syndrome, 62-63
        Zellweger syndrome, 63
    differential diagnosis, 55
    essential, 64-65
    infantile, supraspinal (or central),
        6, 28-29
    medical management of, 65-66,
        261-262

Identifying high risk children, 22-23
Incidence data, 27, 45, 56
Individualized service plans (ISP), 21
Infant hypotonic stage, 6, 28-29,
    64-65
Infantile spinal muscular atrophy,
    59-60
Infants, see Children and infants
Institutional study of behavior,
    215-218
    behavioral incident reports, 216-217
    classification of behaviors, 216-217
Insulin levels, 287-288
    in regulation of adipose tissue lipoprotein lipase, 140-142
IQ (Intelligence quotient), 5, 31, 48,
    148
    effect of obesity on, 10
Interdisciplinary management, 9-10
Investigation of 23 cases, 69-88

Job placement for P-W persons, 159

Kallmann syndrome, 51
Ketogenic diet, 91-92, 105-120, 262
    changes in body composition,
        105-108, 110-114
    cholesterol and triglyceride levels,
        109
    disadvantages, 114
    effect of exercise, 106-108
    hyperphagia controlled by, 114,
        117-119
    long term results, 108-114
    uric acid excretion, 113
    urinary nitrogen excretion, 109
    weight loss, 110-113

Laboratory findings, 58
Language skills, 180
Laurence-Moon-Biedl syndrome, 6,
    84
Learning disabilities, 31-33, 48,
    315-316
Life expectancy, 122, 128
Lipids and lipoproteins, 287
Lipoprotein lipase levels, 30, 114-117,
    138-143
    elevations in, 137-143

predisposing factor for development of obesity, 141
research needs, 313
Living arrangements, group homes, 13, 157-159, 235-236, 257, 315
Living skills, independent, 32
Lordosis, 6
Lower motor unit conditions
  benign congenital myopathies, 60
  differential diagnosis of P-W syndrome, 59-62
  infantile spinal muscular atrophy, 59-60
  muscular dystrophies, 60-61
  neuromuscular glycogenosis, 60
  peripheral neuropathies, 61-62
Luteinizing hormone-releasing hormone (LH-RH) stimulation test, 80, 283-284

Maintenance of programmed weight loss, 201-213
  caloric restriction, 201-203
  contingency-contracting, 201-202, 205, 209-210
  during vacations, 210
  family support, 210-211
  long term, 202
  punishment for food stealing, 203, 210
  results, 206-208
  self-monitoring, 201-203, 208-209
  weight loss program, 203, 211
Malformations, patterns of, 49-51
Maternal and Child Health Programs, 17-19
Maternal and paternal ages, 71-74, 85
Maternity and Infant Care (MIC), 18
Medical management, 261-267
  health maintenance, 261
Medical problems, 13, 42-44
Medication
  antipsychotic and sedative drugs, 267
  behavior-modifying drugs, 267
Memories of P-W syndrome patients, 10
  short term memory difficulties, 33, 48, 315
  compared to other retarded children, 161-177
  short term memory scanning, 169-173
Memory impairment experiments, 161-177
  letter comparison tasks, 173-176
  picture recognition tasks, 161-169
  short term memory scanning, 169-173
Mental development, 79-80
Mental retardation, 5-6
  behavioral and cognitive disabilities, 147-159
  cognitive development, 147-148
  diagnosis, 31-33
  dysfunctional CNS performance, 31-33
  federal programs for, 17-18
  intellectual functioning, 32-33
  reaction of parents, 247
  reinforcement procedures, 151-152
  research centers, 18
  training in independent living skills, 32
  treatment tactics, 148-154
Metabolism, body composition and substrate utilization, 106-108
Metyrapone test, 285
Morphogenesis, abnormalities of, 49-51
Mongolism, 27
Mortality, 7, 8, 22-23
Motor disorders, 59-62, 299
  benign congenital myopathies, 60
  infantile spinal muscular atrophy, 59-60
  lower motor unit conditions, 59-62
  muscular dystrophies, 60-61
  myasthenia gravis, 61
  neuromuscular glycogenosis, 60
  peripheral neuropathies, 61-62
Mouths, small triangular, 5, 33, 49
Muscles
  exercises for strength and coordination, 300
  infantile spinal muscular atrophy, 59-60
  lack of tone, 5
Muscular dystrophy, 6, 60-61
Myasthenia gravis, 6, 61
Myopathies, benign congenital nonprogressive, 60
Myopia, 35
Myotonic dystrophy, congenital or early onset, 63-64

National Institutes of Health (NIH), 18
National workshops, 12–13
Neonatal intensive care units, 22–23
Neurological abnormalities, 59–62, 261–262
  observations in 23 cases, 79
Neuromuscular disorders, 6, 48, 60
Neuromuscular glycogenosis (GLY II), 60
Nutritional management of children, 91–103
  early intervention most successful, 92–93, 102
  environmental control, 91
  exchange system, 93, 97
  family support, 93, 97, 102, 210–211
  hyperphagia and, 117–119
    daily nutrient intake, 118–119
  individualized low calorie balanced diet, 91–102
  ketogenic diet, 91–92, 105–120
  prevention of obesity, 93
  protein-sparing modified fast, 91–92
  results of, 93–97
  vitamin supplements, 97
  weight control, 95–96
  weight gain on low energy intake, 314
  weight reduction approaches, 91
  See also Dietary management

Obesity, 5, 6–8
  in adults, 273, 275
  appetite-suppressing medications, 7, 262
  characteristics of P-W syndrome, 5–7
  in children and adolescents, 121
  crash and fad diets, 262
  diagnosis, 30–31, 273, 314
  effect on family members, 233–234
  excessive, 5
  experimental diets, 7
  failure to thrive stage and, 6–7, 30–31
  gastric bypass surgery, 7, 123–133, 263
  interdisciplinary management, 9–10
  ketogenic diet to control, 105–120
  low calorie diet with behavioral controls, 7–8, 91–103, 263
  medical management, 262–263
  onset of, 30
  in persons not obese, 30–31, 273, 314
  second stage of P-W syndrome, 6, 57–58
  surgical treatment, 121–135
  symptoms essential for diagnosis, 30–31
  weight gain in untreated P-W syndrome, 30–31, 273
  weight gain on low energy intake, 314
Occupational therapists, 9
Office of Maternal and Child Health (OMCH), 17, 19–23
Ophthalmoplegia, 60
Oral pathology, 34
Orthopedic problems, 5–6, 265–266
  congenital hip dislocation, 6, 35, 265
  fractures, 265–266
  uneven leg length, 265
Oxandrolone therapy, for growth retardation, 277–278, 314

Pain, decreased sensitivity to, 27, 35, 266
Parents
  associations for, 10–13
  need support and guidance, 93, 102
  See also Family relationships
Pathogenesis of P-W syndrome, 45, 47–51
  abnormalities of CNS performance, 47–49
  abnormalities of growth, 47
  abnormalities of morphogenesis, 49–51
Patient care, individualized therapy, 52
Peer support groups, 149
  value of, 315
Penis, micropenis in early childhood, 263
Peripheral neuropathies, 61–62
Personality problems, 7
Pharmacological studies, 314

Phenylketonuria (PKU), screening program for, 20
Physical education, 154
   See also Exercises
Physical growth, 45, 269-280
   See also Growth and development
Physical therapy, 261-262
Pickwickian syndrome, 263
Picture recognition tasks, 161-169
Polydactyly, 6
Pompe's disease, 60
Prader-Willi syndrome
   abnormalities, 6
   behavioral and cognitive disabilities, 147-159
   definition, 55
   discovery of, 5
   effect on individual and family, 229-244
   historical perspective, 1-15
   publicizing, 237
Prader-Willi Syndrome Association, 11-13, 237
   support for family, 235-236
Prader-Willi Syndrome Workshop, 12, 27
   federal funding, 19, 23
Pregnancy and birth history, 34, 38, 56-57, 74
   birth size, 22-23, 271-272
   delivery problems, 34, 271-272
   fetal movements, 5, 74
   identification of high risk patients, 23
   neonatal intensive care units, 22-23
   origins of birth defects, 46-47
Prenatal morphogenesis, localized defects, 50
Preventive measures, 45, 93, 96
Prognosis, 237
Prolactin, 286
Puberty, incomplete, 5, 282-284

Questionnaires
   on diagnostic criteria, 28, 37-44
   on family relationships, 230, 239-244

Reading problems, 31
Recreational programs, 13, 252, 300

Recurrence risk, 52
Reinforcements, use of, 151-152, 185
Relaxation training, 219-228
   biofeedback measurements, 221-226
   imagination-controlled technique, 222-223
   measurements, 221-222
   meditation training, 221
   monitoring frontalis muscle activity, 221-222
   prevention of temper tantrums, 219-228
   relaxation exercises, 220-221
Research programs, 10, 45-46
   directions in future research, 313-316
   epidemiological, 314
   etiology and pathogenesis, 52-53
   federal aid for, 17
   negative results, 314
Respiratory problems, 122
Retinitis pigmentosa, 6
Running away problem, 157

Scoliosis, 6, 34, 49, 265, 293-298
   bracing and surgical treatment, 294, 298
   diagnosis, 34
   examination technique, 294-296
   exercise program for, 309-311
   incidence of, 27, 293, 298
   progressive, 294
   x-ray examination, 294, 297
Second phase (obese) of P-W syndrome, 6, 57-58
Seizure disorders, 35, 267
Sexual development, 29, 289
   delayed puberty and, 282
   first phase, 58
Sheltered workshops, 13, 158
Short stature, 5, 33, 47, 289
   delayed bone age and, 281
   height growth in P-W syndrome, 47, 273-277
   oxandrolone treatments, 265
   physical growth in P-W syndrome, 269-280
Siblings, impact of P-W syndrome, 253-256
Skeletal maturation process, 289

Skin problems, 33, 266
  bruising, 266
  decreased pain sensitivity, 266
  skin picking, 266
Social disorder, P-W syndrome, 236–237
Social relationships, 152–153
  with peers, 149
Social Security Act, Supplemental Security Income-Disabled Children's Program, 21–22
Social work intervention, 13, 245–257
  family support services, 10
  impact of P-W syndrome on siblings, 253–256
  parental needs, 246–253
  parental response to diagnosis, 246–249
  stress and pressures on parents, 251–253
  value conflicts, 249–251
Special Olympics program, 154, 304
Speech and language problems, 9–10, 35, 179–183
  articulation skills, 180–182
  comprehension skills, 180
  evaluation process, 179–180
  language skills, 180
  speech-sound production skills, 180–182
    nasal air emission distortions, 181–182
    other articulation deficits, 182
  treatment strategies, 182
Spinal cord lesions, 62
Stages of P-W syndrome, 6
  first (infant hypotonic) stage, 6, 8, 55–68
  second (obese) stage, 6, 57–58
Stigmata, 70, 75–78
Strabismus, 6, 34, 267
Stress for parents, 251–253
  professional intervention, 252–253
  relaxation training, 219–228
Sugar, effect on behavior, 99, 314–315
Summer camps, 13
Summit syndrome, 51
Supplemental Security Income-Disabled Children's Program, 21–22

Surgical treatment, 121–135
  gastric bypass, 123–124, 130–131
  effect on growth and development, 131–132
  gastroplasty, 123–124
  metabolic complications, 130
  of morbid obesity, 121–135
  postoperative care, 132–133
  postoperative weight loss, 122, 133
  small intestinal bypass, 122–123
Symptoms, 4–5, 28–36, 56–58
  essential for diagnosis, 28–33
  first phase, 56–58
  See also under Diagnosis

Temper tantrums, 7, 34, 152
  relaxation training for controlling, 219–228
  suggestions for handling, 155–156
Testes, undescended, 263–264
Testosterone levels, 282, 284, 289
Thyroid function studies, 287
Thyrotropin-releasing hormone (TRH) stimulus, 286–287
Title V programs, 19
Treatment
  behavioral approach to, 185–199
    exercise program, 191
    food selection, 191
    meal program, 187–189
    violations and contingencies, 190–191
  method, 187–192
  not appropriate for children, 197
  self-help skills, 195
  weight reduction program, 185–199, 201–213
  children and infants, 148–154
  early intervention with diet therapy, 92–97
  first phase of P-W syndrome, 65–66
  interdisciplinary management, 9–10
  weight gain in untreated P-W syndrome, 273–274
Triglycerides, 287
  adipose tissue composition, 114–117
  ketogenic diet and, 109, 113
  uptake and storage, 137, 142
Turner syndrome, 278

University Affiliated Facilities
(UAFs), 18-20
identifying high risk children, 23
University of Oregon, Health Sciences
Center, 19, 21
University of Washington
Child Development and Mental Retardation Center, 7, 9-10,
18-19
Prader-Willi Syndrome Clinic, 9,
12, 28
Urinary estrogen studies, 284
Urinary specific gravity, 287

Value conflicts, 249-251
Violent outbursts, 34
See also Temper tantrums
Vitamin supplements, 97
Vocational training, 13
Vomit, lack of ability to, 27, 34, 132

Weight
gain on low energy intake, 314

in untreated persons with P-W syndrome, 273
Weight control programs, 95-97
need for severe caloric restrictions, 97
See also Dietary management
Weight loss
following surgical treatment, 122, 125-128, 133
on ketogenic diet, 110-113
slower weight loss more effective, 211
Weight-Watchers, 159
Werdnig-Hoffmann disease, 6, 59
Workshops, sheltered, 13, 158

Young adults, behavioral and cognitive disabilities, 157-159

Zellweger syndrome, 63
Zinc deficit, 313